Neuroimaging

Editor

LASZLO L. MECHTLER

NEUROLOGIC CLINICS

www.neurologic.theclinics.com

Consulting Editor
RANDOLPH W. EVANS

February 2020 • Volume 38 • Number 1

ELSEVIER

1600 John F. Kennedy Boulevard • Suite 1800 • Philadelphia, Pennsylvania, 19103-2899

http://www.theclinics.com

NEUROLOGIC CLINICS Volume 38, Number 1
February 2020 ISSN 0733-8619, ISBN-13: 978-0-323-75435-4

Editor: Stacy Eastman
Developmental Editor: Donald Mumford

Neurologic Clinics (ISSN 0733-8619) is published quarterly by Elsevier Inc., 360 Park Avenue South, New York, NY 10010–1710. Months of issue are February, May, August, and November. Periodicals postage paid at New York, NY, and additional mailing offices. Subscription prices are $326.00 per year for US individuals, $696.00 per year for US institutions, $100.00 per year for US students, $408.00 per year for Canadian individuals, $843.00 per year for Canadian institutions, $427.00 per year for international individuals, $843.00 per year for international institutions, $210.00 for foreign students/residents, and $100.00 for Canadian students/residents. To receive student/resident rate, orders must be accompanied by name of affiliated institution, date of term, and the *signature* of program/residency coordinator on institution letterhead. Orders will be billed at individual rate until proof of status is received. Foreign air speed delivery is included in all *Clinics* subscription prices. All prices are subject to change without notice. **POSTMASTER:** Send address changes to *Neurologic Clinics*, Elsevier Health Sciences Division, Subscription Customer Service, 3251 Riverport Lane, Maryland Heights, MO 63043. **Customer Service: Telephone: 1-800-654-2452 (U.S. and Canada); 314-447-8871 (outside U.S. and Canada). Fax: 314-447-8029. E-mail: journalscustomerservice-usa@elsevier.com (for print support); journalsonlinesupport-usa@elsevier.com (for online support).**

Reprints. For copies of 100 or more of articles in this publication, please contact the Commercial Reprints Department, Elsevier Inc., 360 Park Avenue South, New York, New York, 10010-1710; Tel.: +1-212-633-3874; Fax: +1-212-633-3820, and E-mail: reprints@elsevier.com.

Neurologic Clinics is also published in Spanish by Nueva Editorial Interamericana S.A., Mexico City, Mexico.

Neurologic Clinics is covered in *Current Contents/Clinical Medicine, MEDLINE/PubMed (Index Medicus), EMBASE/Excerpta Medica, and PsycINFO, and ISI/BIOMED.*

Contributors

CONSULTING EDITOR

RANDOLPH W. EVANS, MD
Clinical Professor, Department of Neurology, Baylor College of Medicine, Houston, Texas, USA

EDITOR

LASZLO L. MECHTLER, MD, FAAN, FEAN, FASN
Professor of Neurology and Oncology, Medical Director, Dent Neurologic Institute, Roswell Park Comprehensive Cancer Center, The State University of New York, University at Buffalo, Past President of the American Society of Neuroimaging, Buffalo, New York, USA

AUTHORS

BELA AJTAI, MD, PhD
Dent Neurologic Institute, Amherst, New York, USA

ANDREI V. ALEXANDROV, MD, RVT
Semmes-Murphey Professor and Chairman, Department of Neurology, The University of Tennessee Health Science Center, Memphis, Tennessee, USA

JOHN A. BERTELSON, MD, FAAN
Associate Professor of Neurology, Texas Tech Health Sciences Center, Lubbock, Texas, USA; Assistant Professor of Neurology and Psychiatry, The University of Texas at Austin Dell Medical School, Austin, Texas, USA

PATRICK M. CAPONE, MD, PhD
Assistant Professor of Neurology, Virginia Commonwealth University, Richmond, Virginia, USA; Department of Neurology and Medical Imaging, Winchester Medical Center, Winchester Neurological Consultants, Inc., Winchester, Virginia, USA

SHASHVAT M. DESAI, MD
Instructor, Neurology, University of Pittsburgh, Pittsburgh, Pennsylvania, USA

LORAND EROSS, MD, PhD, FIPP
Head, Department of Functional Neurosurgery, Center of Neuromodulation, National Institute of Clinical Neurosciences, Budapest, Hungary

JOSEPH V. FRITZ, PhD
Chief Executive Officer, Dent Neurologic Institute, Partner, NeuroNetPro, Amherst, New York, USA

ZSOLT GARAMI, MD
Medical Director, Vascular Ultrasound Lab, Assistant Professor of Radiology in Clinical Cardiothoracic Surgery, Houston Methodist Hospital, Weill Cornell Medical College, Houston, Texas, USA

RYAN HAKIMI, DO, MS, FNCS, NVS
Director, Neuro ICU and Inpatient Neurology Services, Director, Greenville Memorial Hospital-TCD Laboratory, Prisma Health-Upstate, Associate Professor, University of South Carolina School of Medicine Greenville, Greenville, South Carolina, USA

YATHISH HARALUR, MD
Director of Stroke and Neurovascular Services, Neuro-Hospitalist Program, Mississippi Baptist Medical Center, Jackson, Mississippi, USA

RAYMOND Y. HUANG, MD, PhD
Department of Radiology, Brigham and Women's Hospital, Boston, Massachusetts, USA

ASHUTOSH P. JADHAV, MD, PhD
Associate Professor, Neurology, University of Pittsburgh, Pittsburgh, Pennsylvania, USA

DARA G. JAMIESON, MD
Clinical Associate Professor of Neurology, Weill Cornell Medicine, New York, New York, USA

JOSHUA P. KLEIN, MD, PhD
Vice Chair, Clinical Affairs, Department of Neurology, Brigham and Women's Hospital, Associate Professor of Neurology and Radiology, Harvard Medical School, Boston, Massachusetts, USA

ZOLTAN KLIMAJ, MD
Resident, MR Research Center, Semmelweis University, Budapest, Hungary

ELAD I. LEVY, MD, MBA, FACS, FAHA
Professor and L Nelson Chair of Neurological Surgery, Department of Neurosurgery, Jacobs School of Medicine and Biomedical Sciences, University at Buffalo, Buffalo, New York, USA

DAVID S. LIEBESKIND, MD
Professor, Neurology, University of California, Los Angeles, Los Angeles, California, USA

K. INA LY, MD
Stephen E. and Catherine Pappas Center for Neuro-Oncology, Massachusetts General Hospital, Boston, Massachusetts, USA

JOSEPH C. MASDEU, MD, PhD
Nantz National Alzheimer Center, Houston Methodist Hospital, Director, Nantz National Alzheimer Center and Neuroimaging, Houston Methodist Neurologic Institute, Professor of Neurology, Weill Medical College of Cornell University, Houston, Texas, USA

JENNIFER W. McVIGE, MA, MD
Dent Neurologic Institute, Amherst, New York, USA

LASZLO L. MECHTLER, MD, FAAN, FEAN, FASN
Professor of Neurology and Oncology, Medical Director, Dent Neurologic Institute, Roswell Park Comprehensive Cancer Center, The State University of New York, University at Buffalo, Past President of the American Society of Neuroimaging, Buffalo, New York, USA

NANDOR K. PINTER, MD
Imaging Research Scientist, Dent Neurologic Institute, Amherst, New York, USA; Department of Neurosurgery, The State University of New York, University at Buffalo, Buffalo, New York, USA

JONATHAN RILEY, MD
Assistant Professor, Department of Neurosurgery, Jacobs School of Medicine and Biomedical Sciences, University at Buffalo, Buffalo, New York, USA

GABRIELLA SZATMARY, MD, PhD
Director of Neuro-Ophthalmology, Neuroimaging Hattiesburg Clinic, Hattiesburg, Mississippi, USA; Assistant Professor, University of Mississippi Medical Center, Jackson, Mississippi, USA

KUNAL VAKHARIA, MD
Chief Resident, Department of Neurosurgery, Jacobs School of Medicine and Biomedical Sciences, University at Buffalo, Buffalo, New York, USA

LAWRENCE R. WECHSLER, MD
Professor, Neurology, University of Pittsburgh, Pittsburgh, Pennsylvania, USA

PATRICK Y. WEN, MD
Center for Neuro-Oncology, Dana-Farber Cancer Institute, Boston, Massachusetts, USA

Contents

> MRI is a commonly used diagnostic tool in neurology, and all neurologists should possess a working knowledge of imaging fundamentals. An overview of current and impending MRI techniques is presented to help the referring clinician communicate better with the imaging department, understand the utility and limitations of current and emerging technology, improve specificity and appropriateness when ordering MRI studies, and recognize key findings.

> Pregnant women may have exacerbation of preexisting neurologic disorders or new-onset neurologic symptoms for which brain or spinal cord imaging is appropriate. Primary headaches in early pregnancy can be diagnosed and treated without imaging. Headaches later in pregnancy or in the peripartum period may need to be evaluated by brain and/or vascular imaging. Cerebrovascular complications have distinctive imaging but overlapping presentations. Mass lesions can enlarge, producing neurologic symptoms, late in pregnancy. Imaging may be necessary to diagnose neurologic disorders in pregnancy and the peripartum period. MRI is preferred during pregnancy; imaging involving ionizing radiation and/or contrast should be avoided.

> Neuroimaging provides a window on the biological events underlying dementia. Amyloid PET is positive in Alzheimer disease (AD) and some cases of diffuse Lewy body disease, but negative in the frontotemporal dementias (FTDs). Tau PET using the current tracers shows the greatest signal in AD and a lesser signal in FTD. Quantifying volume loss with MRI and measuring metabolism with fluorodeoxyglucose PET helps separate different causes of dementia and follow their progression. Brain inflammation can be assessed with PET. Some of these techniques, still investigational, are likely to find their clinical niche in the near future.

> The 2016 World Health Organization Classification of Tumors of the Central Nervous System (CNS) incorporated well-established molecular markers

diagnosis and can aide in acute treatment decision making and guide information on prognosis. Features that are delineated include the parenchyma and the blood vessels. Parenchymal characteristics include early ischemic changes, established infarct and tissue at risk (penumbra), and hemorrhage. Vessel pathology includes arterial and venous steno-occlusive disease and vascular malformations. In the presence of a vessel occlusion, vessel imaging can assess collateral flow. This article outlines the role of neuroimaging as applied to patients presenting with acute stroke.

Deep brain stimulation is the most advanced and effective neuromodulation therapy for Parkinson disease, essential tremor, and generalized dystonia. This article discusses how imaging improves surgical techniques and outcomes and widens possibilities in translational neuroscience in Parkinson disease, essential tremor, generalized dystonia, and epilepsy. In movement disorders diffusion tensor imaging allows anatomic segment of cortical areas and different functional subregions within deep-seated targets to understand the side effects of stimulation and gain more data to describe the therapeutic mechanism of action. The introduction of visualization of white matter tracks increases the safety of neurosurgical techniques in functional neurosurgery and neuro-oncology.

Transcranial Doppler ultrasonography (TCD) is a noninvasive, bedside, portable tool for assessment of cerebral hemodynamics. Modern TCD head frames allow continuous hands-free emboli detection for risk stratification and assessment of treatment efficacy in several cardiovascular diseases. Identifying a focal stenosis, arterial occlusion, and monitoring the treatment effect of intravenous tissue plasminogen activator can easily be accomplished by assessing TCD waveforms and determining prestenotic and poststenotic mean flow velocities. TCD is an excellent screening tool for vasospasm in aneurysmal subarachnoid hemorrhage. The use of intraoperative TCD during carotid endarterectomy and stenting allows optimal intraoperative hemodynamic management. Other applications are also discussed.

NEUROLOGIC CLINICS

RELATED SERIES

Neuroimaging Clinics
Psychiatric Clinics
Child and Adolescent Psychiatric Clinics

THE CLINICS ARE AVAILABLE ONLINE!
Access your subscription at:
www.theclinics.com

Preface

Neuroimaging

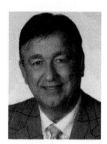

Laszlo L. Mechtler, MD, FAAN, FEAN, FASN
Editor

With its disciplined process of relating lesion visualization to symptoms, neuroimaging is central to neurology and used by most of its subspecialties. Neurologists possess unique insights into the appropriate use of imaging and are well positioned to contribute important advances in neurodiagnostics. For these reasons, an understanding of neuroimaging makes us better neurologists. Neurologists who make urgent point-of-care decisions are particularly inclined to interpret directly from images; examples include neurohospitalists, stroke specialists, critical care neurologists, interventional neurologists, neurooncologists, and practitioners who use teleneurology.

Advances in the burgeoning field of functional neuroimaging require a greater depth of neuroscience training and will certainly benefit from the active involvement of clinical and research neurologists who are also trained in neuroimaging. I hope to see in the future the establishment of efficient multidisciplinary "neuro" departments that merge neurology, neurosurgery, clinical neurophysiology, neuroradiology, nuclear neurology, and neurorehabilitation, according to which the equipment would be purchased and run on a service basis. This arrangement would optimize patient care, improve training, and expand opportunities for research. The evolution of anatomic and especially functional neuroimaging will dictate the need for neurologists to be sitting at the same table as our esteemed neuroradiology colleagues.

To achieve any success in neuroimaging training efforts, a healthy respect for the complexity of imaging technology is needed that encompasses recognizing how artifacts can mimic pathology, understanding how certain techniques can mask or highlight pathology, and learning the process for unbiased interpretation of images while concisely addressing the clinical question. Experienced neuroimagers find the mix of clinical neurology and imaging to be fulfilling and believe that such an integrated career can be an incentive for medical students to choose neurology as a specialty. Given the predictions of a dangerous shortfall in the US neurology workforce, this lure should not be taken lightly.

Neurol Clin 38 (2020) xi–xii
https://doi.org/10.1016/j.ncl.2019.10.001
0733-8619/20/© 2019 Published by Elsevier Inc.

neurologic.theclinics.com

As the editor of 2 previous issues on neuroimaging in *Neurologic Clinics*, I would like to thank Dr Randolph Evans for bestowing and entrusting me with another.. Either Dr Evans believes in me or he is hoping I'll get it right the third time. I would like to thank Donald Mumford, developmental editor of *Neurologic Clinics* at Elsevier, for his support of the field of neuroimaging. I am indebted to all the authors who contributed their time and efforts to this issue. I would also like to thank my executive assistant, Amanda McFayden, for her tireless help in organizing and coordinating this issue.

In my first issue, I thanked my family; in the second issue, I thanked my parents, and now I would like to acknowledge the great neuroimaging minds that have taught and guided me in my 35-year career as a neuroimaging neurologist. This includes Drs William Kinkel, Jack Greenberg, Lawrence Jacobs, Joseph Masdeu, Vernice Bates, and Joseph Fritz. I can only hope that I have shared that knowledge with the scores of neurologists, fellows, residents, and students that have trained at the DENT Neurologic Institute and at annual meetings of the American Academy of Neurology and the American Society of Neuroimaging, the latter of which I am proud to have served as President.

It is my hope that you enjoy reading the latest neuroimaging issue of *Neurologic Clinics* as much as we enjoyed putting it together for you.

Laszlo L. Mechtler, MD, FAAN, FEAN, FASN
Dent Neurologic Institute
Roswell Park
Comprehensive Cancer Center
State University of
New York at Buffalo
3980 Sheridan Drive
Buffalo, NY 14226, USA

E-mail address:
lmechtler@dentinstitute.com

Neuroimaging for the Neurologist
Clinical MRI and Future Trends

Nandor K. Pinter, MD[a,b], Joseph V. Fritz, PhD[c,d],*

KEYWORDS

- Neuroimaging • MRI • Emerging MRI techniques

KEY POINTS

- MRI is a versatile technology that continually introduces new methods for visualizing anatomic and physiologic characteristics.
- Neurologists should be sufficiently versed in available and upcoming MRI methods to communicate effectively with imaging departments and, minimally, enable cursory review of images.
- Extensive resources are available for neurologists to develop more detailed skills and expand their scope of contribution to the growing field of neuroimaging.

INTRODUCTION

MRI is central to neurologic diagnosis and treatment planning, with a rich history of innovations drawing on knowledge and insights from clinical neuroscience experts.[1–3] Recent advances in physiologic imaging, quantitative methods, informatics, artificial intelligence, and scan-time reduction are yielding more information with which to make early clinical diagnoses, but also resulting in greater complexity and the need for strong multidisciplinary communication among subspecialty professionals.

At least a rudimentary technical literacy of MRI is important for all clinicians who regularly refer patients for MRI. Although there are only a few procedure codes to consider when ordering an MRI, there should be an appreciation for the clinical detail required to select from the many MRI scanning protocols, sequences, and parameters that should be tailored precisely to answer the clinical question for that individual patient.[4] Furthermore, knowledge of fundamentals enables the ordering provider to ask about the availability of special techniques that may improve conspicuity of suspected

Disclosure Statement: N.K. Pinter and J.V. Fritz are consultants for Philips Healthcare.
^a Dent Neurologic Institute, 3980A Sheridan Drive, Suite 101, Amherst, NY 14226, USA;
^b Department of Neurosurgery, State University of New York at Buffalo, Buffalo, NY, USA;
^c Dent Neurologic Institute, 3980 Sheridan Drive, Suite 501, Amherst, NY 14226, USA;
^d NeuroNetPro, Amherst, NY, USA
* Corresponding author. 3980 Sheridan Drive, Suite 501, Amherst, NY 14226.
E-mail address: jfritz@dentinstitute.com

Neurol Clin 38 (2020) 1–35
https://doi.org/10.1016/j.ncl.2019.08.002   neurologic.theclinics.com
0733-8619/20/© 2019 Elsevier Inc. All rights reserved.

pathologic condition, set expectations for the patient experience, and take advantage of readily available images to enhance shared decision making with patients. Ultimately, understanding the language of MRI permits a more successful collaboration between patient care and diagnostic imaging professionals.

The purpose of this article is to provide an overview of currently available MRI capabilities, and those in the process of becoming mainstream, to help the practicing clinician achieve these goals. A complete didactic is outside of the scope possible within this article, so the reader is advised to consult readily available papers, books, videos, and illustrations for additional detail on MRI techniques[5–9]; safety considerations related to contrast use, implanted devices or cosmetics[10–13]; and appropriate utilization guidelines used by payers and regulatory agencies.[14–16]

FUNDAMENTALS AND APPLICATIONS OF COMMON MRI SEQUENCES

An MRI imaging study comprises multiple series, each representing unique views tailored to the referring indications. Acquisition techniques are often referred to as sequences, a term derived from the sequential process of generating, receiving, and reconstructing signals from protons in tissue. A virtually unlimited number of permutations of technical parameters are available, leading to the versatility and complexity of MRI.

The primary goal in manipulating sequence parameters is to optimize contrast and anatomic views that improve lesion conspicuity. The timing parameters repetition time (TR), echo time (TE), and inversion time (TI) control tissue contrast; flip angle can reduce imaging time or offer an additional way to control the so called T1 weighting; matrix size, slice thickness, field of view, slice orientation, and whether the acquisition is 2-dimensional (2D; slice by slice) or 3-dimensional (3D; contiguous volume imaging) determine resolution and, therefore, detectability of small structures or lesions. Use of a gadolinium-based contrast agent (GBCA) reduces T1 and T2 relaxation time constants for affected tissue, thereby increasing pixel intensity of T1-weighted images, and reducing the intensity in T2-weighted images. T1-weighted images are generally performed before and after GBCA. The interconnectedness of its many parameters adds to the complexity of MRI, in which acquisition strategies constantly trade signal-to-noise ratio, resolution, scan time, and artifact mitigation.

A glossary of some of the more frequently used parameter terminology is presented in **Table 1**. **Table 2** summarizes sequences typically used for brain and spine imaging. **Table 3** lists some common artifacts.[17]

Basic Structural Scans

T1-weighted and T2-weighted sequences form the anchor for structural MRI using variations of Spin Echo (SE) or Field Echo (FE) sequences. Both SE and FE, as well as their accelerated versions Fast Spin Echo (FSE) and Fast Field Echo (FFE) rely on precise timing of excitations (TR) and readout (TE). An additional parameter called the Flip Angle (FA) can be varied to control the orientation of tissue magnetization, allowing trade-off between maximum signal, shorter scan time and more contrast control. **Fig. 1** illustrates the change in tissue contrast as TR and TE parameters are varied to control the degree of T1, T2, and proton density (PD) weighting. In general, T2 and T1 weightings produce reversed contrast between fat, white matter, gray matter, and cerebrospinal fluid (CSF) (dark to bright in T2 weighting, bright to dark in T1 weighting). Anomalies to this contrast ordering can occur with certain sequences. For example, T2-weighted fast spin echo (FSE) images may exhibit brighter than expected fat signal owing to the complex interaction of the many refocusing pulses with the tissue. In T1-weighted images, the typically bright fat signal may be intentionally suppressed

Table 1 Basic terminology	
Term	**Definition**
Larmor Frequency	Natural precessional frequency of a proton that permits detection and localization of protons in tissues. Proportional to the magnetic field determined by the Bo (B zero, main static field of an MRI, eg, 1.5 T or 3 T), plus any temporarily applied gradient fields used for spatial encoding, plus any tissue effects that change the local field around the proton (eg, chemical structure or susceptibility)
RF pulse or RF excitation	Radiofrequency pulse, also known as the B1 field, tuned to the Larmor frequency that is used to excite the net magnetization of protons toward a perpendicular (measurable) orientation to the Bo field
Echo	Data that are obtained after RF excitation and represent a single "view." Multiple echoes or views are needed to reconstruct an image, similar to multiple projections obtained in CT
Receiver coil	The antenna that is applied to the patient anatomy being scanned. Receiver arrays consist of multiple coil elements to improve signal-to-noise ratio and, together with parallel imaging, speed up scans
TR	Repetition time, or the time between RF pulses that allows for tissues to realign with the magnetic field. Selected to determine T1 weighting. Also a primary determinant of scan time.
TE	Echo time. Time from excitation to echo readout. Selected to control T2 contrast
T1	A tissue property that represents the rate of recovery for excited tissue to realign with the main magnetic field
T2	A tissue property that represents the rate of dephasing (signal loss) in the transverse plane after excitation
T2*	Field echo version of T2, but also accounts for signal lost by not using a refocusing pulse (ie, T2* includes susceptibility effect)
Phase-encode (PE) direction	One of the 2 directions in an image. Specifies the direction in which the phase of the proton signal is used to decode position. The number of phase-encode steps, together with the field of view in the PE direction, determines resolution, is a primary determinant in scan time, and is the direction in which motion and wrap artifacts propagate
Frequency-encoding (FE) direction	A user-defined parameter that specifies the direction in which the magnetic field is changed to encode proton location by its Larmor frequency. Represents one of the 2 directions in an image, and is the direction in which chemical shift artifacts propagate
TI	Inversion time is the time delay parameter in an inversion recovery sequence. It is used to time the point at which certain tissue is nulled based on its T1 before initiating an imaging sequence, or to create a greater contrast in T1-weighted images. A short TI is used in STIR to null fat; a long TI is used in FLAIR to null CSF; and a midrange TI is used to stretch T1 contrast, for example, in high-resolution T1-weighted hippocampal imaging
Matrix	Specifies the in-plane resolution, or number of pixels that cover the field of view in the PE and FE directions (eg, 256 × 192). The matrix size in the PE direction determines the number of views required, and hence is a major determinant in scan time

(*continued on next page*)

Table 1
(continued)

Term	Definition
Field of view	The spatial extent of the imaging volume in the PE and FE directions (eg, 25 cm × 25 cm)
Slice thickness	Determines the voxel dimension in the slice direction
Pixel and voxel resolution	The area of the picture element in an image, or the volume of a voxel (pixel area times slice thickness). Higher resolution means smaller voxels and therefore less signal (fewer protons per voxel), but improved detail (less partial volume averaging)
Bandwidth	Specifies the range of precessional frequencies used for Frequency Encoding. Equates to how quickly a readout signal is acquired. Choosing a high bandwidth is advantageous in speed and reducing chemical shift artifact, but disadvantageous because of a decrease in signal-to-noise ratio
Echo train length (ETL)	The ETL specifies the number of FSE or FFE echoes during a single excitation period, reducing scan time proportionally
Parallel imaging, SENSE factor	Uses sensitivity profiles from individual elements of array coils to reduce scan time

Table 2
Common sequences used for brain and spine imaging

Spin echo (SE) and fast spin echo (FSE)	Routine structural imaging. Fast spin echo (also known as turbo spin echo) obtains multiple views (echo train) within a single repetition to proportionally reduce imaging time. • Proton density weighting (long TR, short TE) • T1 weighting (short TR. short TE) • T2 weighting (long TR, long TE)
Field echo (FE) and fast field echo (FFE)	Same as SE and FSE (TSE) except for eliminating a "refocusing" pulse to correct for loss of signal owing to magnetic field inhomogeneity. • Creates T2*-weighted images that enhance tissue susceptibility effects (eg, blood products) • Increases acquisition speed using shorter TR and lower flip angle, useful in 3D imaging
Inversion recovery	Manipulates T1 tissue contrast with an inversion pulse "TI" seconds before a conventional imaging sequence • Medium TI = greater T1 tissue contrast (phase-sensitive IR = PSIR) • Short TI or short tau IR = STIR for fat suppression and high lesion conspicuity • Fluid-attenuated IR = FLAIR for CSF suppression
Chemical shift–based fat-suppression methods	Different magnetic properties of fat and water cause their frequencies to differ, allowing for manipulation of fat and water signals. • Chemical shift or fat sat uses a prepulse tuned to the resonant frequency of fat • Out-of-phase FE imaging, water-fat separation, and Dixon methods use field echo sequences and specific TEs tuned to the different fat and water frequencies to add or subtract water and fat signals
Diffusion-weighted imaging	Relatively restricted movement of fluids causes bright signal. • Apparent diffusion coefficient (ADC) image provides quantitative value for rate of diffusion (bright DWI owing to restricted diffusion will be dark on ADC because the diffusion is low) • Diffusion tensor images map diffusion boundaries, such as along white matter tracts

(continued on next page)

Table 2 *(continued)*	
Perfusion-weighted imaging (PWI)	• Dynamic susceptibility contrast (DSC) collects T2* images while GBCA contrast perfuses tissue. Dynamic contrast enhancement (DCE) uses dynamic T1 images. Typically calculate CBF, CBV, MTT, and/or TTP maps from pixel-by-pixel dynamic changes • Arterial spin labeling is a noncontrast perfusion technique using MRI pulses to mimic a GBCA bolus
Susceptibility-weighted imaging	A T2* acquisition with special postprocessing to enhance and quantify susceptibility effects. Generally used to accentuate conspicuity of, and differentiate, blood products and calcification
Driven Equilibrium or Fast Recovery FSE (DRIVE, FRFSE, RESTORE)	Additional RF pulse to speed T1 recovery. Improves brightness of long T1 tissue such as CSF. Typically used to create high-contrast, high-resolution T2-weighted images such as cranial nerve imaging
Magnetic resonance angiography (MRA)	Differentiates blood vessels from surrounding static tissue using sequences sensitive to flow. • Time-of-flight MRA uses a very short TR to create an excessively T1-weighted image (little signal). Inflowing blood that does not experience the short TR is relatively bright. • Phase-contrast MRA quantifies blood flow using special sequences sensitive to user-defined ranges of flow velocities, and is typically used for slow/venous imaging • Contrast-enhanced MRA uses very fast, heavily weighted T1 sequences timed to the injection of a contrast agent. Used for speed, a more accurate representation of vessel lumen, and dynamic visualization of flow
Whole-body imaging	Stitches together and creates projections of fat-suppressed STIR or DWI images that are sensitive to either diffusion restriction (hypercellularity) or long T2/short T1 pathology. Used as an oncology screen
Functional MRI (fMRI)	Uses Blood Oxygen Level Dependent (BOLD) technique to identify areas of the brain that correlate oxygenation-related signal changes and neural activity. The paradigm-driven method uses a dynamic acquisition during timed patient activities, and correlates signal changes to activity to determine areas of activation. Newer "resting state" functional imaging (rs-fMRI) correlates naturally occurring oxygenation changes across brain regions to identify functional connectivity. fMRI can be used with DTI to identify eloquent tissue and fiber tract connections as part of presurgical planning
Magnetic resonance spectroscopy	Identifies relative levels of metabolites such as lactate, NAA, creatine, choline, and myoinositol. Low NAA implies cell death, high choline implies hyperactive metabolism (tumor), myoinositol is associated with dementia. Image maps typically display colorized metabolite ratios

Table 3 **Common MRI artifacts**	
Artifact	**Description and Comments**
Echo train blurring	Blurring in sequences with short TE and a long echo train. Caused by T2 signal loss while collecting multiple echoes
Wrap, aliasing	Anatomy from one edge of the field of view in the PE direction is misplaced to the opposite side of the field of view. When using parallel imaging to shorten scan time, which effectively stitches together smaller fields of view, the artifact can appear toward the middle of the image

(continued on next page)

Table 3
(continued)

Artifact	Description and Comments
Susceptibility	Signal loss and distortion associated with interfaces between tissues and objects with differing magnetic field properties, such as bone, air, metal, and soft tissue. Also the basis for susceptibility-weighted imaging of blood products
Chemical shift	Misplacement of fat signal along the FE direction, causing a bright/dark band at edge of fat-containing tissue
Pulsation and ghosting	Motion, including variable blood flow, creates replication "ghosting" along the phase-encode direction
MRA TOF artifacts: turbulent flow and venetian blind artifacts	Blood flow turbulence causes dephasing and exaggeration of stenosis; in multi-slab 3D TOF MRA, boundaries between slabs may exhibit abrupt signal changes
Nonuniform fat suppression	Caused by magnetic field distortion from susceptibility effects, equipment malfunction, or at the boundaries of the useable field of view for a given scanner
STIR suppression of gadolinium enhancement	Suppression of GBCA enhancement because of inappropriate use of STIR for fat suppression in postcontrast study
Gibbs/edge ringing	Replication of sharp boundaries when image resolution in PE direction is too low in a high-contrast area of an image, such as the CSF-cord interface in T2-weighted spine imaging

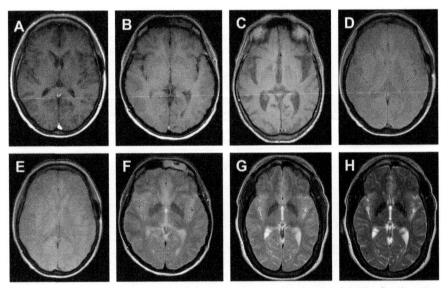

Fig. 1. Effect of sequence parameters on image contrast. In (*A*) through (*D*), TE is fixed at 10 ms while TR is set at 400 ms, 1000 ms, 1800 ms, and 3000 ms, respectively. This shows white matter signal decreasing and gray matter and CSF signal increasing as image appearance shifts from typical T1-weighted contrast (*A*) to typical proton density contrast (*D*). In images (*E*) to (*H*), TR is fixed at 3000 ms while TE is set at 10 ms, 70 ms, 90 ms, and 150 ms. The signal of white matter and deep gray matter structures decreases while the signal of CSF remarkably increases as image appearance shifts from a proton density contrast (*E*) to typical T2-weighted contrast (*H*).

through the use of a "chemical saturation" technique; this may be done, for example, to differentiate fat from contrast agent enhancement, or to eliminate an artifact that can misrepresent the location of fatty tissue resulting from a phenomenon called chemical shift. **Fig. 2** demonstrates that structural imaging can itself offer functional insights.

Acquisition of some sequences in different imaging planes is not only helpful in visualizing the anatomy but also provides a check against certain artifacts that propagate along specific directions (eg, pulsatile flow can "ghost" in the phase-encode direction). Axial, sagittal, coronal, or oblique orientations are generally standardized to anatomic landmarks to provide consistency in interpretation, and when comparing series within or between studies.

3D acquisitions are high signal-to-noise ratio, time-efficient scans that offer versatile tissue contrast. An important benefit of a 3D scan is the ability to separately optimize the acquisition orientation and the anatomic view by using postprocessing rather than individual acquisitions to generate multiplanar reformatted views (**Fig. 3**).

Long TE field echo imaging generates are known as T2*-weighted rather than T2-weighted images. They are more sensitive to signal changes from magnetic field disturbances, whether from equipment or tissue interaction. Although this sensitivity does produce vulnerability to artifacts, T2* sequences offer certain advantages, such as blood product visualization (eg, hemosiderin and calcification are dark).

The concept of susceptibility-weighted imaging to view blood products has long existed using this basic T2*-weighted field echo sequence. However, today the term susceptibility-weighted imaging (SWI) has evolved to represent a more sophisticated version of a long TE field echo sequence, using "phase data" normally ignored in classic magnitude reconstructions to enhance subtle areas of susceptibility changes.

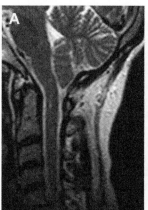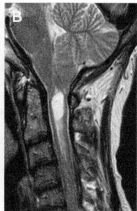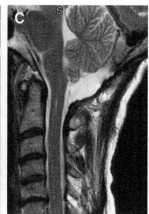

Fig. 2. Evolution of Chiari malformation and cervical syrinx in a 58-year-old patient. Sagittal T2-weighted sequence (*A*) shows cerebellar tonsils extending 3.5 mm below the foramen magnum and a subtle hyperintensity in the center of the spinal cord at C1 (A, *arrowhead*). Four years later (*B*), the tonsils extend 5 mm below the foramen magnum, consistent with Chiari I malformation; a large syrinx with surrounding edema developed at C1–C2 (*B*, *arrowheads* and *bracket*). (C) shows follow-up after decompressive surgery, with resolution of the syrinx. This case illustrates the interplay between structural changes and CSF flow dynamics in the evolution of syrinx and Chiari malformation, and calls attention to the role of functional diagnostics in the evaluation of abnormalities of the craniocervical junction.

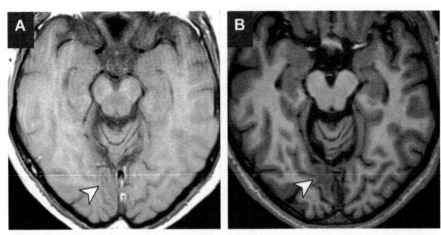

Fig. 3. Significance of 3D imaging in epilepsy diagnostics. (*A*) A 2D T1 scan with 4 mm slice thickness; (*B*) an axial reformat of a 3D T1 scan acquired in sagittal plane. Although the 2D acquisition has higher in-plane resolution (0.9 × 0.9 mm), the worse gray-white contrast and the flow artifact running in lateral (phase) direction from the straight sinus make the occipital focal cortical dysplasia (*arrowhead*) difficult to detect compared with the axial reformat that has slightly lower in-plane resolution (1 × 1 mm).

Standard variations include 2D, 3D, and thick slab "projection" views (minimum-intensity projections), along with display of "phase maps" that are used to differentiate blood products from calcifications. Compared with conventional T2* imaging, SWI is superior in venous imaging, amyloid angiopathy, trauma, and various causes of microbleeds (**Fig. 4**). Newer developments seek to quantify the degree of susceptibility and relate that value to oxygenation.[18]

3T magnetic resonance systems are often preferred over 1.5 T and lower field strengths for neuroimaging because of advantages in signal-to-noise ratio, higher-resolution scanning, and improved lesion conspicuity. However, 3T does require higher-power RF pulses, which increases the rate of heat buildup in a patient. Specific absorption rate (SAR) limitations are built into MRI systems to ensure patient safety, but can result in slower scans. For this reason, 3T MRI sequences have been adjusted to minimize the use of high-power pulses, such as greater use of use of 2D and 3D field echo sequences.

T2*-related distortion from metal or pulsatile flow tend to be greater, however, and 3T MRI further exacerbates these artifacts. In contrast, spin echo (SE) or turbo spin echo (TSE) sequences (T1, T2, or PD contrast) offer better signal-to-noise ratio and tend to self-correct for artifacts caused by tissue interactions with the magnetic field, and blood flow tends to create signal voids that minimize pulsatility artifacts while providing helpful views of major vessel lumens and aneurysms. In recent years, special sequence methodologies have been created to increase the speed of 3D SE sequences through longer echo trains and novel approaches to reduce the SAR effect of many refocusing pulses. 3D field echo sequences remain the norm for T1-weighted 3D acquisitions, although 3D TSE sequences are becoming more popular for long TE, T2-weighted imaging.

The following sections provide an overview of other structural and physiologic imaging techniques, selected to highlight certain practical aspects that the authors consider important based on their experience. The discussions are not intended to

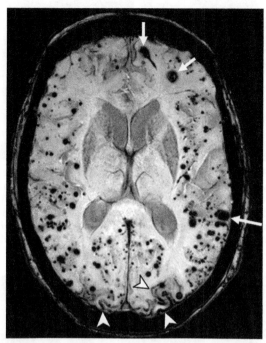

Fig. 4. Severe amyloid angiopathy on SWI showing innumerable hemorrhages in cortical and subcortical localization in both hemispheres. There is a striking contrast between the appearance of the spared basal ganglia and thalami and of the heavily affected peripheral parenchyma. Larger hemorrhagic foci are seen in the left frontal and temporal lobes (*arrows*). Areas of superficial siderosis are also noted in the posterior parietal lobes (*arrowheads*), resulting from prior subarachnoid hemorrhage of superficial lesions.

be comprehensive, but rather to provide clinically useful takeaway points and ignite interest in current and future methods.

Inversion Recovery and Fluid-Attenuated Inversion Recovery

Fluid-attenuated inversion recovery (FLAIR), or more specifically T2 FLAIR, has become an essential part of brain evaluation because the suppression of CSF signal produces excellent contrast between lesions and white matter. With a few exceptions, lacunar infarcts in the basal ganglia being one, it is superior to T2-weighted images in lesion visualization.

Improving contrast by eliminating CSF signal has always been important for clinical scanning and until as recently as the mid 2000s, proton density (PD) was the primary technique used for this purpose because of its relative "dark CSF" appearance (see **Fig. 1**). Starting in the mid 2000's, FLAIR has become the primary sequence for detection and monitoring of demyelinating lesions.[19,20] Advances in technology for 3D FSE techniques have resulted in the ability to perform time-efficient 3D FLAIR, which offers superior signal, reduced artifacts, and improved resolution compared to 2D scans.-**Figs. 5** and **6** illustrate advantages of 3D FLAIR.

FLAIR is a variation of the inversion recovery (IR) technique, which manipulates tissue contrast based on T1 characteristics; short tau IR (STIR) suppresses T1 fat, dual IR

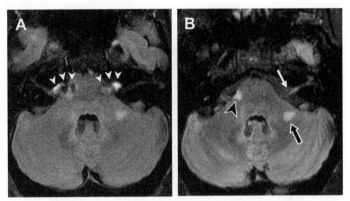

Fig. 5. On 2D FLAIR (*A*), prominent CSF pulsation artifacts are seen in the cerebellopontine angles (*white arrowheads*), obscuring a demyelinating lesion in the right lateral aspect of the pons, which becomes visible on 3D FLAIR (*B, black arrowhead*). With 3D acquisition the fluid attenuation in cerebellopontine cisterns is homogeneous, allowing sharp visualization of not only the pons, but the 7th and 8th cranial nerves as well (*B, white arrow*). A second lesion is seen in the middle cerebellar peduncle on the right, which is also more conspicuous on 3D (*B, black arrow*).

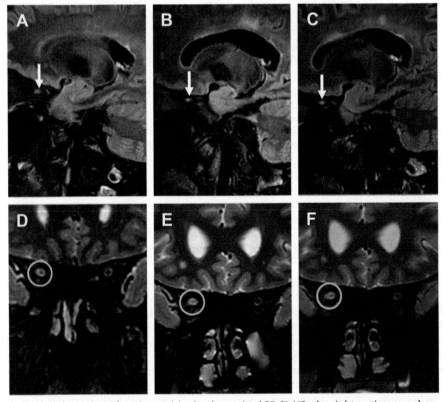

Fig. 6. Serial imaging of optic neuritis. On the sagittal 3D FLAIR, the right optic nerve shows a short, segmental hyperintensity that stands out against the background (*arrow* in *A–C*). On coronal fat-suppressed T2-weighted images, the affected nerve is depicted with smaller caliber and higher signal intensity compared with the normal left optic nerve (*circled area* in *D–F*). During the course of the longitudinal follow-up, the abnormality shows up consistently on both sequences and is more conspicuous on the 3D FLAIR. This draws attention to the broad utility of 3D FLAIR in imaging of multiple sclerosis.

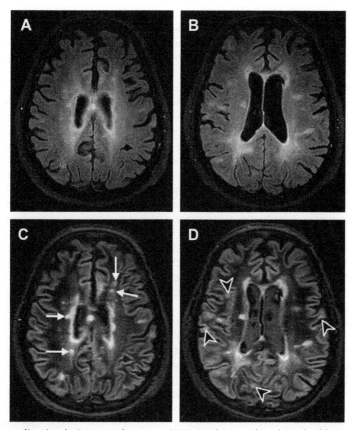

Fig. 7. Demyelinating lesions are shown on 3D FLAIR (*top row*) and 3D double inversion recovery (DIR, bottom row) in multiple sclerosis.(*A–C*) and (*B–D*) image pairs show the same slices. Increased lesion contrast is seen on the DIR images, which allows for an improved differentiation of deep white matter lesions (*white arrows* in *C*) as well as juxtacortical and cortical lesions (*arrowheads* in *D*).

uses multiple inversion pulses to suppress both CSF and white matter (**Fig. 7**), and phase-sensitive IR (PSIR) uses a midrange inversion time (TI) to stretch the T1 contrast of tissues.

Diffusion-Weighted Imaging

The diffusion-weighted sequence has high sensitivity to very slow flow, causing signal loss from normal extracellular fluid diffusion, and relatively bright signal in areas of abnormally restricted fluid motion. The flow sensitivity is controlled by a parameter known as the "b-value". At a b-value of zero, the image is essentially a conventional T2*-weighted image. At a b-value of 1000, normal tissue diffusion causes significant loss of signal. The b1000 image is typically referred to as the diffusion-weighted image. The b0 and b1000 images can be mathematically combined to calculate an apparent diffusion coefficient (ADC) image, which provides a numerical value for each pixel that equates to tissue diffusion. The purpose of an ADC image is to isolate the diffusion effect from other T2* effects that can cause the diffusion-weighted image to be bright (this is known as T2 shine-through). Bright pixels on a diffusion-weighted image should correspond to pixels with low diffusion coefficient values (dark pixels) on ADC, as long as the bright diffusion-weighted area is related to diffusion restriction and not T2 shine-through (**Fig. 8**). It is crucial that ADC is the "reality check" for diffusion-weighted imaging (DWI), meaning that **DWI cannot be reliably interpreted without the ADC map**.

DWI is very useful in differential diagnostics. It provides relevant information quickly and is generally easy to interpret. Abnormalities that will typically appear with high signal intensity on the DWI b1000 image and with corresponding low signal on ADC ("DWI positive") are associated with restriction in normal motion of the water molecules. Examples include: cytotoxic edema in acute infarcts when the water moves from the large extracellular space (where it is relatively free to move along white matter tracts) into the smaller intracellular space where its motion is confined in every direction; pus (ie, thick cellular debris) in an abscess where there is no real water diffusion; hypercellularity in some tumors with the most well-known example being primary central nervous system lymphoma; accumulation of material such as cholesterol and keratinous content in an epidermoid blood or even acute venous thrombosis; or again, cytotoxic edema in acute demyelinating plaques.[21,22] Other scenarios when DWI can be positive (ie, it shows restricted diffusion compared with normal tissue) include metabolic encephalopathies and degenerative disorders, such as Creutzfeld-Jakob disease, hypoglycemia, carbon-monoxide (CO) poisoning, hepatic encephalopathy, or osmotic demyelination syndrome, to name only a few.[23]

The opposite, increased diffusion, appears dark *or* bright on b1000 and *always* bright on ADC. Any tissue that has a buildup of freely moving water content will show high signal on ADC relative to normal parenchyma: from arachnoid cysts to liquefaction in chronic infarcts to cystic components in tumors to vasogenic edema (see **Fig. 8**).

Diffusion tensor imaging (DTI) is a reconstruction of directional diffusivity from multiple DWI sequences that probe proton mobility in several directions. Images representing average diffusivity and fractional anisotropy (FA) maps are created to characterize the magnitude of diffusion, its prominent direction, and directional distribution (tensor) within each voxel. The pixel FA value quantifies the ellipsoidal nature of diffusion, ranging from 0 for spherical (isotropic) diffusion in which there are no boundaries, to 1 for voxels that exhibit linear diffusion, such as along intact white matter tracts. Cautious use of functional MRI (fMRI) and DTI can provide a helpful visualization of eloquent tissue and related interconnections for presurgical planning or assessing the mass effect of a tumor (**Figs. 9** and **10**). Although the terms "pathways" and "tracts" are used, these color-coded images are representations of FA in the image voxels, which are large compared with real fiber size and thus are only a rough estimate of the real pathways. Quantitative FA maps may have value in determining the degree of white matter injury.[24–26]

DWI typically uses echo planar imaging (EPI), a very fast "single-shot" (1 minute) version of a field echo sequence. In general, EPI methods are very sensitive to susceptibility-related geometric distortion and signal loss at bone, air, tissue and metal interfaces (**Fig. 11**). Thus, the brain typically has a distorted shape on DWI images compared with other structural scans, with areas of artifactual high signal ("false positive") and signal loss along the frontal skull, the temporal bone, in the posterior fossa, and along any metal implants. This will make it difficult (and often impossible) to detect abnormalities in the brainstem, in the vicinity of surgical clips, in the presence of orthodontic appliances, adjacent to ventriculoperitoneal shunts or deep brain stimulation electrodes, and even in uncomplicated cases in the basal areas of the temporal lobes and in the orbital frontal cortex. EPI-based DWI can be replaced by TSE

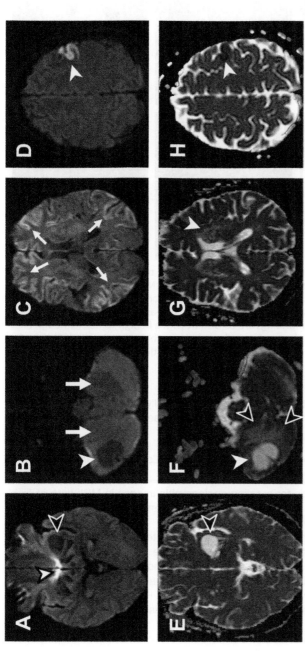

Fig. 8. DWI b1000 (top row) and corresponding ADC images (bottom row) from 4 cases. (A–E) Giant Virchow-Robin space in the area of the left basal ganglia (black arrowhead). The signal of the abnormality follows CSF on every sequence. Susceptibility artifact is creating high signal and distortion on DWI (white arrowhead). (B–F) Cystic tumor in the right cerebellar hemisphere (white arrowheads). Its appearance is similar to that of the enlarged peri-vascular space in (A–E); however, there is vasogenic edema in the parenchyma, which is prominent on ADC (F, black arrowheads). On DWI the edema appears as only a mild increase of white matter signal compared with the normal left side (B, white arrows) owing to T2 shine-through. (C–G) Diffuse cortical diffusion restriction is seen on the DWI image in both frontal lobes, parietal lobes, and insula, typical for Creutzfeld-Jakob disease (arrows). ADC is less demonstrative of these findings. In the basal ganglia increased diffusion is seen on ADC, owing to the high number of enlarged perivascular space (L'etat crible, white arrowhead in G). (D and H) An acute cortical infarct with diffusion restriction as demonstrated by the high DWI signal and corresponding marked ADC hypointensity.

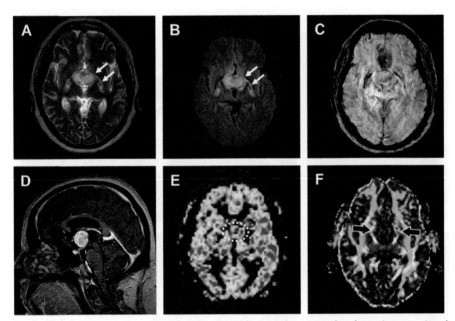

Fig. 9. Multiparametric imaging of a chordoid glioma. The tumor has hyperintense signal on T2-weighted image (*A, red dashed circle*) and FLAIR (*B*). No blood products or calcification are found on SWI (*C*), and homogeneous contrast enhancement is seen on 3D T1 (*D*). The 2D pCASL scan is unremarkable, without evident increased perfusion (*E*). The overall morphology and the perfusion findings are consistent with a benign tumor. Although bilateral minimal edema is seen in the basal ganglia and diencephalon (*arrows in A, B*) the adjacent white matter tracts are displaced and no true destruction is found on the fractional anisotropy map (*F, arrows*).

methods to mitigate artifacts, but results in a substantially longer scan (5–6 minutes). Decisions on applicability of DWI or which variation to use depend on relevant clinical information.

Magnetic Resonance Angiography: Time-of-Flight and Contrast-Enhanced Magnetic Resonance Angiography

There are 3 distinct methods for creating angiographic images in MRI: time-of-flight (TOF) magnetic resonance angiography (MRA), contrast-enhanced (CE) MRA, and phase-contrast (PC) MRA.

TOF MRA relies on bright signal from blood that enters an imaging volume that has low signal because of short TR saturation. There are 2D and 3D variations. 3D TOF MRA results in greater signal and resolution and is the usual scan for intracranial arterial imaging. 2D TOF is better for slow, venous flow, which tends to blend in with static background tissue in 3D volumes. However, 2D TOF has relatively poorer signal-to-noise ratio and resolution and is less commonly used than PC MRA or CE MRA.

Vessel lumen size can be estimated from the cross-section of the bright pixels, but only with caution because TOF works best with laminar flow and the flowing blood loses signal when turbulent flow occurs—one typical example being the carotid syphon. In general, TOF has a high negative predictive value but a low positive predictive value. For this reason it is widely accepted for aneurysm imaging, but less so for

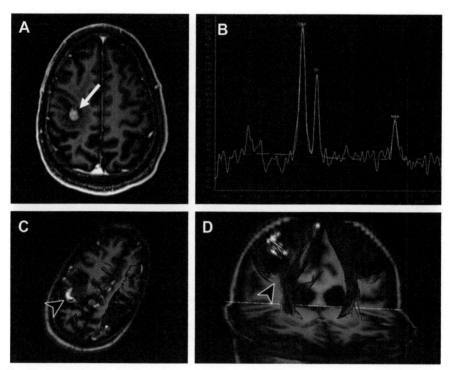

Fig. 10. Presurgical evaluation of an anaplastic astrocytoma shows a right posterior frontal mass with central contrast enhancement (*A, arrow*) and abnormal spectrum with elevated choline and decreased Cr and NAA in the same area (*B*). In (*C*) and (*D*) the fMRI motor activation map and tractography of the corticospinal tracts are shown, merged with the non-enhanced 3D T1 image. The most prominent activation during the left finger tapping paradigm is seen just posterior to the tumor, in the displaced and infiltrated precentral gyrus (*C, arrowhead*). The tractography shows fewer "tracts" on the right and abruption of the corticospinal pathways (*arrowhead* in *D*). The abnormal findings on DTI likely resulted from the combination of vasogenic edema and disruption of white matter microstructure owing to tumor infiltration.

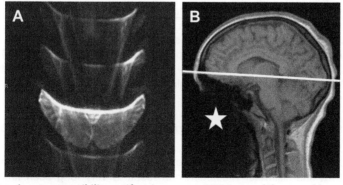

Fig. 11. Prominent susceptibility artifact is seen on DWI image (*A*), caused by orthodontic appliance in a young patient. Sagittal T1 (*B*) shows the angulation of the axial DWI (*white line*) and a large area of signal void overlying the oral cavity and facial tissue (*asterisk*), also caused by susceptibility for magnetic field changes. The DWI artifact might be reduced if the slices are aligned more parallel with the frontal skull base.

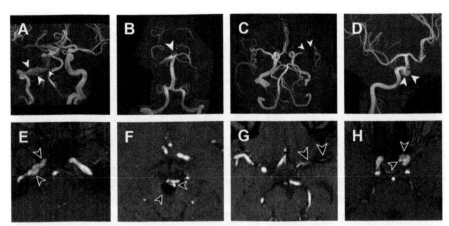

Fig. 12. 3D maximum-intensity projection images and corresponding to time-of-flight (TOF) MRA source images from 4 cases. (*A–E*) Fibromuscular dysplasia of the right internal carotid artery. (*B–F*) Basilar tip aneurysm following coiling. The arrowheads in (*F*) point out the residual flow in the basilar tip and the large susceptibility artifact caused by the coils. (*C–G*) Stent in the left middle cerebral artery (MCA) after acute stroke. No flow signal is seen in the MCA, which is again caused by susceptibility artifact and not the complete lack of flow, evident by the intact signal in the peripheral MCA branches. For stent evaluation, therefore, CT angiography is recommended. (*D–H*) Saccular aneurysm on the intracavernous segment of the left internal carotid artery (ICA). This location is more frequent than one would expect.

imaging of intracranial stenosis. It overestimates the degree of stenosis, and CT angiography is more reliable in that regard. The TOF scan consists of about 150 to 160 images (source images), which are then used to create 3D reconstructions (a virtual cast of vasculature) with a method called maximum-intensity projection (MIP). MIP images are routinely created for evaluation, but the final conclusion should never be made solely on MIP images because the reconstruction parameters are arbitrary and can (and almost always will) change the appearance of some vessels, potentially leading to false-negative or false-positive findings. The final decision should always be based on the source images (**Fig. 12**).

CE MRA uses fast 3D imaging after contrast agent injection to differentiate blood from static tissue. The technique requires proper timing between bolus injection and imaging, which can be more difficult for patients with vascular disease, and repeated CE MRAs in the same session are not recommended. An advantage of CE MRA is the ability to use cine views to visualize flow characteristics. CE MRA tends to be the preferred MRA technique for carotid imaging, as long as the patient is able to tolerate the contrast agent.

Imaging of Cranial Nerves: Driven Equilibrium, Constructive Interference in Steady State, and Other Useful Sequences

Heavily T2-weighted sequences that seek high contrast between CSF and parenchyma with a submillimeter resolution can result in very long scan times (many views, very long TR to allow full CSF signal recovery). Driven equilibrium techniques, such as DRIVE (driven equilibrium), RESTORE, or forced recovery FSE, help reduce scan time by using a somewhat shorter TR together with additional pulses to force longitudinal recovery. To further reduce scan time when the focus is on high CSF contrast and not parenchymal detail, a very long echo train length can be used, which blurs short T2 tissue but leaves resolution intact for a long T2 CSF signal. Although the scan duration is still long (5–6 minutes) and should only be used with strong clinical justification, these high-resolution scans are excellent in visualizing small tissues bathed by CSF, such as cranial nerves. DRIVE is popular for vestibular nerve imaging to evaluate for potential vestibular schwannoma, and also useful in imaging of trigeminal nerve and other cranial nerves (CN3, CN6, CN9–12). **Fig. 13** demonstrates the use of DRIVE in the evaluation of neurovascular compression in trigeminal neuralgia, when coregistered with a TOF MRA.[27]

Another well-known sequence in this space is CISS (constructive interference in steady state),[28] which has a T1 component and thus can be used to assess abnormal contrast enhancement, and is helpful in inflammatory or cancerous processes involving cranial nerves or the Meckel cave. However, even without special scans the cranial nerves are often visible on a high-resolution 3D T1 (the CE scans can be

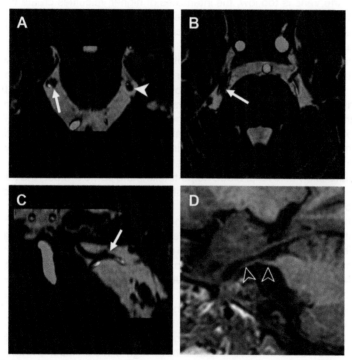

Fig. 13. Fusion of 3D DRIVE and TOF MRA images is shown in coronal, axial, and sagittal planes (A–C, respectively). The merging of the two image series is easily performed on a clinical postprocessing workstation. This visualization makes it easier to understand and interpret the relation between arteries and nerves and is useful in the evaluation of neurovascular conflict. In this patient, the trigeminal nerve on the right is compressed by the superior cerebellar artery and the anterior inferior cerebellar artery as highlighted by the arrow in (A–C). On the coronal image, the cross-section of the compressed nerve is elliptical in contrast to the rounded shape of the unaffected nerve on the left (*white arrowhead* in A). On the high-resolution sagittal 3D T1 (0.9 mm isotropic, D) the trigeminal nerve is clearly seen (*black arrowheads*); however, the small arteries are not visualized, thus the assessment of the neurovascular contact is not possible (compare C with D).

particularly satisfying for imaging the mandibular and maxillary nerves) or 3D FLAIR (can be surprisingly good for the abducens nerve). When a clinical question concerning a cranial nerve is left unanswered after a routine MRI, a second look on the image set is often good enough to find the answer and can spare the time, stress, and cost of an additional MRI examination- naturally, such additional investigation relies on a clear clinical question and good communication between the clinician and the radiologist.

Phase-Contrast Angiography

Phase-contrast angiography (PCA) is generally used for imaging of venous flow and is often referred to as magnetic resonance venography (MRV) in clinical practice. Its velocity sensitivity allows for visualization of the slower venous blood flow, making it a good alternative to contrast-enhanced (CE) computed tomography (CT). Flow sensitivity is defined by the parameter *velocity encoding* or "Venc," which specifies the expected velocity range. This property of PCA has two important practical implications: (1) if the Venc is too high, it will be difficult to differentiate variations of much slower normal venous flow representative of anatomic or physiologic variations; (2) if the Venc is too low, the intensities of higher velocities create variable intensity artifacts because their flow is misrepresented into the expected range (eg, if the Venc encodes velocities from 0 to 10 cm/s, an actual velocity of 16 cm/s "wraps around" and maps to 6 cm/s).

A typical case is the unilateral hypoplasia of the transverse sinus, when the sinus with the smaller caliber has slower venous flow that does not show up on PCA with a high Venc and mimics thrombosis. Concurrent hypoplasia of the internal jugular vein may also be present. This false positivity can be overcome easily by lowering the Venc to 5 to 10 cm/s whereby slower flow becomes visible; with this simple step one can both eliminate the possibility of a potentially life-threatening condition and spare further imaging tests. However, this lower Venc image becomes less clean as new flow-related artifacts appear. Although presaturation suppression of arterial blood helps to eliminate some artifact, the lower Venc is mostly used as an additional scan after the regular PCA scan, and only in dubious cases.

When there is a high likelihood of sinus thrombosis or occlusion of a small vein a 3D PCA must be done, as it creates a high-resolution image of the intracranial venous system. The 3D scans, however, take 5 to 6 minutes. Therefore, the 3D imaging should be done only in cases with high likelihood of thrombosis. Arteries are more prominent on 3D PCA, and proper interpretation requires experience.

Conversely, to quickly rule out a large sinus thrombosis when it is a less likely cause, such as in a patient with headaches, two fast, low-resolution 2D PCA sequences with 1 or 2 thick slices (20–40 mm, also called a "slab") and with low Venc can be applied, one in sagittal and another in axial plane, over the main venous sinuses. These 15- to 25-second scans have high clinical value, showing evident flow signal in the sinuses in healthy cases, allowing for a quick "rule-out" of large thrombosis.

An important source of false-positive results when using MRI to rule out sinus thrombosis is to misdiagnose arachnoid granulations as thrombus (**Fig. 14**). In most cases the morphology and signal characteristics makes the diagnosis evident, and with the proper amount of supervised training and experience this should be an error easy to avoid; however, this mistake still occurs in clinical routine. The importance of differentiating arachnoid granulations from thrombosis cannot be overstated because false-positive studies can result in unnecessary diagnostic tests and therapeutic interventions.

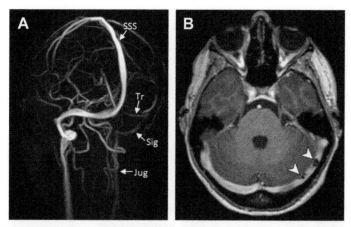

Fig. 14. MIP reconstruction of 3D PCA (*A*) shows low-intensity flow signal in the left transverse (Tr) and sigmoid (Sig) sinuses and in the left jugular vein (Jug). Normal flow is seen in the contralateral identical vessels and in the superior sagittal sinus (SSS). These findings are due to anatomic variation, most likely unilateral hypoplasia or slow flow. However, the contrast-enhanced T1-weighted (*B*) images show two well-defined, rounded filling defects in the transverse sinus (*arrowheads*). These are characteristic to arachnoid granulations, but in the presence of the PCA findings they may be mistaken for sinus thrombosis, although their presence is coincidental.

Of note, principles of PC MRA also apply to quantitative flow (Q-flow) imaging. Q-flow is often used in the diagnosis of normal pressure hydrocephalus, in which dynamic 2D or 3D dynamic acquisitions, gated to the cardiac cycle, measure and visualize CSF flow through the cerebral aqueduct.[29]

Fat-Suppression Techniques for Contrast-Enhanced Studies of the Spine

CE spine examinations should always be performed with fat suppression. Much can be gained and little will be lost. Without eliminating the signal from the adipose tissue, abnormal contrast enhancement can be completely missed, as it can be masked by the (equally high-intensity) signal of fat (**Fig. 15**). A widely used fat-suppression technique in spine is fat saturation ("fat sat", also known as chem sat), whereby a selective saturation pulse is applied at the beginning of the T1 pulse sequence to spoil the fat signal.[30] The end result will be a T1-weighted image minus the fat. This method can be sensitive to magnetic field inhomogeneities, but less so with the introduction of multitransmit magnetic resonance technology.[1]

Since CE T1 scans are done with fat saturation, should the same be done for precontrast scans? Ideally, yes: for good comparison it is preferred if both pregadolinium and postgadolinium scans are done with fat suppression. However, it is also generally important to have fat information; however, doing T1 scans both without and with fat sat in all relevant planes would add 5 to 15 minutes to the examination. Furthermore, it may be difficult to determine the relevant scan planes before adding gadolinium.

An alternative to conventional fat saturation and a good practical solution for this conflict is the Dixon method, which collects sufficient information in a single acquisition to decode multiple image representations: "fat," "water," "water plus fat," and "water minus fat" images.[31] This sequence is robust in its ability to produce homogeneous images of these four distinct types. Its drawback is that it tends to be

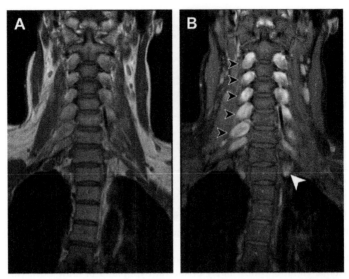

Fig. 15. Multiple cervical schwannomas are shown on contrast-enhanced T1 without fat suppression (*A*) and with fat suppression (*B*). The contrast-enhancing lesions are much more conspicuous in *B* (*black arrowheads*), demonstrating the importance of fat suppression in contrast-enhanced spine studies. The lesion at Th1–2 on the left is only visible in *B*, while completely obscured by fat signal in *A* (*white arrowhead*).

acquired at lower resolution than conventional T1 fat-saturated images owing to scan time.

As mentioned earlier, STIR is a popular fat suppression technique that is utilized widely in spine imaging to detect bone marrow edema. It is critical to note that STIR should never be used after GBCA injection, because the signal of the contrast agent will be nulled along with the fat resulting from its short T1 time (**Fig. 16**). This practically means that if one tries to create a contrast-*enhanced* STIR by administrating GBCA, inevitably a contrast-*reduced* image will be created.

Perfusion

The classic approach to measure relative tissue perfusion is dynamic susceptibility contrast (DSC) and to a lesser extent dynamic contrast enhancement (DCE), with applications in stroke, tumor, dementia, and multiple sclerosis.[32,33] In both methods, a contrast agent bolus is injected and a dynamic scan is obtained. As contrast reaches tissue, a T2* sequence undergoes susceptibility-related signal loss (DSC), or a T1-weighted sequence undergoes signal enhancement (DCE). The characteristics of the dynamic pixel-by-pixel flow pattern can be mathematically converted to cerebral blood volume (CBV), cerebral blood flow (CBF), mean transit time (MTT), and time to peak (TTP) maps and displayed as perfusion images (**Fig. 17**).

Arterial spin labeling (ASL) is a more repeatable alternative, since it does not require gadolinium injection. It replaces the exogenous GBCA agent with a simulated contrast bolus in the form of a separate MRI excitation (endogenous contrast) to blood vessels entering the imaging volume.[34] In clinical practice, ASL proves to be a heavily operator-dependent technique because of physiologic and anatomic variations, and therefore requires close attention and individual case-based quality

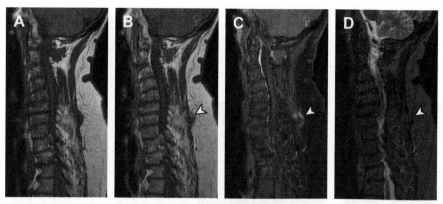

Fig. 16. Severe chronic degenerative disease of the cervical spine is seen on nonenhanced T1-weighted image (*A*). An area of abnormal contrast enhancement is noted in the soft tissue adjacent the C7 spinous process, indicating ongoing inflammatory process (*B–D, arrowhead*). This abnormality is difficult to distinguish on the regular contrast-enhanced T1-weighted image without fat suppression (*B*), while it is very conspicuous on contrast-enhanced T1 with fat saturation (*C*). However, on contrast-enhanced STIR (*D*), the lesion "disappears" owing to the suppression of the gadolinium signal along with fat signal, demonstrating why it is unwise to perform STIR following the administration of gadolinium-based contrast agent.

control.[35] This is most obvious in the elderly and in patients with cardiovascular or cerebrovascular disease, but occurs in younger and healthy individuals as well, resulting from variations of vascular anatomy. This naturally has consequences on the workflow, both in scanning and in interpretation. **Fig. 18** illustrates how normal anatomic variations can affect ASL results and may lead to the underestimation of cerebral perfusion. It also highlights the importance of planning the

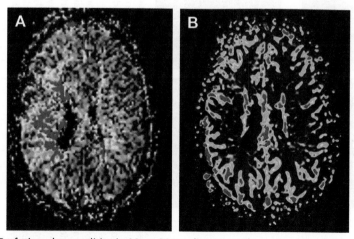

Fig. 17. Perfusion abnormalities in Moya-Moya disease on dynamic susceptibility contrast–based perfusion. Prominent delay is seen on the mean transit time map (*A*) in the right hemisphere, indicating that blood arrives via collaterals to this area. The cerebral blood volume map (*B*) however shows no regional rCBV deficit, suggesting that the collateral supply is well functioning.

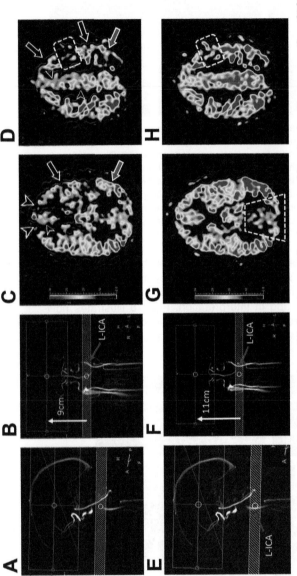

Fig. 18. 3D pseudocontinuous ASL (pCASL) images from a patient with chronic stage of carbon monoxide poisoning. Two consecutive pCASL scans from the same exam are shown in the top row (A–D) and in the bottom row (E–H). The sagittal and coronal PCA surveys (A, B and E, F) show how pCASL was planned. The yellow box is the imaging volume and below it the striped white slab is the labeling plane. (C–G) and (D–H) image pairs show the identical slices of the color cerebral blood flow (CBF) maps. The CBF maps are visualized using the same scale. In the first run the labeling distance was 9 cm (B, white arrow), in accordance with the recommendation by the 2015 ISMRM consensus paper. Extensive low signal is seen in the left middle cerebral artery (MCA) territory (black and orange arrows in C, D) and in both anterior cerebral artery (ACA) territories (arrowheads). On the second run the labeling plane was moved 2 cm lower, to achieve a more symmetrical labeling of the carotid arteries. The imaging volume is the same. Most of the "hypoperfused" areas "fill up" and show normal and more symmetric signal. The only remaining true hypoperfusion is in the posterior left frontal lobe, indicated by dashed rectangle in (D) and (H). The more symmetric and perpendicular ICA labeling has likely led to better labeling efficiency and resulted in higher signal on the left, despite the 2-cm longer labeling distance (11 cm, white arrow in F). Relatively lower signal is seen in the posterior circulation bilaterally, marked by the white trapezoid in (G). This difference between the posterior cerebral artery (PCA) territories and ICA territories is often observed in cases when the PCAs arise from the basilar artery, and may be due to less efficient labeling of blood in the vertebral arteries, or perhaps longer arterial transit time. This phenomenon can be confusing and may be misinterpreted as posterior parietal hypoperfusion. Its clinical importance is that posterior parietal hypoperfusion on ASL has been described in early Alzheimer's disease; therefore, extra attention is needed with regard to anatomic variations when applying ASL in neurodegenerative cases in clinical practice. A unilateral fetal PCA may further complicate the situation, as its territory shows a signal similar to that in ICA territories, whereas the contralateral regular PCA may still show relatively lower signal.

ASL scans individually based on the vascular anatomy. The use of PCA survey images is a quick and effective way to map internal carotid artery anatomy and should always be performed before ASL scans. In the future, artificial intelligence–powered automated vessel labeling will likely be applied to maximize labeling efficiency by mapping the patient's vascular anatomy, identifying the ideal arterial segments, and selectively labeling each vessel with individual labeling planes that are optimized for vessel geometry.

MRI perfusion tends to provide relative, nonquantitative estimates of regional perfusion, as opposed to nuclear medicine or even CT, which has been better at truly quantitative perfusion. Although not yet available commercially, ASL quantification would represent an important clinical advance. Indeed, without this feature, proper interpretation is hampered, which is one area where ASL has to improve to become a widely used clinical technique (**Fig. 19**).

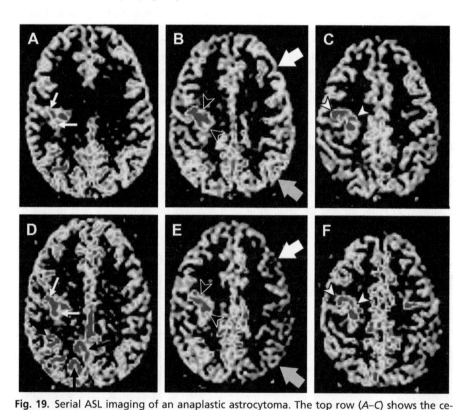

Fig. 19. Serial ASL imaging of an anaplastic astrocytoma. The top row (*A–C*) shows the cerebral blood flow map from the baseline scan; the bottom row (*D–F*) is the follow-up 2 months later, after chemotherapy. (*A–D*), (*B–E*), and (*C–F*) are identical slices. In (*E*) and (*F*) the CBF in the center of the lesion is lower and the extent of the highest perfusion is smaller compared with the baseline images, which might indicate therapeutic response (compare *black and white arrowheads* on the identical slices). However, in (*D*) there is higher CBF compared with baseline (*arrows* in *A* versus *D*). There is similarly higher signal in the right posterior cortical areas (*black arrows* in *D*), suggesting a measurement artifact. On closer look asymmetrical signal distribution is seen with higher signal on the right, most conspicuously on (*D*) and (*E*): compare the signal distribution in the 2 hemispheres in (*A*) and (*B*) (symmetric) versus (*D*) and (*E*) (*black arrows*). The conflict could be resolved by the quantification of ASL, which could eliminate the anatomical bias and operator dependency.

Functional MRI and Spectroscopy, and Quantitative MRI

Functional MRI relies on subtle susceptibility changes related to blood oxygenation. A dynamic 3D T2*-weighted FE sequence is obtained to monitor signal changes pixel by pixel. In the paradigm method, a correlation is drawn between regional signal changes and tasks that stimulate functional regions of the brain. Paradigm fMRI is most used in assessing regions of eloquent brain surrounding brain tumors, and as a replacement for a WADA test. Multiple paradigms are typically used to identify motor and language centers. Special training is required to ensure the patient understands and abides by the task instructions given during the examination. In resting state fMRI (rs-fMRI), inherent correlations between regional oxygenation (activity) changes are used to infer neural network connectivity.[36] Although the postprocessing is complex, the acquisition itself is effectively no different from a conventional MRI from a patient and scan-time perspective.

Proton spectroscopy has been in the sequence arsenal since the early days of MRI. Spectra from individual locations can be displayed, as well as colorized images representing a choice of metabolites, such as N-acetyl aspartate (NAA), choline, creatine, lactic acid, and myoinosotol. The normal shape of an magnetic resonance spectroscopy plot follows "Hunter's angle," whereby NAA, creatine, and choline peaks line up in descending order from right to left. The magnetic resonance spectroscopy plot in **Fig. 10** illustrates elevated choline and depressed NAA peaks (inverted Hunter's angle) in a malignant tumor.

New Types of Physiologic Imaging and Amide Proton Transfer

Physiologic MRI of the brain has been an area of research focus since the early 1990s. Structural scans still provide the core of every imaging study, and postprocessing of structural images to obtain tissue volume information can improve clinical insights, as illustrated in **Figs. 20** and **21**. Still, structural imaging tends to show end results of

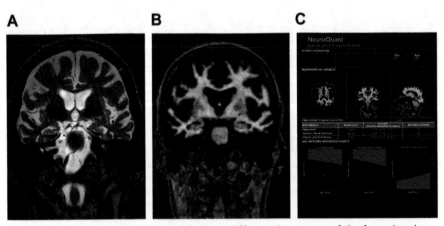

Fig. 20. Coronal T2-weighted image (A) shows diffuse enlargement of the frontal and temporal sulci, as well as the body and temporal horns of the lateral ventricles. (B) shows the color segmentation of the 3D T1 image in coronal plane, at the same slice position as (A). The hippocampi are marked in yellow. The age-related atrophy report (C) provides the absolute combined volumes of the hippocampi and lateral ventricles, their proportion in the intracranial volume, and the normative percentile compared with a database of healthy age-matched controls. At the bottom of the report, these values are visualized.

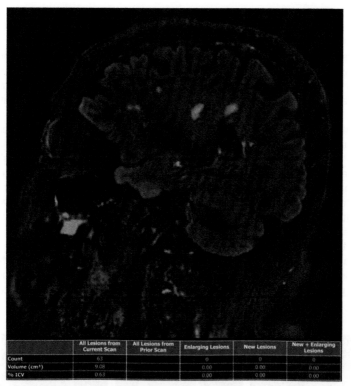

	All Lesions from Current Scan	All Lesions from Prior Scan	Enlarging Lesions	New Lesions	New + Enlarging Lesions
Count	63		0	0	0
Volume (cm³)	9.08		0.00	0.00	0.00
% ICV	0.63		0.00	0.00	0.00

Fig. 21. The automated lesion quantification in multiple sclerosis provides a colored segmentation map of FLAIR hyperintensities and assigns color based on the lesion location. In the report, the lesion distribution and overall lesion volume are shown. On follow-up examinations the difference is also provided, simplifying interpretation and reducing reading time.

pathophysiological changes. Attempts to track the circulation, oxygen extraction, protein metabolism, membrane turnover, and other mechanisms in the brain are intended to reveal disease processes at early stages. As a result, techniques such as perfusion MRI, fMRI, quantitative flow and dynamic studies, magnetic resonance spectroscopy, and DTI have grown in popularity.[37,38]

A relatively new group of physiologic imaging techniques in the clinical research and early clinical implementation is chemical exchange saturation transfer (CEST), whereby magnetization transfer (proton exchange) between a target molecule and water is used to indirectly assess differences in regional distribution of that molecule.[39,40] When a saturation pulse is applied for the target molecule's frequency, the water signal will be reduced proportionally to the proton exchange and this signal change will be visualized on an "asymmetry map." This will replace as a focal intensity change on the CEST image, but is not an absolute measurement of the amount of the substance.

There are multiple different CEST techniques, each specified for a certain molecule (eg, glucose, glycosaminoglycans, amine proton, or creatine).[41,42] Amide proton transfer (APT) is the type of CEST that generates contrast based on the concentration of endogenous mobile proteins and tissue pH.[43] It has been studied in brain tumor diagnostics with promising results: it was shown to discriminate between low-grade and high-grade gliomas,[44] predict isocitrate dehydrogenase status[45] in gliomas, help guide brain biopsy,[43] differentiate between true progression and pseudoprogression,[46] distinguish between metastasis and glioblastoma,[47] and explored in other areas such as hypoxic ischemic injury.[48]

APT imaging is available commercially, and relative to spectroscopy is very simple to run. Lesions appear as an obvious focal spot against a background of homogeneous normal tissue that does not exhibit conventional resolution and contrast variations of classic MRI scans (**Figs. 22** and **23**). It is noteworthy that even the ventricles do not stand out because the water signal is distributed evenly.

Applications for APT are still under investigation. More studies are needed to fully understand its diagnostic power in tumor diagnostics and therapy monitoring. Also, it is an EPI sequence and cannot be used in the posterior fossa or on the skull base in most cases. It often has prominent EPI artifacts along the skull and postoperative areas (which may render it less useful in tumor cases), and intravascular artifacts may cause uncertainty in interpretation as well. Based on early experience with serial imaging, its reproducibility is variable. Its variability to pH changes can be a weakness and a strength. Clinical studies and further engineering work are expected to clarify solutions to many of these issues.

APT is a good candidate to become a clinically useful technique. It already has a role in tumor imaging. It is unlikely that APT will remain the only CEST player in clinical practice given its physiological target substrate represents a narrow focus. Rather,

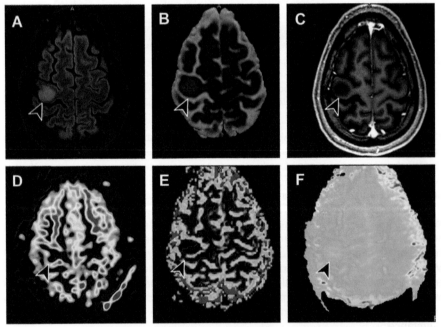

Fig. 22. Multiparametric imaging of a low-grade glioma with brain perfusion and amide proton transfer (APT) imaging. The infiltrative tumor is located in the right precentral gyrus (*black arrowhead*), exhibiting hyperintense signal on FLAIR (*A*), increased diffusion on ADC (*B*), and no abnormal contrast enhancement (*C*). The 3D pCASL-derived CBF map (*D*) and the DSC-derived rCBV map (*E*) show no increased perfusion compared with the normal parenchyma. Subtle signal increase is seen on the APT (*F, arrowhead*). The physiologic findings are consistent with a low-grade tumor and are in accordance with the structural scans.

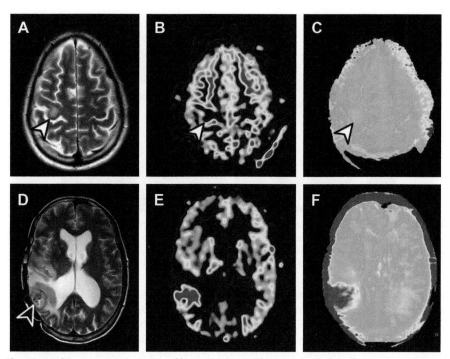

Fig. 23. Multiparametric imaging of brain tumors with arterial spin labeling and amide proton transfer (APT). The top row shows a low-grade glioma in the right precentral gyrus (*white arrowhead*) with homogeneous high T2 signal (*A*), without increased CBF on the 3D pCASL scan (*B*) and without abnormal signal increase on 3D APT (*C*). The bottom row demonstrates a recurrent glioblastoma with heterogeneous structure on T2 (*D, black arrowhead*) and markedly elevated CBF (*E*) as well as APT (*F*) signal.

it may eventually be recognized as the first of a bigger CEST portfolio. A clinically useful and versatile tool of the future may be a CEST map: a sequence that acquires and combines different CEST contrasts (amide proton, glucose, etc), providing a comprehensive picture of brain metabolism, which could be used in conjunction with other physiologic techniques and perhaps even tailored for specific diseases.

Fast Imaging Methods

An important limitation of MRI is its inherently long scan time. Although diagnostic insight is improved by maximizing signal-to-noise ratio, resolution, and obtaining multiple tissue contrasts and views, the total scan time will increase. As a result, motion artifact becomes more likely as patients become uncomfortable, tolerance to complete the study is reduced, and affordability becomes a factor as scanner capacity decreases. These practical constraints limit the acceptable duration of a scan. To overcome this constraint, MRI technology is increasingly integrating new algorithms and hardware with innovations in data science and artificial intelligence. As such innovations are implemented, new parameters, complexities, and artifacts are inevitably introduced, which will require clinical optimization, education, and practical adjustments.

Compressed sensing and spiral imaging are two fast MRI methods that are currently the subject of extensive research and development. Spiral imaging is not yet

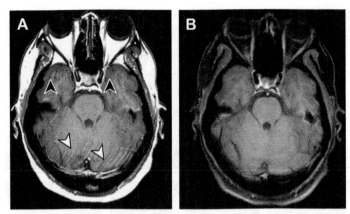

Fig. 24. Cartesian T1 spin echo (*A*) shows typical flow artifacts in phase direction, originating from the transverse sinuses (*white arrowheads*) and from the internal carotid arteries (*black arrowheads*). These artifacts are completely missing from the spiral acquisition (*B*), creating a clearer image of the cerebellum, the temporal poles, and the parasellar regions.

commercially available as of the date of this writing, but research has shown promising results in T1-weighted brain and spine imaging, DWI, ASL, and TOF MRA.[49–56] Compared with standard TSE or SE scans, it can achieve higher signal-to-noise ratio under shorter scan time, dramatically reduce classic flow artifacts, and has inherent fat suppression using the Dixon method (**Figs. 24–26**). These examples also

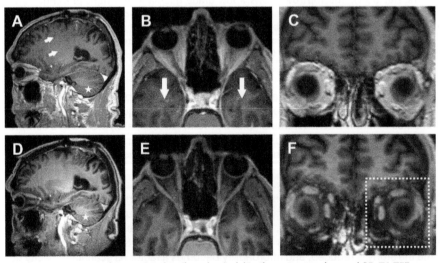

Fig. 25. Comparison of Cartesian (*A–C*) and spiral (*D–F*) contrast-enhanced 3D T1 TFE scans. The spatial resolution is 0.94 mm isotropic for both scans. The spiral is shorter (3:30 min vs 4:45 min), has higher SNR (*A and D, asterisk*) and flow artifact mitigation (*A and B, arrows*), resulting in higher image quality. It also uses Dixon for fat suppression, which can be exploited in many clinical scenarios, such as the imaging of the orbits, which normally requires additional fat-saturated scans before and after administration of GBCA. By using spiral 3D T1 the fat-suppressed orbital images can be reconstructed from the brain 3D dataset (*F, dashed rectangle*), eliminating the need for running additional sequences. Thus, a significant amount of time can be saved in clinical workflow.

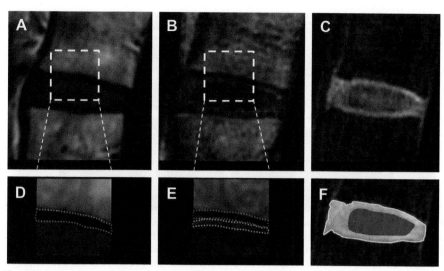

Fig. 26. Comparison of a standard Cartesian T1-weighted scan (*A*) and a spiral T1-weighted research scan using Dixon technique (*B, C*). In (*A*) the endplate appears as one dark band, while on the in-phase spiral image (*B*) it is separated into an upper darker and lower brighter layer, which may represent the real endplate and the annulus fibrosus, respectively. These structures are blown up and highlighted in (*D*) and (*E*); blue dotted line delineates the endplate and white dotted line the annulus on (*E*). The water-only image of spiral scan (*C*) shows an outer brighter and a central darker component, likely representing the annulus fibrosus and the nucleus pulposus of the intervertebral disc. These are highlighted in yellow and red in (*F*). This more detailed image of the intervertebral disc and the vertebral body may provide useful diagnostic information in the early phase of the evolution of degenerative spine disease, as it may visualize annular tear, endplate changes, and early formation of disc herniation.

demonstrate that fast or efficient imaging protocols can either increase the capacity of an MRI or permit additional scrutiny in the same patient time slot. A current disadvantage of spiral imaging is that image blurriness and EPI artifacts must yet be overcome.

Compressed sensing is currently offered commercially. It operates with a sparse data sampling and iterative reconstruction methodology that mimics newer CT reconstruction algorithms, and has been shown to produce 25% to 30% reduction in scan time under certain conditions (**Figs. 27–29**).[57,58] However, compressed sensing comes with a slight change of image character that will require user acclimation. It cannot be applied to EPI scans, and to date requires individual protocol optimization to maintain image quality. Because its speedup relies on eliminating information redundancy in data acquisition, its performance relies on the greater signal-to-noise ratio achieved at higher field strength MRI systems and efficient coil technology. Compressed sensing is well positioned to reduce scan time without compromising diagnostic quality of high-resolution images. Ongoing development and clinical optimization are expected to further reduce examination time and mitigate artifacts.

It is likely that a combination of different approaches, rather than any of these individual techniques alone, will be needed to make dramatic improvements in clinical MRI scan times. Today, a typical brain examination consists of 5 or more structural scans and lasts for 15 to 30 minutes. A full spine and brain examination can be as long as 1 hour. The real difference will be when a brain MRI examination becomes as fast as a brain CT (ie, less than 1 minute) without sacrificing image quality. This lofty goal does not seem unrealistic given the strong interest and current state of research

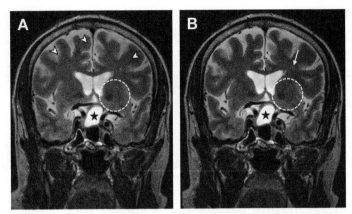

Fig. 27. Comparison of sensing (SENSE) and compressed sensing (C-SENSE) accelerated T2-weighted images. (*A*) is acquired using regular SENSE, with 2:30 min scan time. (*B*) uses C-SENSE, with 1:26 min scan time. Mild motion artifacts are seen in (*A*) (*arrowheads*), which are reduced in (*B*). The overall appearance of the basal ganglia is more consistent in (*B*) (compare the circled areas). The size and signal characteristics of the small white matter lesion in the left frontal lobe is unchanged (*B, white arrow*). The intrasellar-suprasellar cystic abnormality (*asterisk*) and the parasellar structures show the same signal and edge definition on the 2 scans. The overall clinical diagnostic utility is not affected by using C-SENSE.

in this area. Such increased speed will require concomitant innovations in practical implementation, including how to move patients in and out efficiently, reading a higher volume of MRI examinations, quality control, and new hardware that may be required to support the new workflow. It is worth noting that although the 1-minute high-

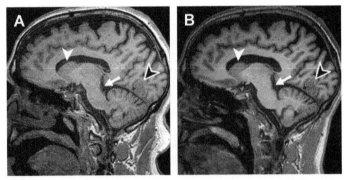

Fig. 28. Comparison of SENSE and C-SENSE accelerated 3D T1 (MPRAGE) images. (*A*) 3D T1 with SENSE acceleration (SENSE factor = 2.2), 0.9 mm isotropic voxels, with a scan time of 4:18 min. (*B*) 3D T1 with C-SENSE acceleration (C-SENSE factor = 3.5), 1 mm isotropic voxels, and scan time of 3:02 min. Image denoising applied by the C-SENSE algorithm is apparent in (*B*) in white matter resulting in a generally better gray-white contrast, which makes the occipital abnormality easier to detect (*black arrowhead*). However, edges in (*B*) are less sharp compared with (*A*), as seen on the superior border of the caudate nucleus (*white arrowhead*), along the posterior border of the pons (*arrow*), and in the cortex. This may have resulted from the slightly larger voxel size and from the iterative image reconstruction used for denoising in C-SENSE. In this regard the image quality of C-SENSE MRI images are similar to computed tomographic images that are reconstructed with iterative algorithms: the images appear smoother and have a "plastic-like" character.

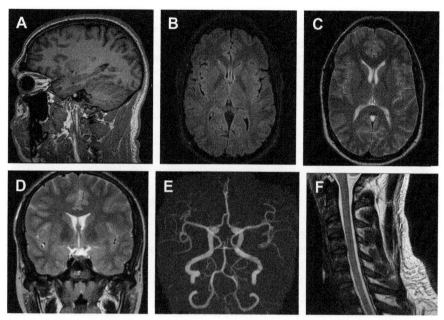

Fig. 29. C-SENSE accelerated head and spine imaging in a rapid headache protocol on 3T. The total exam length is 16:07 min with the following individual scan times: sagittal 3D T1 (*A*): 3:37 min; axial 3D FLAIR (*B*): 4:00 min; axial 2D T2 TSE (*C*): 1:24 min; coronal 2D TSE (*D*): 1:26 min; 3D TOF MRA (*E*): 3:46 min; sagittal 2D TSE of the cervical spine (*F*): 1:54 min.

resolution MRI examination does not yet exist in routine practice, some of the listed new techniques already save substantial scan time that allows for additional physiologic data to be collected in conventional time slots; this benefit may have an even greater positive impact on neuroradiology than the sheer exam time reduction.

SUMMARY

The review of some of the clinical and fundamental principles of MRI presented in this article serves as only a basic foundation in this increasingly complex field. More rigorous study of neuroimaging is vital for all neurologists, at a minimum to understand the language and logic of neuroradiology, thus improving communication and patient care. It is increasingly important for the ordering neurologist to understand advantages and disadvantages of routine and specialty sequences, and to be able to perform at least cursory review of images. Furthermore, a wide spectrum of additional advantages occurs as training and experience in imaging interpretation increases.[3] With its disciplined process of relating lesion visualization to symptoms, MRI skills arguably make for better neurologists. Certain subspecialties, such as stroke specialists, critical care neurologists, interventional neurologists, and practitioners who use teleneurology tend to rely their own image review to make treatment decisions. Neuroimaging is a logical component of comprehensive neuroscience group practices, and neurologists trained in neuroimaging can offer tremendous value in such organizations.[59]

Ultimately, it takes time to develop an in-depth understanding of technical aspects of imaging, translate physiologic and pathologic processes into pixels through those physical principles, and integrate this new knowledge into clinical scenarios. There are precedents and resources for neurologists seeking to develop more advanced skills, including rotations, preceptorships, remote didactics, professional conferences, and formal fellowship programs through societies such as the American Society of Neuroimaging, the American Academy of Neurology, the American Society of Neuroradiology, the Radiologic Society of North America, and the United Council for Neurologic Subspecialties.

REFERENCES

1. Viallon M, Cuvinciuc V, Delattre B, et al. State-of-the-art MRI techniques in neuroradiology: principles, pitfalls, and clinical applications. Neuroradiology 2015; 57(5):441–67.
2. Fritz JV. Neuroimaging trends and future outlook. Neurol Clin 2014;32(1):1–29.
3. Mechtler L, Fritz J. Why neuroimaging plays a critical role in shaping the future of neurology. Pract Neurol 2016;16:17–20.
4. Fritz JV. What neurologists need to know about MRI sequences. Paper presented at: American Academy of Neurology Annual Meeting. Philadelphia, April 30, 2014.
5. Mamourian A, Lembo J, Mamourian M. Top ten MR artifacts. Oxford (England): Radiology Boards Prep; 2015.
6. Mamourian AC. Practical MR physics and case file of MR artifacts and pitfalls. Oxford (England): Oxford Univesity Press; 2010.
7. Hornack JP. The basics of MRI. 2019. Available at: https://www.cis.rit.edu/htbooks/mri/. Accessed April 22, 2019.
8. The MRI Registry Review Program. Medical imaging consultants. 2019. Available at: http://www.micinfo.com/courses/mrrrp/index.xml?ss=course_detail. Accessed April 22, 2019.
9. Currie S, Hoggard N, Craven IJ, et al. Understanding MRI: basic MR physics for physicians. Postgrad Med J 2013;89:209–23.
10. Shellock F. MRISafety.com. 2019. Available at: http://www.mrisafety.com/. Accessed April 24, 2019.
11. Korutz AW, Obajuluwa A, Lester MS, et al. Pacemakers in MRI for the neuroradiologist. AJNR Am J Neuroradiol 2017;38(12):2222–30.
12. Ramalho J, Semelka RC, Ramalho M, et al. Gadolinium-based contrast agent accumulation and toxicity: an update. AJNR Am J Neuroradiol 2016;37(7):1192–8.
13. Chehabeddine L, Al Saleh T, Baalbaki M, et al. Cumulative administrations of gadolinium-based contrast agents: risks of accumulation and toxicity of linear vs macrocyclic agents. Crit Rev Toxicol 2019;1–18. https://doi.org/10.1080/10408444.2019.1592109.
14. Weiner SL, Ru R, Javan R, et al. Health care economics: a study guide for neuroradiology fellows, part 1. AJNR Am J Neuroradiol 2018;39(1):2–9.
15. Buethe J, Nazarian J, Kalisz K, et al. Neuroimaging wisely. AJNR Am J Neuroradiol 2016;37(12):2182–8.
16. Appropriate use criteria. Centers for Medicare and Medicaid Services. 2016. Available at: www.cms.gov/Medicare/Quality-Initiatives-Patient-Assessment-Instruments/Appropriate-Use-Criteria-Program/index.html. Accessed September 21, 2019.
17. Bernstein MA, Huston J, Ward HA. Imaging artifacts at 3.0T. J Magn Reson Imaging 2006;24:735–46.

18. Haake EM, DelProposto ZS, Chaturvedi S, et al. Imaging cerebral amyloid angiopathy with susceptibility-weighted imaging. AJNR Am J Neuroradiol 2007;28(2): 316–7.

19. McNamara C, Sugrue G, Murray B, et al. Current and emerging therapies in multiple sclerosis: implications for the radiologist, part 2—surveillance for treatment complications and disease progression. AJNR Am J Neuroradiol 2017;38(9): 1672–80.

20. Arevalo O, Riascos R, Rabiei P, et al. Standardizing magnetic resonance imaging protocols, requisitions, and reports in multiple sclerosis: an update for radiologist based on 2017 magnetic resonance imaging in multiple sclerosis and 2018 Consortium of Multiple Sclerosis Centers Consensus Guide. J Comput Assist Tomogr 2019;43(1):1–12.

21. Fernanda RLC, Hygino da Cruz LC Jr, Doring M, et al. Diffusion-weighted imaging and demyelinating diseases: new aspects of an old advanced sequence. Am J Roentgenol 2014;202(1):W34–42.

22. Davoudi Y, Foroughipour M, Torabi R, et al. Diffusion weighted imaging in acute attacks of multiple sclerosis. Iran J Radiol 2016;13(2):e21740.

23. Osborn AG, Salzman KL, Jhaveri MD, et al. Diagnostic imaging: brain. 3rd edition. Philadelphia (PA): Elsevier; 2015.

24. Ptak T, Sheridan RL, Rhea JT, et al. Cerebral fractional anisotropy score in trauma patients: a new indicator of white matter injury after trauma. Am J Roentgenol 2003;181(5):1401–7.

25. Edlow BL, Copen WA, Izzy S, et al. Longitudinal diffusion tensor imaging detects recovery of fractional anisotropy within traumatic axonal injury lesions. Neurocrit Care 2016;24(3):342–52.

26. Li XH, Wu F, Zhao F, et al. Fractional anisotropy is a marker in early-stage spinal cord injury. Brain Res 2017;1672:44–9.

27. Haller S, Etienne L, Varoquaux AD, et al. Imaging of neurovascular compression syndromes: trigeminal neuralgia, hemifacial spasm, vestibular paroxysmia, and glossopharyngeal neuralgia. AJNR Am J Neuroradiol 2016;37(8):1384–92.

28. Besta R, Shankar YU, Kumar A, et al. MRI 3D CISS- a novel imaging modality in diagnosing trigeminal neuralgia - a review. J Clin Diagn Res 2016;10(3):ZE01–3.

29. Yamada S, Tsuchiya K, Bradley W, et al. Current and emerging MR imaging techniques for the diagnosis and management of CSF flow disorders: a review of phase-contrast and time–spatial labeling inversion pulse. AJNR Am J Neuroradiol 2015;36(4):623–30.

30. Delfaut EM, Beltran J, Johnson G, et al. Fat suppression in MR imaging: techniques and pitfalls. Radiographics 1999;19:373–82.

31. Pokomey AL, Chia JM, Pfeifer CM, et al. Improved fat-suppression homogeneity with mDIXON turbo spin echo (TSE) in pediatric spine imaging at 3.0T. Acta Radiol 2017;58(11):1386–94.

32. Lapointe E, Li DKB, Traboulsee AL, et al. What have we learned from perfusion MRI in multiple sclerosis? AJNR Am J Neuroradiol 2018;39(6):994–1000.

33. Gaddikeri S, Gaddikeri RS, Tailor T, et al. Dynamic contrast-enhanced MR imaging in head and neck cancer: techniques and clinical applications. AJNR Am J Neuroradiol 2016;37(4):588–95.

34. Alsop DC, Detre JA, Golay X, et al. Recommended implementation of arterial spin labeled perfusion MRI for clinical applications: a consensus of the ISMRM perfusion study group and the European consortium for ASL in dementia. Magn Reson Med 2015;73(1):102–16.

35. Li Y, Mao D, Li Z, et al. Cardiac-triggered pseudo-continuous arterial-spin-labeling: a cost-effective scheme to further enhance the reliability of arterial-spin-labeling MRI. Magn Reson Med 2018;80(3):969–75.
36. Lv H, Wang Z, Tong E, et al. Resting-state functional MRI: everything that nonexperts have always wanted to know. AJNR Am J Neuroradiol 2018;39(8):1390–9.
37. Zhou M, Scott J, Chaudhury B, et al. Radiomics in brain tumor: image assessment, quantitative feature descriptors, and machine-learning approaches. AJNR Am J Neuroradiol 2018;39(2):208–16.
38. Zaharchuk G, Gong E, Wintermark M, et al. Deep learning in neuroradiology. AJNR Am J Neuroradiol 2018;39(10):1776–84.
39. Ward KM, Aletras AH, Balaban RS. A new class of contrast agents for MRI based on proton chemical exchange dependent saturation transfer (CEST). J Magn Reson 2000;143:79–87.
40. Zhou J, van Zijl PC. Chemical exchange saturation transfer imaging and spectroscopy. Prog Nucl Magn Reson Spectrosc 2006;48:109–36.
41. Jones KM, Pollard AC, Pagel MD. Clinical applications of chemical exchange saturation transfer (CEST) MRI. J Magn Reson Imaging 2018;47(1):11–27.
42. Pankowska A, Kochalska K, Łazorczyk A, et al. Chemical exchange saturation transfer (CEST) as a new method of signal obtainment in magnetic resonance molecular imaging in clinical and research practice. Pol J Radiol 2019;84:e147–52.
43. Shanshan J, Eberhartc C, Zhanga Y, et al. Amide proton transfer-weighted MR image-guided stereotactic biopsy in patients with newly diagnosed gliomas. Eur J Cancer 2017;83:9–18.
44. Choi YS, Ahn SS, Seung-Koo L, et al. Amide proton transfer imaging to discriminate between low- and high-grade gliomas: added value to apparent diffusion coefficient and relative cerebral blood volume. Eur Radiol 2017;27:3181–9.
45. Jiang S, Zou T, Eberhart CG, et al. Predicting IDH mutation status in grade ii gliomas using amide proton transfer-weighted(APTw) MRI. Magn Reson Med 2017;78:1100–9.
46. Ma B, Blakeley JO, Hong X, et al. Applying amide proton transfer-weighted MRI to distinguish pseudoprogression from true progression in malignant gliomas. J Magn Reson Imaging 2016;44:456–62.
47. Yu H, Lou H, Zou T, et al. Applying protein-based amide proton transfer MR imaging to distinguish solitary brain metastases from glioblastoma. Eur Radiol 2017;27(11):4516–24.
48. Zheng Y, Wang X. The applicability of amide proton transfer imaging in the nervous system: focus on hypoxic-ischemic encephalopathy in the neonate. Cell Mol Neurobiol 2018;38:797–807.
49. Li Z, Schär M, Wang D, et al. Arterial spin labeled perfusion imaging using three-dimensional turbo spin echo with a distributed spiral-in/out trajectory. Magn Reson Med 2016;75(1):266–73.
50. Ahn CB, Kim JH, Cho ZH. High-speed spiral-scan echo planar NMR imaging-I. IEEE Trans Med Imaging 1986;5(1):2–7.
51. Meyer CH, Hu BS, Nishimura DG, et al. Fast spiral coronary artery imaging. Magn Reson Med 1992;28(2):202–13.
52. Pipe JG, Robison RK. Simplified signal equations for spoiled gradient echo MRI. Paper presented at: Proceedings of the 18th Annual Meeting of ISMRM, Stockholm, 2010.
53. Nishimura DG, Irarrazabal P, Meyer CH. A velocity k-space analysis of flow effects in echo-planar and spiral imaging. Magn Reson Med 1995;33(4):549–56.

54. Wang D, Zwart NR, Pipe JG. Joint water-fat separation and deblurring for spiral imaging. Magn Reson Med 2018;79(6):3218–28.
55. Li Z, Karis JP, Pipe JG. A 2D spiral turbo-spin-echo technique. Magn Reson Med 2018;80(5):1989–96.
56. Li Z, Hu HH, Miller JH, et al. A spiral spin-echo MR imaging technique for improved flow artifact suppression in T1-weighted postcontrast brain imaging: a comparison with cartesian turbo spin-echo. AJNR Am J Neuroradiol 2016; 37(4):642–7.
57. Sartoretti T, Reischauer C, Sartoretti E, et al. Common artefacts encountered on images acquired with combined compressed sensing and SENSE. Insights Imaging 2018;9:1107–15.
58. Worters P, Sung K, Stevens K, et al. Compressed-sensing multi-spectral imaging of the post-operative spine. J Magn Reson Imaging 2013;37(1):243–8.
59. Fritz JV. The practice of neuroimaging within a neurology office setting. Neurol Clin Pract 2013;3(6):501–9.

Imaging of Neurologic Disorders in Pregnancy

Dara G. Jamieson, MD[a],*, Jennifer W. McVige, MA, MD[b]

KEYWORDS

- Pregnancy • Headache • Eclampsia • Cerebral venous thrombosis
- Reversible cerebral vasoconstriction syndrome • Ischemic stroke
- Intraparenchymal hemorrhage • Lymphocytic hypophysitis

KEY POINTS

- Pregnant women may have the exacerbation of preexisting neurologic disorders or the new onset neurologic symptoms, necessitating brain or spinal cord imaging.
- Headaches during the last trimester and the immediate postpartum period may indicate cerebrovascular disease or expansion of a mass lesion and appropriate imaging should be strongly considered.
- MRI is the preferred imaging modality during pregnancy, and the use of ionizing radiation and/or contrast should be avoided, if possible.

INTRODUCTION

Pregnancy is associated with multiple physiologic changes that can cause an exacerbation of preexisting neurologic conditions or the onset of new neurologic disorders.[1] Neuroimaging is often crucial in the differentiation between acute disorders requiring immediate intervention and less concerning chronic or benign conditions; however, neuroimaging can be problematic during pregnancy because of concern for the fetus. Certain neurologic complaints, most obviously the new onset of focal neurologic deficits, mandate neuroimaging during pregnancy and the postpartum period. A headache is most concerning in the third trimester and the postpartum period.[2] Differentiating between common, non–life-threatening types of headaches (primary headaches) and secondary headaches due to conditions that require neuroimaging and specific treatment is extremely important because some pregnancy-related disorders causing headache can be life-threatening. Headache may be the initial symptom of multiple cerebrovascular disorders of pregnancy, including cerebral venous thrombosis (CVT), reversible cerebral vasoconstriction syndrome

The authors have no relevant disclosures.
[a] Weill Cornell Medicine, Department of Neurology, 525 East 68th Street, New York, NY 10065, USA; [b] Dent Neurologic Institute, 3980 Sheridan Drive, Amherst, New York 14226, USA
* Corresponding author.
E-mail address: dgj2001@med.cornell.edu

Neurol Clin 38 (2020) 37–64
https://doi.org/10.1016/j.ncl.2019.09.001
0733-8619/20/© 2019 Elsevier Inc. All rights reserved.

neurologic.theclinics.com

(RCVS), and hypertensive disorders of pregnancy, as well as expanding cerebral mass lesions.

NEUROIMAGING SAFETY IN PREGNANCY

When the clinical examination and history indicate a need for emergent neuroimaging during pregnancy and the peripartum period, the risk and benefit to mother and fetus must be examined. There are known and potential fetal and maternal risks involving exposure to ionizing radiation, high magnetic fields, contrast dye, increased temperatures, and loud noises which must be weighed against the benefits of diagnosis. Therefore, deferring elective neuroimaging until after delivery is advised, if appropriate. However, if neuroimaging is indicated, the type of imaging and adapting the procedure to maintain lowest possible risk is recommended.[3]

Neuroimaging with Computed Tomography

Computed tomography (CT) imaging involves risks related to ionizing radiation exposure, as well as iodinated contrast dye administration. The risk of ionizing radiation is considered by evaluating both deterministic and stochastic effects. Deterministic effects involve the results of ionizing radiation exposure related to a dose above a determined threshold, which may produce apoptosis and failure of cellular replication, resulting in damage such as cataract, infertility, telangiectasias, and dermal necrosis.[4] Stochastic effects involve the chance events of ionizing radiation damaging a single cell, regardless of dose, which then goes on to induce mutagenic effects, producing carcinogenesis.[4,5] However, the American College of Obstetricians and Gynecologists (ACOG) Committee recommends that use of a CT scan should not be withheld if clinically indicated; however, an MRI scan should be considered a safer alternative if it is appropriate for diagnosis and can be obtained in a timely manner. The ACOG Committee Opinion lists radiation dose as 0.001 to 0.01 mGy (milligray; unit of absorbed dose) for a head and neck CT, which places it in the "very low-dose examinations (<0.1 mGy)" category.[3,6]

CT radiation is highly collimated; therefore, risk to the fetus with neuroimaging of the head and neck is significantly lower due to increased scatter compared with CT imaging of the pelvis, abdomen, and lower chest in which the beam is located closer to the uterus.[4] Shielding the abdomen during imaging of the head and neck "does not significantly reduce the minimal fetal radiation exposure but may help to alleviate maternal anxiety."[5] The risk of childhood cancer is less than 1:1000 for most radiologic procedures; however, the risk of fetal carcinogenesis increases by a factor of 2 with larger doses of fetal milligray exposure, such as with a pelvic CT, although the absolute risk is low (1:250).[7,8] Therefore, dose considerations and positioning in the scanner are important. In addition, both the rate of absorption and the gestational age have been shown to correlate with conceptus injury. Radiation exposure less than 50 mGy has not been associated with fetal injury or side effects; however, radiation levels higher than this can cause concern, depending on the gestational age of the fetus. It is imperative that the mother be counseled about these risks and benefits before the procedure.[3]

The low-osmolality iodinated contrast dye used in CT scans can cross the human placenta to the fetus. There are no available data to suggest potential harm to the fetus through maternal intravenous (IV) administration; however, no well-controlled studies have been performed in pregnant women. In the past, there were reports of hypothyroidism in newborns after receiving fat-soluble iodinated contrast in utero but not with water-soluble contrast. Regardless, a thyroid evaluation is recommended in newborns exposed to iodinated contrast in utero.[9] There is a small amount of contrast excreted in breast milk; however, there are no studies that show harm to the fetus. A 12-hour to 24-hour period of interruption in breast feeding may be recommended but is not mandatory.[10]

NEUROIMAGING WITH MRI

The potential theoretic risks of MRI to a developing fetus include exposure to a static magnetic field (associated with possible cellular changes), pulsed radiofrequency (associated with increased heat), and varying gradient-echo electromagnetic fields (associated with increased noise), as well as gadolinium contrast.[7] A study by Ray and colleagues[11] (2016) showed that, compared with controls, fetal exposure to MRI in the first trimester of pregnancy did not reveal an increased risk of harm to the fetus or to the growing child early in their life. In addition, the American College of Radiology found no evidence that fetal exposure to MRI on a 1.5-T or 3-T magnet caused harm to the fetus.[10] The emerging technique of fetal MRI with single-shot fast spin-echo T2-weighted imaging, with diffusion-weighted imaging (DWI) and other sequences in development, emphasizes that an MRI can be used safely in pregnancy, when clinically indicated.[12] During the first trimester, MRI scanning should be avoided unless clinically imperative, although inadvertent exposure does not appear harmful.[13]

The use of gadolinium-based contrast agents (GBCAs) in MRI should be avoided unless the risk outweighs the benefit to the fetus and mother. Conceptus exposure to a gadolinium-enhanced MRI was not associated with a higher incidence of congenital anomalies at any gestational age in a large recent study; however, the number of first trimester patients was underpowered and the comparison group may not have been optimal.[11] There was, however, an increased risk of "a broad set of rheumatologic, inflammatory and infiltrative skin conditions as well as stillbirth and neonatal death." As stated, this study has some limitations so the information should be interpreted with caution and, therefore, the American College of Radiology recommends that gadolinium contrast should only be used if there is a critical situation and the potential risk outweighs the benefit.[10,11] There is a low amount of gadolinium that is transferred into the breast milk of a lactating mother; therefore, the risk of exposure to the fetus is believed to be low. As with iodinated contrast, a 12-hour to 24-hour period of interruption in breast feeding may be recommended but is not mandatory. In 2017, the US Food and Drug Administration required a new class warning and other safety measures for all GBCAs because of concerns about gadolinium remaining in patients' bodies, including the brain, for months to years after receiving the injection. However, gadolinium retention has not been directly linked to adverse health effects in patients with normal renal function. Of the 2 chemical structures of GBCAs, linear GBCAs result in more frequent and more durable retention than do macrocyclic GBCAs.[14] Especially during pregnancy, a brand of GBCA with less retention in tissues should be used.

IMAGING OF HEADACHES IN PREGNANCY

Brain imaging is not needed for most pregnant women who present with symptoms consistent with primary headaches, as described in the *International Classification of Headache Disorders*, 3rd edition.[15] Neuroimaging is not indicated with a clear diagnosis of tension-type headache, or with migraine headache, an especially common complaint in the first trimester.[16] Migraines are common in women of reproductive age and approximately 5% of pregnancies are affected by a new onset or new type of headache, which is most often migraine.[17] Although both migraine and tension-type headache are common in pregnancy and the postpartum period, the frequency and severity of migraine headaches tend to decrease during the later months of pregnancy owing to the shifting ratio of maternal estrogen to progesterone.[18] About 40% of postpartum women are thought to have headaches, often in the first weeks after delivery. Migraine headaches often resume soon after delivery, especially if the woman is not breastfeeding; however, cerebrovascular disorders associated with pregnancy causing headaches are more likely to occur in the 6 weeks after delivery than they are during pregnancy itself. Secondary headaches associated with pregnancy can be due to life-threatening disorders and about half of all secondary headaches in the postpartum period are related to hypertensive disorders of pregnancy. In a study of pregnant women receiving inpatient neurologic consultation, more than one-third of women had secondary headaches, especially in women without a prior headache history. The absence of a prior headache history, elevated blood pressure, fever, and seizures should prompt neuroimaging and monitoring for vascular causes of headaches.[19] Brain imaging is advised in patients whose history and examination suggest secondary headaches, associated with an underlying central nervous system or systemic disorders. Studies have shown that emergent neuroimaging for headache during pregnancy revealed an underlying secondary headache cause in 25% to 27% of pregnant women, which can be essential for proper diagnosis and treatment.[20,21] The European Headache Federation published a list of "Red Flags for Headache in Pregnancy" that can be helpful in determining which patients require emergent neuroimaging.[22] Conditions that increase concern for a secondary headache in a peripartum woman include a significant change in the descriptive symptoms of the headache; poor or no response to the usual effective headache treatments; the presence of persistent or unusual visual, motor, or sensory symptoms accompanying the headache; and altered mental status associated with the headache. The presence of these symptoms indicates the need for prompt imaging studies, generally an MRI.[19,23]

SECONDARY HEADACHES

Many of the secondary headaches most commonly associated with pregnancy are caused by cerebrovascular disease, especially in the later stages of pregnancy or in the weeks after delivery.[24] Hypertensive disorders of pregnancy, CVT, posterior reversible encephalopathy syndrome (PRES), and RCVS are heralded by a headache, with or without other neurologic complaints. Headache may also be prominent in arterial dissection, acute ischemic stroke, and intracranial hemorrhage. Pregnancy-related changes in the pituitary, both vascular and inflammatory, may be associated with a secondary headache. Even some nonvascular secondary headaches associated with pregnancy, such as a postdural puncture headache (PDPH), a type of postpartum headache related to obstetric anesthesia, may have superimposed cerebrovascular conditions.

Postdural Puncture Headache

A PDPH typically occurs after spinal or epidural anesthesia, occurring in about 1% of postpartum women. Inadvertent dural puncture during insertion of an epidural catheter may cause a characteristically positional headache with the diagnosis made based on the clinical description. However, MRI with contrast is indicated to confirm the diagnosis with the characteristic enhancement of the dura and outer layer of arachnoid (pachymeningeal enhancement) along with sagging of the cerebellar tonsils and brainstem due to decreased cerebral spinal fluid volume[5,25] (**Fig. 1**). Cerebrovascular complications of dural puncture may necessitate treatment more complicated

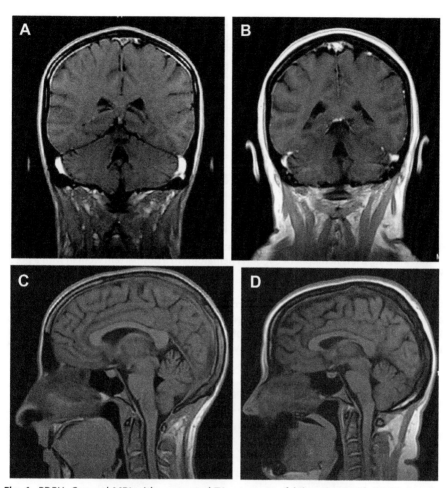

Fig. 1. PDPH. Coronal MRI with contrasted T1 sequence of (*A*) patient with PDPH showing pachymeningeal enhancement compared with (*B*) image without intracranial hypotension.-Sagittal MRI T1 sequence of (*C*) patient with PDPH showing sagging of the cerebellar tonsils compared with (*D*) image without intracranial hypotension.

than the usual hydration and epidural blood patch. Downward traction may lead to unilateral or bilateral subdural hematomas (**Fig. 2**) or thrombosis of cerebral veins with subarachnoid blood in the area of the venous thrombosis[26,27] (**Fig. 3**). Either CT myelography or an MRI of the spine may localize the cerebrospinal fluid (CSF) leak; however, further investigation of a postpartum PDPH beyond head imaging is generally not indicated. Although spontaneous low pressure headaches or PDPHs are associated with low cerebral spinal fluid pressure causing positional exacerbation of the headache, hemorrhage into an enlarged or neoplastic pituitary can also cause headaches with distinct positional components (**Fig. 4**).

CEREBROVASCULAR DISORDERS IN PREGNANCY

The risk of cerebrovascular disorders in pregnancy is greatest after delivery, at a time when the mother does not have the close obstetric follow-up as present in the later

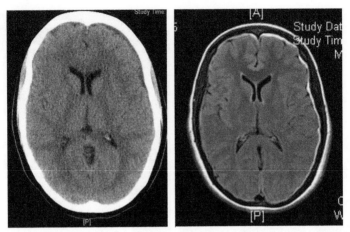

Fig. 2. PDPH with SDH. A CT scan and a fluid-attenuated inversion recovery (FLAIR) sequence on MRI showing a left hemispheric subdural hematoma in a postpartum woman with a postdural puncture headache.

stages of her pregnancy. A substantial proportion of pregnancy-related cerebrovascular disease occurs in the postpartum period after discharge from the hospital, up to 6 weeks after delivery, so the period of vulnerability and need for investigation of neurologic complaints may occur when women may not receive medical follow-up.[28]

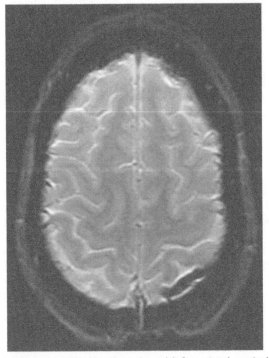

Fig. 3. CVT thrombosed vein. MRI of a thrombosed left parietal cortical vein seen on the susceptibility-weighted imaging (SWI) sequence.

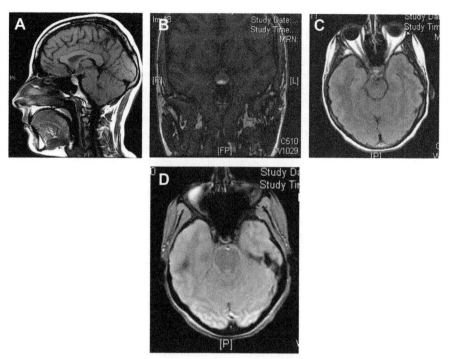

Fig. 4. Pituitary bleed. A 33-year-old woman, 31 weeks pregnant, developed headaches worsened with bending over or coughing. She denied visual changes. An MRI showed hemorrhage into her pituitary gland on saggital T1 (*A*), coronal (*B*), axial FLAIR (*C*) and GRE (*D*) sequences. No pituitary lesion was found on follow-up imaging after delivery.

Kamel and colleagues[29] evaluated the risk of primary thrombotic events after pregnancy compared with the same period 1 year later and found that the risk was markedly higher within 6 weeks after delivery, with an absolute risk difference of 22.1 events per 100,000 deliveries, modestly but significantly higher during the period of 7 to 12 weeks after delivery, for an absolute risk difference of 3.0 events per 100,000 deliveries. Risks of thrombotic events were not significantly increased beyond the first 12 weeks after delivery. An elevated risk of thrombosis persisted until at least 12 weeks after delivery, with a lower increase in risk beyond 6 weeks. However, the greatest cerebrovascular risk appears to be in the first 10-day period after hospital discharge.[30] During this entire postpartum period, new significant neurologic complaints, of both headache and focal neurologic symptoms, should be evaluated with brain imaging, without the constraints of fetal concerns.

Cerebral Venous Thrombosis

The increased risk of CVT during later stages of pregnancy and up to 8 weeks postpartum is caused by multiple pregnancy-related factors, including iatrogenic intracranial hypotension from anesthetic dural puncture, hypercoagulability, and dehydration.[31,32] Headache, change in mental status or alteration in level of consciousness, intracranial hypertension leading to papilledema with potential visual loss, focal or generalized seizures, and focal neurologic deficits due to venous infarcts can all be due to CVT.[33] The incidence of both hemorrhagic and ischemic stroke associated with pregnancy, especially CVT, is increasing, with prepregnancy hypertension in older pregnant women contributing to this alarming increase in cerebrovascular complications of pregnancy.[34] An increased rate of CVT in pregnancy has a less clear relationship to increasing maternal age than does arterial thrombosis or hemorrhage, and, unlike hypertensive disorders of pregnancy, CVT does not seem to be more common in women with migraine. An MRI of the brain and magnetic resonance venography (MRV), without need for contrast injection, are used to evaluate pregnant women with suspected CVT.[35] Contrast injection for MRI of the brain or MRV of the brain may increase diagnostic yield to evaluate suspected postpartum CVT. Time of flight (TOF) MRV assesses flow in large draining cerebral veins and the dural sinuses; however, MRV can miss thrombosis of isolated cortical veins, which may herald future thrombosis and is better seen on susceptibility-weighted imaging (SWI) or gradient-recalled echo (GRE) sequences on MRI (see **Fig. 3**). Interruption of flow-related signal usually indicates CVT; however, low-flow pressure in cerebral veins and dural sinuses can also cause a dropout of TOF-related signal. The presence of thrombus in cerebral veins and sinuses is also associated with the absence of normal hypointense flow voids on brain MRI T1-weighted and T2-weighted sequences or hypointense signal abnormality on SWI or GRE (**Fig. 5**). In MRI with and after delivery, contrast-enhanced sequences improve the diagnostic utility in the diagnosis of CVT.[36,37] Cerebral venous infarction due to CVT is associated with more severe periinfarct edema than with arterial infarction and is associated with a hyperintense signal on T2-weighted and fluid-attenuated inversion recovery (FLAIR) sequences. The localization of cerebral edema overlaps arterial territories, especially notable with involvement in bilateral hemispheres, and both anterior and posterior arterial territories. A noncontrast head CT scan can reveal a hyperdense thrombus in the dural sinus or cortical vein; however, the finding may be subtle, so an MRI is preferred for the diagnosis of CVT. With contrast injection after delivery, the CT scan can show an empty delta sign due to the lack of flow outlining a triangular filling defect caused by a clot in the superior sagittal sinus and the dural sinus torcula. CT venography, with the need for iodinated contrast injection, can be used in postpartum period. In cases of CVT complicated by intracranial hypertension, diffuse cerebral edema can be seen on both MRI and CT imaging. Other brain imaging findings associated with intracranial

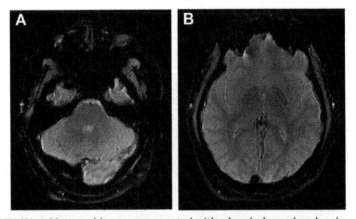

Fig. 5. CVT MRI. A 20-year-old woman presented with a headache and neck pain worsening over several days without focal neurologic complaints. An MRI scan of the head showed multiple small acute infarcts on DWI. The GRE sequence (A,B) showed extensive venous thrombosis involving the superior sagittal, right transverse, and sigmoid sinuses. Despite anticoagulation, she lost vision owing to increased intracranial pressure.

hypertension, such as flattening of the posterior globes, protrusion of the globes, enlarged subarachnoid space around the optic nerves, and an empty sella, may be seen with CVT (**Fig. 6**). Cases of CVT associated with PRES have been reported, indicating a continuum between the various forms of cerebrovascular disease found in pregnant women.[38] Bleeding into a venous infarct can present as an intraparenchymal hemorrhage (IPH) and CVT should be considered in a peripartum woman with an IPH of unclear cause.

Hypertensive Disorders of Pregnancy: Preeclampsia; Eclampsia; or Hemolysis, Elevated Liver Enzymes, and Low Platelet Count Syndrome

Preeclampsia, the most common hypertensive disorder of pregnancy, occurs in approximately 5% pregnancies. Preeclampsia is a syndrome that includes acute blood pressure elevation during the second half of pregnancy and up to approximately 8 weeks postpartum. Preeclampsia can progress to eclampsia in 1% to 2% of cases in which new-onset, generalized seizures occur.[23] Blood pressure elevation in hypertensive disorders of pregnancy is accompanied signs and symptoms of end-organ hypertensive damage, such as headaches, vision changes, seizures, abdominal pain, peripheral edema, and proteinuria. Other manifestations of end-organ damage include hemolysis, elevated liver function tests, and decreased platelets as part of the hemolysis, elevated liver enzymes, and low platelet count (HELLP) syndrome. Proteinuria is not required for diagnosis of preeclampsia, reflecting the high variability in disease presentation and progression based on the various organs (eg, brain, liver, spleen, kidneys) affected by the new onset of an often precipitous elevation in blood pressure.[39] These accompaniments to the acutely elevated blood pressure are not always present in a woman with preeclampsia or eclampsia, with the exception of the complaint of headache, which is almost universally present in hypertensive disorders of pregnancy. Preeclampsia, eclampsia, or HELLP syndrome is often heralded by the new onset of headache later in pregnancy, as can occur with migraine.[40] Hypertensive disorders of pregnancy are more common in woman with migraine headaches before pregnancy; however, migraine is not associated with blood pressure elevation, the hallmark of hypertensive disorders of pregnancy. The neurologic manifestations of hypertensive disorders of pregnancy are caused by disordered cerebral vascular autoregulation, with

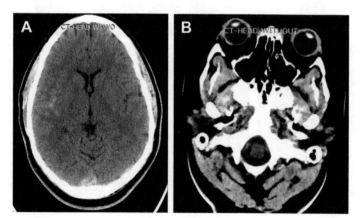

Fig. 6. CVT CT. Subtle signs of CVT on uncontrasted CT scanning include (A) hyperdensity in the region of venous sinuses (at the torcula) and subarachnoid blood (in the right Sylvian fissure), and (B) exophthalmos due to increased intracranial pressure.

endothelial damage and capillary leakage causing cerebral edema. Certain circulating angiogenic factors released by the placenta are associated with preeclampsia and may reflect the severity of outcome of hypertensive disorders of pregnancy.[41] There are no pathognomonic imaging findings associated with these conditions on either brain MRI or head CT scan in the early stages of the blood pressure elevation, and the diagnosis should be made on clinical suspicion alone. Nevertheless, noncontrast brain MRI should be performed to rule out other causes of headache, particularly PRES and RCVS.[42,43] These cerebrovascular complications of pregnancy, representing a continuum of disorders with overlapping presentations, are variably associated with elevated blood pressure. Acute elevation in blood pressure is generally, but not always, seen with the imaging diagnosis of PRES (**Fig. 7**) Untreated, preeclampsia, eclampsia, or HELLP syndrome can result in ischemic and hemorrhagic strokes, as well as progression to PRES and RCVS (**Fig. 8**) The clinical and imaging presentations of RCVS are generally not associated with elevated blood pressure; however, RCVS can be part of the spectrum of hypertensive disorders of pregnancy and can lead to ischemic or hemorrhagic strokes. Interestingly, hypertension as a complication of pregnancy increases a woman's risk of ischemic stroke in her future, unrelated to future pregnancies.[44]

Posterior Reversible Encephalopathy Syndrome

PRES is a characteristic imaging syndrome that can present clinically with a pressure-like dull holocephalic headache, encephalopathy, visual changes, and seizures. Patchy parietooccipital or diffuse hemispheric hyperintensities

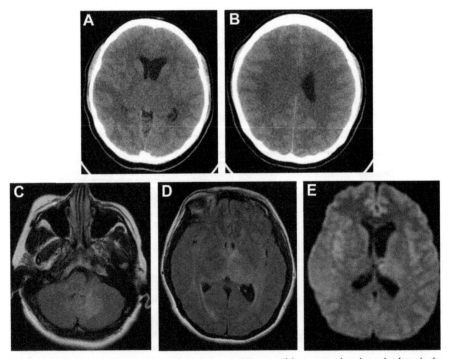

Fig. 7. PRES without elevated blood pressure. A 28-year-old woman developed a headache and dizziness 4 weeks after delivery, without elevated blood pressures. The CT (*A, B*) and MRI (*C, D, E*) scan showed imaging changes of PRES.

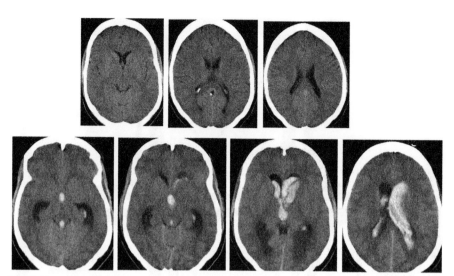

Fig. 8. Preeclampsia IPH. A 42-year-old developed a severe headache and elevated blood pressures a week after an uneventful delivery. A CT scan was obtained as shown. Pain medication was given and she was sent home. She presented the next day unresponsive with the MRI showing a basal ganglia hemorrhage extending into the ventricles. No underlying lesion was found on autopsy.

on T2-weighted and FLAIR sequences, and T1-weighted sequence hypointensities, are imaging characteristics; however, PRES can involve all areas of the brain and, in rare cases, can include the brain-stem and spinal cord. Imaging with a CT scan of the head reveals 9 patchy posterior or diffuse hypodensities in the bilateral cerebral hemispheres (**Fig. 9**). These changes do not follow a particular arterial distribution, differentiating them from cerebral arterial infarction, but potentially confusing them with the localization of venous infarction associated with CVT. Recognition of the clinical symptoms and the significance of the elevated blood pressure, if present, should lead to the timely initiation of treatment with the resolution of clinical symptoms and imaging findings. Imaging consistent with PRES is often found in women with preeclampsia, eclampsia, or HELLP syndrome, as well as with a multitude of other conditions, some of which are not associated with elevated blood pressure. Pregnancy-related PRES is usually a complication of preeclampsia or eclampsia but can be found in normotensive women[45] (see **Fig. 7**). The underlying pathophysiology of this spectrum of disorders with the radiological presentation of PRES is thought to be due to loss of cerebral autoregulation, increased capillary leakage resulting in vasogenic edema predominantly in the parietal and occipital lobes. However, imaging changes can be diffuse in the brain, brainstem, and spinal cord.[46] Brain imaging is crucial with a noncontrast brain MRI being the imaging modality of choice in pregnant women with symptoms of headache and blurred vision suspicious for a PRES-related disorder (**Fig. 10**). Untreated PRES, associated with or separate from preeclampsia, eclampsia, or HELLP syndrome, can lead to strokes, both ischemic and hemorrhagic. As with the hypertensive disorders of pregnancy, there is an overlap in physiologic mechanisms of PRES and RCVS, and cases of concurrent conditions are reported.[42,47,48] The presence of vasospasm in patients with PRES has been documented by catheter angiography and magnetic resonance angiography (MRA), emphasizing the overlap between the various types of cerebrovascular syndromes in pregnancy.[49]

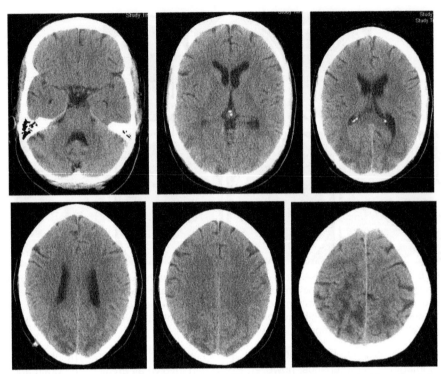

Fig. 9. Preeclampsia CT. A 45-year-old woman, 36 weeks pregnant, presented in active labor with a blood pressure of 182/88. She complained of a headache and blurred vision, and then had a generalized tonic-clonic seizure. A CT scan of the brain showed posterior hypoattenuation consistent with PRES in all cerebral sections shown. A healthy baby was delivered by emergent sectioning and blood pressure was controlled. She was discharged to home on antihypertensive medication.

Reversible Cerebral Vasoconstriction Syndrome or Postpartum Cerebral Angiopathy

RCVS is a clinical and radiographic syndrome, of multiple etiologies, that is associated with a headache of generally abrupt onset and reversible multifocal vasoconstriction in large and medium size arteries.[50–52] The vasospastic disorders of postpartum angiopathy, Call Fleming syndrome, drug induced cerebral vasospasm, and benign cerebral angiopathy are part of an RCVS spectrum.[53] The cause of RCVS may be unknown or be related to exposure to vasoactive substances such as medications or illicit drugs. The presence of circulating angiogenic factors may explain the increased risk of RCVS in the postpartum.[54] In uncomplicated cases not associated with progression to an ischemic or hemorrhagic stroke, a CT or MRI scan of the brain, may be unrevealing. Vasospasm, with beading, may be seen on MRA, CT angiography (CTA), or cerebral catheter angiography; although, MRA, the preferred imaging modality in pregnant patients, may only reveal subtle or nonspecific changes (**Fig. 11**). Contrast-requiring CTA and cerebral angiography can be used in postpartum patients because iodinated contrast in breast milk is not associated with adverse effects in the infant.[55–57] Catheter angiography, is most likely to show a pattern of vasospasm, which needs to be differentiated from the beaded and tapered vessels, with cutoff and ballooning, seen

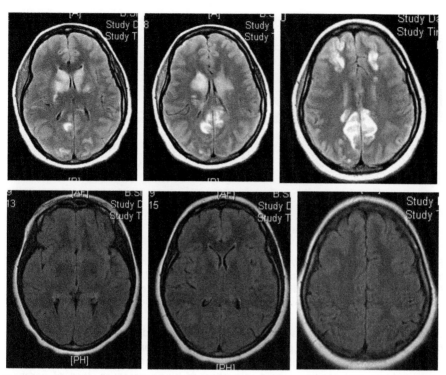

Fig. 10. Preeclampsia MRI. A 19-year-old woman, 31 weeks pregnant, seized with a blood pressure of 190/140. A placental abruption with fetal demise was diagnosed. Her blood pressure and seizures were controlled and a stillborn fetus was delivered. A CT scan (not shown) revealed bilateral parietal medial hypodensities and bilateral internal capsule hypodensities. The MRI showed multifocal changes of PRES on FLAIR imaging (top row), with resolution about a week later (bottom row).

with central nervous system vasculitis. Repeat vascular imaging, generally MRA or CTA, in 3 months is warranted to confirm the resolution of the imaging of cerebral vasospasm, as dictated by the clinical course.

Postpartum RCVS, although generally associated with a favorable outcome, can be complicated by ischemic stroke, IPH, and nonaneurysmal subarachnoid hemorrhage (SAH) (**Fig. 12**). An approximately 2% mortality due to IPH and ischemic stroke has been associated with complicated cases of RCVS.[53,58] SAH associated with RCVS, which may be subtle, is more common than ischemic stroke or IPH and has a more benign outcome because there is no underlying cerebral aneurysm.[59,60] As seen with CVT, the small volume of subarachnoid blood associated with RCVS is usually pericortical, as opposed to intracisternal, and the area surrounding the hemorrhage should be evaluated for a thrombosed cortical vein. Although there is an association of RCVS with PRES and hypertensive disorders of pregnancy, isolated RCVS is usually benign with headache as the only symptom. The RCVS-related headache may be treated with calcium channel blockers, but the removal of the precipitating agent generally leads to clinical and imaging resolution.

Intracranial hemorrhage, both IPH and aneurysmal SAH (as distinct from CVT or RCVS associated SAH), although rare in pregnancy, constitutes the third leading

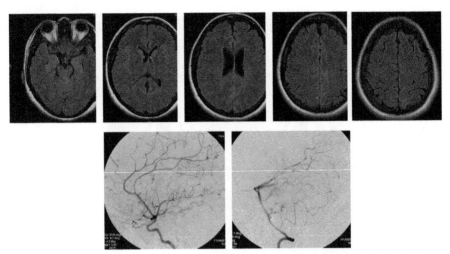

Fig. 11. Postpartum angiopathy or RCVS. A 40-year-old woman had a headache that began immediately before delivery and persisted to postpartum day 7, with normal blood pressure. An MRI showed abnormal FLAIR signal posteriorly (top row) and MRA was nondiagnostic. Multifocal areas of arterial spasm were seen on catheter angiography (bottom row).

cause of nonobstetric-related mortality in pregnant and postpartum women. The causes of hemorrhages in pregnancy are different from the general population and are mainly related to physiologic changes in pregnancy, such as increased blood volume and cardiac output, elevation of blood pressure, loss of cerebral

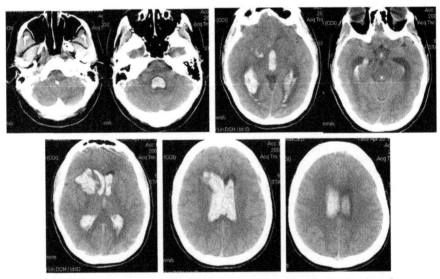

Fig. 12. A 43-year-old woman complained of a continuing headache the day after an uneventful vaginal delivery. Her blood pressures were normal. The next day she complained of a severe headache and immediately became unresponsive with marked blood pressure elevation. A CT scan showed a right basal ganglia IPH with intraventricular extension seen in all images. No underlying lesion was found on autopsy. Postpartum cerebral angiopathy (RCVS) was suspected as a cause of the headache starting the day after delivery.

vascular autoregulation, and vascular wall remodeling. Cerebrovascular structures present before pregnancy, such as arteriovenous malformations (AVMs), cavernomas, and intracerebral aneurysms, are the most common lesions related to IPH.[61] AVM rupture most commonly presents with parenchymal, followed by intraventricular, hemorrhage.[62] The risk of cavernoma-related symptomatic hemorrhages during pregnancy is not increased.[63] The risk of aneurysmal SAH during pregnancy and delivery is lower than in nonpregnant women.[64] Although there may be an increase in aneurysmal size with the hemodynamic changes in pregnancy, the risk of hemorrhagic cerebrovascular disease, presenting with the apoplectic onset of a severe headache, is increased immediately after delivery (**Fig. 13**). More than 50% of aneurysmal SAH occur in the postpartum period.[65] A noncontrasted CT scan of the head has high sensitivity and specificity in detecting acute intracranial blood, including in the intraventricular and subarachnoid spaces, and should be a quick screening study before a more detailed imaging evaluation of cerebral vasculature. Although cerebral catheter angiography provides the most detailed description of a cerebral aneurysm, a CTA has a very high sensitivity and specificity, especially for larger aneurysms that are at high risk for rupture.[66] If fetal safety is a concern due to exposure to ionizing radiation and IV iodinated contrast, MRA can be performed for screening; however, the technique has high sensitivity to motion artifact.[61]

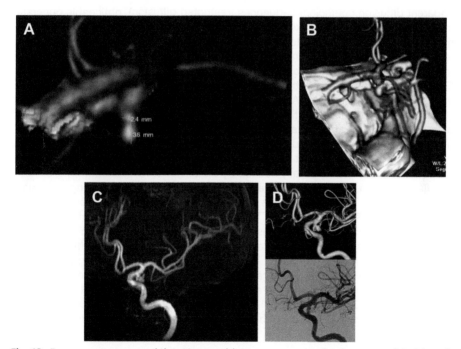

Fig. 13. Pregnancy aneurysm. (*A*) A 40-year-old woman was noted to have a small incidental left posterior communication artery aneurysm measuring 3.6 × 2.4 mm on CTA. (*B*) Two years later, a follow-up CTA study showed that the aneurysm, measured at 3.5 × 2.6 cm, was essentially unchanged. (*C*) At age 44 years she became pregnant with twins. An MRA at 31 weeks showed that the bilobed and irregular aneurysm had grown to 5 × 3.5 cm. (*D*) At 35 weeks, the twins were delivered by sectioning and the aneurysm was successfully coiled.

Arterial Ischemic Stroke

The risk of arterial ischemic stroke is increased around the time of delivery and for up to 8 weeks after delivery. A study by Kuklina and colleagues[34] showed a disturbing increase in the rate of antepartum and postpartum stroke of all causes in the past decade, likely related to an increase in traditional risk factors, including hypertension, as pregnancy is delayed. Pregnancy-specific arterial ischemic stroke risk factors include estrogen-induced hypercoagulability, trophoblastic embolism, amniotic fluid embolism, cardioembolism due to pregnancy-related cardiomyopathies, hypertensive disorders of pregnancy, RCVS, cervical arterial dissection, and paradoxic embolism due to lower extremity deep venous thrombosis in the setting of a right-to-left cardiac shunt. IPH is more common than is acute ischemic stroke in the postpartum period. Although headaches are not typical for patients with ischemic stroke, they are not uncommon in pregnant patients with ischemic stroke and may be the initial reason for obtaining brain imaging.[24] Otherwise, clinical presentations of ischemic stroke in pregnancy do not differ from the usual focal neurologic deficits, change in mental status, and (less commonly) accompanying seizures, seen in the nonpregnant population. Also, neuroimaging is similar to ischemic stroke imaging in the general population. A CT scan of the head reveals loss of grey-white differentiation, sulcal effacement, and hypoattenuation of the infarcted area. Chronic infarcts appear hypodense with associated volume loss. MRI of the brain reveals hyperintense lesions on DWI with correlating hypointense lesions on apparent diffusion coefficient sequences (restricted diffusion), noticeable generally from the first minutes of stroke onset. Later ischemic changes are associated with hyperintensities on T2-weighted and FLAIR sequences and are eventually hypointense on T1-weighted sequence. Pregnancy is only a relative contraindication to the treatment with IV thrombolysis, which should be offered when appropriate. Endovascular intervention with radiation and contrast exposure could be considered during pregnancy if MRA screening shows a large vessel occlusion.[67,68]

Postpartum arterial dissection occurs with tearing of the endothelial lining of extracranial and intracranial arterial vessels, producing associated symptoms of headache or neck pain, and local (eg, Horner syndrome, lower cranial nerve paresis) or cerebral (transient ischemic attack or ischemic stroke) symptoms and signs. Ischemic stroke is usually caused by distal clot embolization from a dissection flap, with a hemodynamic cause from an occlusive dissection being less common. Postpartum arterial dissection seems to be unrelated to the type of delivery and can involve single or multiple, posterior and/or anterior circulation vessels, as well as cardiac and renal arteries. The reason for this postpartum vulnerability is unknown and seems to be unrelated to an underlying connective tissue disorder.[69] Dissection is best visualized by MRA of head and neck during pregnancy, with MRA of the neck with contrast or CTA obtained after delivery, showing characteristic flame-like tapering of a dissection to occlusion in the internal carotid artery (**Fig. 14**). Cross-sectional T1-weighted imaging with fat suppression may show a characteristic crescent-shaped deformity in the wall of the dissected internal carotid artery.

CENTRAL NERVOUS SYSTEM MASS LESIONS
Neoplasms in Pregnancy

An intracranial mass lesion can expand or hemorrhage due to cardiovascular and hormonal changes during pregnancy. Primary brain tumors and metastases can become symptomatic, recur, or progress during pregnancy, and pathology can

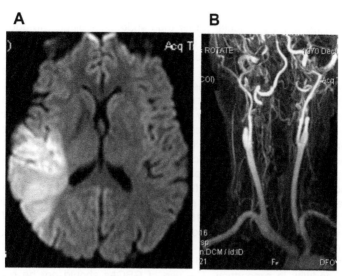

Fig. 14. Internal carotid artery (ICA) dissection. An MRA (*B*) showing bilateral internal carotid artery dissections in a postpartum woman with an acute right middle cerebral infarct on the DWI sequence on MRI (*A*).

progress from low grade to a more aggressive form.[9] Because a standard protocol for the treatment of brain tumors during pregnancy may lead to a favorable outcome, appropriate brain imaging should be used to investigate symptoms suggestive of an intracranial mass lesion. Verheecke and colleagues[70] followed 27 pregnant subjects diagnosed with intracranial tumors, all but one during the last 2 trimesters, who were treated with surgery, radiation, and chemotherapy. With treatment, 21 of the ongoing pregnancies resulted in live births of children without visible congenital malformations. The last trimester carries the greatest risk of symptomatic tumor expansion owing to increases in cardiac output and intravascular volume, which can cause increased vascularity with increased hemorrhage risk. In addition, the use of a spinal or epidural anesthesia, as well as the increased pressure involved with a vaginal delivery in a woman with an intracranial mass, may necessitate neuroimaging. Changes in progesterone, estrogen, and prostacyclins are also related to accelerated tumor expansion owing to the estrogen and progesterone receptors detected on some tumors, leading to headache from increased intracranial pressure.[71] Elevated intravascular volume can increase the risk of hemorrhage into a neoplasm, also causing an acute headache in pregnancy.

Primary brain or metastatic tumors with a significant vascular component are particularly susceptible to hemorrhage-related headaches during pregnancy. Choriocarcinomas are rare but they are derived from the placenta during pregnancy and can metastasize to the central nervous system, presenting with an acute headache and focal neurologic deficits in the setting of tumor hemorrhage.[72] Even benign vascular mass lesions, such as intracranial or spinal hemangioblastomas, can become acutely symptomatic during pregnancy because of vascular mechanisms causing expansion or hemorrhage presenting as IPH.[73,74]

Meningiomas account for 35% of all primary brain tumors and are twice as common in women as in men; however, unlike pregnancies, their incidence increases with age.[75] Meningiomas express progesterone (70%) receptors and estrogen

(30%) receptors on tumor cells; however, the mechanism of pregnancy-related expansion is most likely vascular rather than endocrinological.[76] In addition, hormones in pregnancy can act on the steroid receptors expressed by meningiomas and cause accelerated growth and vascularity.[77] Meningiomas, especially the more vascular (angiomatous) ones, tend to grow rapidly during pregnancy and may become symptomatic due to their mass effect from edema, hypervascularity, and intratumoral hemorrhage and/or necrosis.[78] Parasellar meningiomas may present in the later months of pregnancy with headaches owing to the expanding mass effects of hydrocephalus caused by elevated intracranial pressure, by the distortion of the diaphragm sella, or by parasellar dura irritation. Meningiomas located in the skull base are especially likely to become symptomatic during pregnancy, with visual complaints and cranial nerve palsies, and require surgical resection.[78] The dural venous sinuses can also be affected by mass effect from a meningioma in the parafalcine area. Imaging of the mass, as well as the dural venous sinuses, is indicated with MRI and MRV (**Fig. 15**). Meningiomas may present on MRI during pregnancy as isointense T1-weighted and T2-weighted lesions with a broad dural attachment, adjacent hyperostosis, and normal sellar dimensions. A dural tail may not be seen on an unenhanced scan obtained during pregnancy. MRI is the preferred modality in pregnancy. The use of GBCAs should not be restricted if they will increase diagnostic yield.

Gliomas are the most common primary malignant brain tumor, with glioblastoma accounting for 16% of all primary brain tumors.[75] They can have a diverse presentation, including during pregnancy.[79] A study of pregnant women found that individuals with grade II and III gliomas showed a greater risk of increased growth during the pregnancy, whereas grade I gliomas did not. This was attributed to tumor vascularity and that the higher grade tumors rely on angiogenesis.[80]

Pituitary Lesions in Pregnancy

Normal pregnancy is associated with enlargement of the pituitary, as well as hormonal and vascular changes. Women with known pituitary adenomas should be monitored with imaging, visual field testing, and blood work because the lesions can become symptomatic during pregnancy owing to vascular or endocrine mechanisms.[81] The normal pituitary enlargement seen during pregnancy or pituitary enlargement in the setting of a pituitary adenoma leads to risk of pituitary hemorrhage or infarction. The onset of symptoms with pituitary hemorrhage is usually apoplectic[77,82–84] (see **Fig. 4**). Symptoms of hypopituitarism in Sheehan syndrome generally occur insidiously after a pituitary infarct owing to hypotension or the extreme blood loss associated with delivery. MRI may show enlarged pituitary with central hypointensity on T1-weighted images and hyperintensity on T2-weighted images with irregular enhancement. With time, the pituitary atrophies and a residual empty sella are noted.[85]

Lymphocytic hypophysitis is an inflammatory autoimmune disease of the pituitary gland that characteristically presents as a perisellar expansion of the adenohypophysis, neurohypophysis, or infundibulum, with isodense or hypodense signals on T1-weighted images[86] (**Fig. 16**). Patients, including peripartum women, present with headache, nausea, and vomiting, as well as a bitemporal visual field deficit. Although empiric steroids could be considered if the diagnosis is convincing, the diagnosis is usually made on pathologic examination of a frozen biopsy specimen, so as not to remove a functioning pituitary gland. The diagnosis should be suspected in a peripartum woman with a nonhemorrhagic enlargement of the pituitary, and prompt steroid

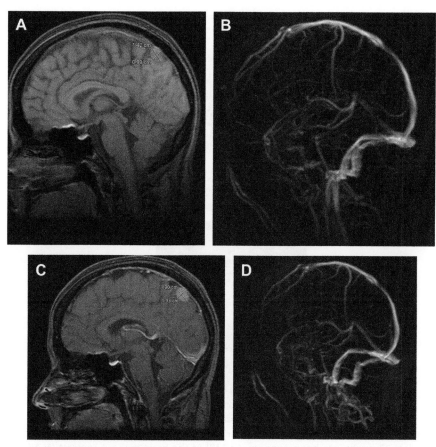

Fig. 15. Meningioma, case study: 28-year-old woman presented at 9 weeks pregnant with visual blurring and severe headache described as a pressure on top of her head. MRI brain showed a rounded extraaxial parafalcine mass on T1W on contrast. MRV showed focal narrowing of the superior sagittal sinus. Postpregnancy MRI with contrast showed the lesion in hyperintense on T1-weighted sequences and that it had increased in size. The narrowing of the superior sagittal sinus on MRV looked similar. (*A*) Three-dimensional PCA MRV during pregnancy. (*B*) MRV during pregnancy. (*C*) Three-dimensional PCA MRV contrast postpartum. (*D*) MRV head postpartum.

treatment after confirmation by pituitary biopsy generally leads to return of the pituitary to its usual size and normal function.[87]

CENTRAL NERVOUS SYSTEM INFLAMMATION AND DEMYELINATION

During pregnancy, hormonal changes alter maternal antiinflammatory responses to protect from rejection of the fetus. As the maternal hormones increase, there is a gradual increase in immune responses to support and protect fetal development and a decrease in the regulatory cells that affect disease pathogenesis. The severity of diseases caused by inflammatory responses (e.g., multiple sclerosis) is reduced and the severity of diseases that are mitigated by inflammatory responses (e.g., influenza and malaria) is increased during pregnancy.[88] For some infectious diseases as a woman progresses through the 3 trimesters, her hormone levels increase, bringing her

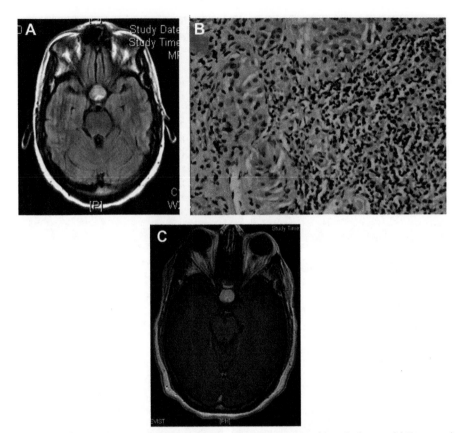

Fig. 16. Lymphocytic hypophysitis. A 34-year-old woman noted headaches and bitemporal vision loss 32 weeks into her pregnancy. An MRI of the brain without contrast (FLAIR) (A) showed a pituitary lesion that was diagnosed as lymphocytic hypophysitis on biopsy (B). She was treated with steroids and had improvement in her vision. A contrast-enhanced study after delivery (C) showed a T1-enhancing pituitary lesion characteristic of lymphocytic hypophysitis.

from a proinflammatory to an antiinflammatory state, which is necessary to support the pregnancy. These changes can cause the onset of a new disease state or even exacerbate a preexisting condition.

Multiple Sclerosis and Other Demyelinating Disorders

Multiple sclerosis is caused by autoimmune inflammatory responses involving demyelination and axonal damage. It affects women more often than men (70%) and occurs more frequently during childbearing years. Demyelinating disorders, including MS, clinically isolated syndrome, neuromyelitis optica spectrum disorder (NMOSD), and acute disseminated encephalomyelitis (ADEM) may presented de novo or may become acutely symptomatic during pregnancy.[89]

During pregnancy, hormone-mediated immune responses are believed to alter relapse rates. A study of female MS subjects followed before, during, and after pregnancy, which was carried out before the common use of disease-modifying therapies (DMTs), found fewer relapses in subjects in the third trimester. There was a subsequent increase in relapse rates postpartum in approximately one-third of the subjects, who returned to their prepregnancy relapse rates. Breast feeding and occurrence of epidural analgesia did not correlate with postpartum relapses.[90,91] A more recent study of the rate of relapse occurrence during pregnancy and the postpartum period found a higher relapse rate during pregnancy, indicating that the use of effective DMTs, with long washout periods before conception, was associated with an increased risk of relapses during pregnancy. For 99 pregnancies in 87 subjects, the relapse rates during pregnancy and the postpartum period were 17.2% and 13.7%, respectively, with most of the relapses occurring during the first and third trimesters. Postpartum relapse occurrence was similar to that previously reported.[92] In an administrative database study, women with MS were at increased risk for infections and preterm delivery but not other adverse pregnancy outcomes, including cerebrovascular disease. Disease activity before delivery was not a strong predictor of outcomes.[93] Pregnancy and breastfeeding after a diagnosis of a clinically isolated syndrome do not increase the risk of developing clinically definite MS.[94]

Neuroimaging findings in pregnancy are similar to nonpregnant patients. An MRI is superior to CT scan for lesion detection and is safer in pregnancy. Typical MRI findings in MS include radiating periventricular or pericallosal, ovoid subcortical, and juxtacortical lesions that are hyperintense in T2-weighted imaging. FLAIR sequences in the brain are hyperintense and there may also be T1-weighted hypointensities or so-called black holes (**Fig. 17**). Optic nerves may also be evaluated and can be hyperintense on T2-weighted or proton-dense sequences with fat and CSF suppression sequences if there is evidence of optic neuritis.[95] There are no specific safety data on patients with MS in regard to neuroimaging.[96] Although GBCAs are routinely used in the diagnosis and follow-up of patients with MS, their use during pregnancy should be avoided, if possible. The lack of contrasted study does not significantly hamper the accuracy of diagnosis and follow-up. In a study using subtraction maps, nonenhanced images (double-inversion recovery,[97] FLAIR) did not miss lesions on follow-up studies compared with T1-weighted contrast-enhanced images. The investigators concluded that "[a]t 3.0 T, use of a gadolinium-based contrast agent at follow-up MRI did not change the diagnosis of interval disease progression in patients with multiple sclerosis."[97]

Khalid and colleagues[98] assessed the change in cerebral lesions and atrophy associated with pregnancy in 16 subjects with MS with prepregnancy and postpartum 1.5-T brain MRI separated by (mean ± SD) 15.4 plus or minus 3.2 months. Pregnancy was associated with an increase in T2-weighted and T1-weighted cerebral lesion load, without whole brain or cortical atrophy. For the short term, pregnancy protects against the brain volume loss, despite an increased lesion load. If there is a significant increase in lesion load during pregnancy and the patient is on disease-modifying agents, alternate causes need to be considered, such as progressive multifocal leukoencephalopathy.[5]

Pregnant women with NMOSD are almost always seropositive for antibodies targeting aquaporin-4–immunoglobulin G,[99] and generally do not have detectable oligoclonal bands in the cerebral spinal fluid. They seem to have a different clinical course than do pregnant women with MS. Although they also have a higher risk for relapses in the first 3 months after delivery, women with NMOSD are also at risk for relapse during pregnancy. They also have higher rates of nondemyelinating complications of pregnancy, such as miscarriage and preeclampsia. Because treatment of NMOSD differs from that of MS, MRI scanning of the brain, spinal cord, and optic nerves, which are areas of involvement with NMOSD, are necessary during pregnancy if the diagnosis is suspected.[89] Incidental

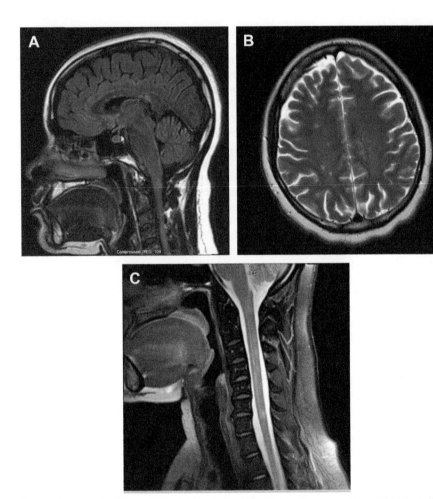

Fig. 17. Case study: 37-year-old woman. Demyelinating lesions were found incidentally on MRI scan, without symptoms of MS, after a fall: (*A*) FLAIR sagittal and (*B*) T2-weighted axial. She was followed throughout a pregnancy and did very well. Two months postpartum she developed weakness, vision changes, and increased falls. Subsequent MRI showed an increase in spinal cord lesions: (*C*) Short-TI Inversion Recovery (STIR) sagittal.

reports of pregnant women with ADEM, generally in association with a viral infection[100,101] and acute hemorrhagic leukoencephalitis,[102] do not indicate any increased vulnerability to a single episode of aggressive demyelination during pregnancy.

SUMMARY

Most pregnancies progress through the postpartum period without any neurologic symptomatology or need for brain or spinal cord imaging. However, when new-onset neurologic symptoms necessitate imaging, MRI without contrast-enhancement is safe and generally diagnostic, and should be obtained during any stage of pregnancy if a neurologic diagnosis or procedure is necessary for the health of the mother. A new-onset headache is concerning in a pregnant woman and an MRI of the brain and/or an MRA of the head and neck and/or MRV should be obtained, especially when a new-onset headache occurs in the peripartum period with focal neurologic symptoms or elevated blood pressure. Mass lesions, both neoplastic and vascular, may enlarge most aggressively in the later months of pregnancy, and MRI should be used to follow these lesions and determine the appropriate time for intervention. Many of the cerebrovascular complications of pregnancy are preventable or easily treatable after appropriate brain imaging of women with complaints of headache in the later stages of pregnancy and in the immediate period after delivery. Elevation of blood pressure in this peripartum period of risk for preeclampsia, eclampsia, or HELLP syndrome should be immediately and appropriately treated in order to avoid the stroke complications of these hypertensive disorders of pregnancy. Conversely, pregnancy may serve as a protective factor in some disorders, such as with MS demyelination and inflammatory flares. Neuroimaging, especially contrast administration, should be avoided in pregnancy if possible. However, if the clinical presentation necessitates neuroimaging for proper care, the risks and benefits to mother and fetus must always be considered.

REFERENCES

1. Toscano M, Thornburg LL. Neurological diseases in pregnancy. Curr Opin Obstet Gynecol 2019;31(2):97–109.
2. Hamilton KT, Robbins MS. Migraine treatment in pregnant women presenting to acute care: a retrospective observational study. Headache 2019;59(2):173–9.
3. Copel J, El-Sayed Y, Heine RP, et al. Committee opinion no. 723: guidelines for diagnostic imaging during pregnancy and lactation. Obstet Gynecol 2017; 130(4):e210–6.
4. Chansakul T, Young GS. Neuroimaging in pregnant women. Semin Neurol 2017; 37(6):712–23.
5. Bove RM, Klein JP. Neuroradiology in women of childbearing age. Continuum (Minneap Minn) 2014;20(1 Neurology of Pregnancy):23–41.
6. Jain C. ACOG committee opinion no. 723: guidelines for diagnostic imaging during pregnancy and lactation. Obstet Gynecol 2019;133(1):186.
7. Tremblay E, Thérasse E, Thomassin-Naggara I, et al. Quality initiatives: guidelines for use of medical imaging during pregnancy and lactation. Radiographics 2012;32(3):897–911.
8. Chen MM, Coakley FV, Kaimal A, et al. Guidelines for computed tomography and magnetic resonance imaging use during pregnancy and lactation. Obstet Gynecol 2008;112(2 Pt 1):333–40.
9. Bonfield CM, Engh JA. Pregnancy and brain tumors. Neurol Clin 2012;30(3): 937–46.
10. Media ACoRCoDaC. American College of Radiology manual on contrast media v. 10.3. American College of Radiology; 2018. Available at: https://www.acr.org/Clinical-Resources/Contrast-Manual.
11. Ray JG, Vermeulen MJ, Bharatha A, et al. Association between MRI exposure during pregnancy and fetal and childhood outcomes. JAMA 2016;316(9): 952–61.
12. Tee LM, Kan EY, Cheung JC, et al. Magnetic resonance imaging of the fetal brain. Hong Kong Med J 2016;22(3):270–8.
13. Patenaude Y, Pugash D, Lim K, et al. The use of magnetic resonance imaging in the obstetric patient. J Obstet Gynaecol Can 2014;36(4):349–63.

14. Administration FaD. FDA Drug Safety Communication: FDA warns that gadolinium-based contrast agents (GBCAs) are retained in the body; requires new class warnings. Available at: https://www.fda.gov/drugs/drugsafety/ucm5892132018.

15. Headache Classification Committee of the International Headache Society (IHS). The International classification of headache disorders, 3rd edition. Cephalalgia 2018;38(1):1–211.

16. Callaghan BC, Kerber KA, Pace RJ, et al. Headaches and neuroimaging: high utilization and costs despite guidelines. JAMA Intern Med 2014;174(5):819–21.

17. Spierings EL, Sabin TD. De novo headache during pregnancy and puerperium. Neurologist 2016;21(1):1–7.

18. Wells RE, Turner DP, Lee M, et al. Managing migraine during pregnancy and lactation. Curr Neurol Neurosci Rep 2016;16(4):40.

19. Robbins MS, Farmakidis C, Dayal AK, et al. Acute headache diagnosis in pregnant women: a hospital-based study. Neurology 2015;85(12):1024–30.

20. Raffaelli B, Neeb L, Israel-Willner H, et al. Brain imaging in pregnant women with acute headache. J Neurol 2018;265(8):1836–43.

21. Ramchandren S, Cross BJ, Liebeskind DS. Emergent headaches during pregnancy: correlation between neurologic examination and neuroimaging. AJNR Am J Neuroradiol 2007;28(6):1085–7.

22. Mitsikostas DD, Ashina M, Craven A, et al. European Headache Federation consensus on technical investigation for primary headache disorders. J Headache Pain 2015;17:5.

23. Edlow JA, Caplan LR, O'Brien K, et al. Diagnosis of acute neurological emergencies in pregnant and post-partum women. Lancet Neurol 2013;12(2): 175–85.

24. Jamieson DG, Cheng NT, Skliut M. Headache and acute stroke. Curr Pain Headache Rep 2014;18(9):444.

25. Nappi RE, Albani F, Sances G, et al. Headaches during pregnancy. Curr Pain Headache Rep 2011;15(4):289–94.

26. Sachs A, Smiley R. Post-dural puncture headache: the worst common complication in obstetric anesthesia. Semin Perinatol 2014;38(6):386–94.

27. Sinha A, Petkov S, Meldrum D. Unrecognised dural puncture resulting in subdural hygroma and cortical vein thrombosis. Anaesthesia 2010;65(1):70–3.

28. Hovsepian DA, Sriram N, Kamel H, et al. Acute cerebrovascular disease occurring after hospital discharge for labor and delivery. Stroke 2014;45(7):1947–50.

29. Kamel H, Navi BB, Sriram N, et al. Risk of a thrombotic event after the 6-week postpartum period. N Engl J Med 2014;370(14):1307–15.

30. Too G, Wen T, Boehme AK, et al. Timing and risk factors of postpartum stroke. Obstet Gynecol 2018;131(1):70–8.

31. Coutinho JM, Ferro JM, Canhão P, et al. Cerebral venous and sinus thrombosis in women. Stroke 2009;40(7):2356–61.

32. Bousser MG, Crassard I. Cerebral venous thrombosis, pregnancy and oral contraceptives. Thromb Res 2012;130(Suppl 1):S19–22.

33. Fam D, Saposnik G, Stroke Outcomes Research Canada Working Group. Critical care management of cerebral venous thrombosis. Curr Opin Crit Care 2016;22(2):113–9.

34. Kuklina EV, Tong X, Bansil P, et al. Trends in pregnancy hospitalizations that included a stroke in the United States from 1994 to 2007: reasons for concern? Stroke 2011;42(9):2564–70.

35. Ganeshan D, Narlawar R, McCann C, et al. Cerebral venous thrombosis-A pictorial review. Eur J Radiol 2010;74(1):110–6.

36. Hinman JM, Provenzale JM. Hypointense thrombus on T2-weighted MR imaging: a potential pitfall in the diagnosis of dural sinus thrombosis. Eur J Radiol 2002;41(2):147–52.
37. Sadigh G, Mullins ME, Saindane AM. Diagnostic performance of MRI sequences for evaluation of dural venous sinus thrombosis. AJR Am J Roentgenol 2016;206(6):1298–306.
38. Petrovic BD, Nemeth AJ, McComb EN, et al. Posterior reversible encephalopathy syndrome and venous thrombosis. Radiol Clin North Am 2011;49(1): 63–80.
39. Tranquilli AL. Introduction to ISSHP new classification of preeclampsia. Pregnancy Hypertens 2013;3(2):58–9.
40. Duhig KE, Shennan AH. Recent advances in the diagnosis and management of pre-eclampsia. F1000Prime Rep 2015;7:24.
41. Rana S, Powe CE, Salahuddin S, et al. Angiogenic factors and the risk of adverse outcomes in women with suspected preeclampsia. Circulation 2012; 125(7):911–9.
42. Fletcher JJ, Kramer AH, Bleck TP, et al. Overlapping features of eclampsia and postpartum angiopathy. Neurocrit Care 2009;11(2):199–209.
43. Fugate JE, Ameriso SF, Ortiz G, et al. Variable presentations of postpartum angiopathy. Stroke 2012;43(3):670–6.
44. Zoet GA, Linstra KM, Bernsen MLE, et al. Stroke after pregnancy disorders. Eur J Obstet Gynecol Reprod Biol 2017;215:264–6.
45. Acar H, Acar K. Posterior reversible encephalopathy syndrome in a pregnant patient without eclampsia or preeclampsia. Am J Emerg Med 2018;36(9): 1721.e3-4.
46. McKinney AM, Short J, Truwit CL, et al. Posterior reversible encephalopathy syndrome: incidence of atypical regions of involvement and imaging findings. AJR Am J Roentgenol 2007;189(4):904–12.
47. Singhal AB. Postpartum angiopathy with reversible posterior leukoencephalopathy. Arch Neurol 2004;61(3):411–6.
48. Fugate JE, Wijdicks EF, Parisi JE, et al. Fulminant postpartum cerebral vasoconstriction syndrome. Arch Neurol 2012;69(1):111–7.
49. Garg RK, Malhotra HS, Patil TB, et al. Cerebral-autoregulatory dysfunction syndrome. BMJ Case Rep 2013;2013 [pii:bcr2013201592].
50. Miller TR, Shivashankar R, Mossa-Basha M, et al. Reversible cerebral vasoconstriction syndrome, part 1: epidemiology, pathogenesis, and clinical course. AJNR Am J Neuroradiol 2015;36(8):1392–9.
51. Miller TR, Shivashankar R, Mossa-Basha M, et al. Reversible cerebral vasoconstriction syndrome, part 2: diagnostic work-up, imaging evaluation, and differential diagnosis. AJNR Am J Neuroradiol 2015;36(9):1580–8.
52. Ducros A, Wolff V. The typical thunderclap headache of reversible cerebral vasoconstriction syndrome and its various triggers. Headache 2016;56(4): 657–73.
53. Ducros A. Reversible cerebral vasoconstriction syndrome. Handb Clin Neurol 2014;121:1725–41.
54. Sheikh HU, Mathew PG. Reversible cerebral vasoconstriction syndrome: updates and new perspectives. Curr Pain Headache Rep 2014;18(5):414.
55. Alons IM, van den Wijngaard IR, Verheul RJ, et al. The value of CT angiography in patients with acute severe headache. Acta Neurol Scand 2015;131(3): 164–8.

56. Ito S. Drug therapy for breast-feeding women. N Engl J Med 2000;343(2): 118–26.
57. Webb JA, Thomsen HS, Morcos SK, Members of Contrast Media Safety Committee of European Society of Urogenital Radiology (ESUR). The use of iodinated and gadolinium contrast media during pregnancy and lactation. Eur Radiol 2005;15(6):1234–40.
58. Singhal AB, Hajj-Ali RA, Topcuoglu MA, et al. Reversible cerebral vasoconstriction syndromes: analysis of 139 cases. Arch Neurol 2011;68(8):1005–12.
59. Geocadin RG, Razumovsky AY, Wityk RJ, et al. Intracerebral hemorrhage and postpartum cerebral vasculopathy. J Neurol Sci 2002;205(1):29–34.
60. Ducros A, Fiedler U, Porcher R, et al. Hemorrhagic manifestations of reversible cerebral vasoconstriction syndrome: frequency, features, and risk factors. Stroke 2010;41(11):2505–11.
61. Hacein-Bey L, Varelas PN, Ulmer JL, et al. Imaging of cerebrovascular disease in pregnancy and the puerperium. AJR Am J Roentgenol 2016;206(1): 26–38.
62. Mohr JP, Kejda-Scharler J, Pile-Spellman J. Diagnosis and treatment of arteriovenous malformations. Curr Neurol Neurosci Rep 2013;13(2):324.
63. Kalani MY, Zabramski JM. Risk for symptomatic hemorrhage of cerebral cavernous malformations during pregnancy. J Neurosurg 2013;118(1):50–5.
64. Kim YW, Neal D, Hoh BL. Cerebral aneurysms in pregnancy and delivery: pregnancy and delivery do not increase the risk of aneurysm rupture. Neurosurgery 2013;72(2):143–9 [discussion: 150].
65. Bateman BT, Olbrecht VA, Berman MF, et al. Peripartum subarachnoid hemorrhage: nationwide data and institutional experience. Anesthesiology 2012; 116(2):324–33.
66. Hacein-Bey L, Provenzale JM. Current imaging assessment and treatment of intracranial aneurysms. AJR Am J Roentgenol 2011;196(1):32–44.
67. Blythe R, Ismail A, Naqvi A. Mechanical thrombectomy for acute ischemic stroke in pregnancy. J Stroke Cerebrovasc Dis 2019;28(6):e75–6.
68. Watanabe TT, Ichijo M, Kamata T. Uneventful pregnancy and delivery after thrombolysis plus thrombectomy for acute ischemic stroke: case study and literature review. J Stroke Cerebrovasc Dis 2019;28(1):70–5.
69. Kelly JC, Safain MG, Roguski M, et al. Postpartum internal carotid and vertebral arterial dissections. Obstet Gynecol 2014;123(4):848–56.
70. Verheecke M, Halaska MJ, Lok CA, et al. Primary brain tumours, meningiomas and brain metastases in pregnancy: report on 27 cases and review of literature. Eur J Cancer 2014;50(8):1462–71.
71. Taylan E, Akdemir A, Zeybek B, et al. Recurrent brain tumor with hydrocephalus in pregnancy. J Obstet Gynaecol Res 2015;41(3):464–7.
72. Mandong BM, Emmanuel I, Vandi KB, et al. Secondary brain choriocarcinoma: a case report. Niger J Med 2015;24(1):81–3.
73. Hallsworth D, Thompson J, Wilkinson D, et al. Intracranial pressure monitoring and caesarean section in a patient with von Hippel-Lindau disease and symptomatic cerebellar haemangioblastomas. Int J Obstet Anesth 2015;24(1):73–7.
74. Capone F, Profice P, Pilato F, et al. Spinal hemangioblastoma presenting with low back pain in pregnancy. Spine J 2013;13(12):e27–9.
75. Dolecek TA, Propp JM, Stroup NE, et al. CBTRUS statistical report: primary brain and central nervous system tumors diagnosed in the United States in 2005-2009. Neuro Oncol 2012;14(Suppl 5):v1–49.

76. Kurdoglu Z, Cetin O, Gulsen I, et al. Intracranial meningioma diagnosed during pregnancy caused maternal death. Case Rep Med 2014;2014:158326.
77. Stevenson CB, Thompson RC. The clinical management of intracranial neoplasms in pregnancy. Clin Obstet Gynecol 2005;48(1):24–37.
78. Lusis EA, Scheithauer BW, Yachnis AT, et al. Meningiomas in pregnancy: a clinicopathologic study of 17 cases. Neurosurgery 2012;71(5):951–61.
79. Zwinkels H, Dörr J, Kloet F, et al. Pregnancy in women with gliomas: a caseseries and review of the literature. J Neurooncol 2013;115(2):293–301.
80. Yust-Katz S, de Groot JF, Liu D, et al. Pregnancy and glial brain tumors. Neuro Oncol 2014;16(9):1289–94.
81. Gilbert AL, Prasad S, Mallery RM. Neuro-ophthalmic disorders in pregnancy. Neurol Clin 2019;37(1):85–102.
82. Woodmansee WW. Pituitary disorders in pregnancy. Neurol Clin 2019;37(1): 63–83.
83. Hayes AR, O'Sullivan AJ, Davies MA. A case of pituitary apoplexy in pregnancy. Endocrinol Diabetes Metab Case Rep 2014;2014:140043.
84. Araujo PB, Vieira Neto L, Gadelha MR. Pituitary tumor management in pregnancy. Endocrinol Metab Clin North Am 2015;44(1):181–97.
85. Kaplun J, Fratila C, Ferenczi A, et al. Sequential pituitary MR imaging in Sheehan syndrome: report of 2 cases. AJNR Am J Neuroradiol 2008;29(5):941–3.
86. Wada Y, Hamamoto Y, Nakamura Y, et al. Lymphocytic panhypophysitis: its clinical features in Japanese cases. Jpn Clin Med 2011;2:15–20.
87. Guo S, Wang C, Zhang J, et al. Diagnosis and management of tumor-like hypophysitis: A retrospective case series. Oncol Lett 2016;11(2):1315–20.
88. Robinson DP, Klein SL. Pregnancy and pregnancy-associated hormones alter immune responses and disease pathogenesis. Horm Behav 2012; 62(3):263–71.
89. Kaplan TB. Management of demyelinating disorders in pregnancy. Neurol Clin 2019;37(1):17–30.
90. Confavreux C, Hutchinson M, Hours MM, et al. Rate of pregnancy-related relapse in multiple sclerosis. Pregnancy in Multiple Sclerosis Group. N Engl J Med 1998;339(5):285–91.
91. Vukusic S, Confavreux C. Multiple sclerosis and pregnancy. Rev Neurol (Paris) 2006;162(3):299–309 [in French].
92. Alroughani R, Alowayesh MS, Ahmed SF, et al. Relapse occurrence in women with multiple sclerosis during pregnancy in the new treatment era. Neurology 2018;90(10):e840–6.
93. MacDonald SC, McElrath TF, Hernández-Díaz S. Pregnancy outcomes in women with multiple sclerosis. Am J Epidemiol 2019;188(1):57–66.
94. Zuluaga MI, Otero-Romero S, Rovira A, et al. Menarche, pregnancies, and breastfeeding do not modify long-term prognosis in multiple sclerosis. Neurology 2019;92(13):e1507–16.
95. Trip SA, Miller DH. Imaging in multiple sclerosis. J Neurol Neurosurg Psychiatry 2005;76(Suppl 3):iii11–8.
96. Mendibe Bilbao M, Boyero Durán S, Bárcena Llona J, et al. Multiple sclerosis: pregnancy and women's health issues. Neurologia 2019;34(4):259–69.
97. Eichinger P, Schön S, Pongratz V, et al. Accuracy of unenhanced MRI in the detection of new brain lesions in multiple sclerosis. Radiology 2019;291(2): 429–35.

98. Khalid F, Healy BC, Dupuy SL, et al. Quantitative MRI analysis of cerebral lesions and atrophy in post-partum patients with multiple sclerosis. J Neurol Sci 2018;392:94–9.
99. Shosha E, Dubey D, Palace J, et al. Area postrema syndrome: frequency, criteria, and severity in AQP4-IgG-positive NMOSD. Neurology 2018;91(17): e1642–51.
100. Macerollo A, Dalfino L, Brienza N, et al. Life-threatening ADEM in an immunocompetent pregnant woman with concomitant asymptomatic Cytomegalovirus infection. J Neurol Sci 2016;364:53–5.
101. Zeb Q, Alegria A. Acute disseminated encephalomyelitis (ADEM) following a H3N3 parainfluenza virus infection in a pregnant asthmatic woman with respiratory failure. BMJ Case Rep 2014;2014.
102. George IC, Youn TS, Marcolini EG, et al. Clinical reasoning: acute onset facial droop in a 36-year-old pregnant woman. Neurology 2017;88(24):e240–4.

Neuroimaging of Diseases Causing Dementia

Joseph C. Masdeu, MD, PhD

KEYWORDS

• Alzheimer disease • Neurodegeneration • Tau • Amyloid β • Neuroimaging • PET

KEY POINTS

- Neuroimaging provides a window on the biological events underlying dementia.
- Amyloid PET is positive in Alzheimer disease (AD) and some cases of diffuse Lewy body disease, but negative in the frontotemporal dementias (FTDs).
- Tau PET using the current tracers shows the greatest signal in AD and a lesser signal in FTD.
- Quantifying volume loss with MRI and measuring metabolism with fluorodeoxyglucose PET helps separate different causes of dementia and follow their progression.
- Some of these techniques, still investigational, are likely to find their clinical niche in the near future.

INTRODUCTION

Neuroimaging comprises a powerful set of instruments to diagnose various disorders that cause dementia, clarify their neurobiology, and monitor their treatment. MRI depicts volume changes, as well as abnormalities in functional and structural connectivity. PET allows the quantification of regional cerebral metabolism, abnormal brain deposition of β-amyloid and tau, as well as brain inflammation. This article not only reviews neuroimaging tools that are currently used in the clinic to diagnose and manage diseases causing dementia but also discusses some neuroimaging procedures that are still investigational, because it is likely that they will soon enter clinical practice.

The landscape of imaging diseases that cause dementia is changing rapidly. Until the 2012 approval by the US Food and Drug Administration (FDA) of florbetapir to

Funding: This work was supported by the Nantz National Alzheimer Center, Houston Methodist Stanley H. Appel Department of Neurology, and by the Houston Methodist Research Institute
Conflicts of Interest: Dr J.C. Masdeu is a consultant for General Electric Healthcare and has received research support from this company, from Eli Lilly (AVID Radiopharmaceuticals), and from Merck.
Nantz National Alzheimer Center, Houston Methodist Neurological Institute and Weill Medical College of Cornell University, 6560 Fannin Street, Scurlock 802, Houston, TX 77030, USA
E-mail address: jcmasdeu@houstonmethodist.org

image brain β-amyloid (abeta) deposition, neuroimaging in patients with slowly progressive cognitive impairment leading to dementia was being used in the clinic mostly to detect tumors, hydrocephalus, or vascular lesions, all apparent on MRI simply by inspecting images, without the need to quantify them. However, neurodegenerative disorders cause subtle changes on MRI, but remarkable changes on PET, using metabolism,[1] amyloid beta (abeta),[2] or tau[3,4] PET markers. Slowly these tools are becoming part of the clinical armamentarium to define the presence of early Alzheimer changes in patients with mild cognitive impairment (MCI) or to differentiate Alzheimer disease (AD) from frontotemporal dementia (FTD).[4,5]

More importantly, these tracers are being used to image the brain abnormalities that antecede the first symptoms because treatment at this stage has the potential to prevent or delay the clinical onset.[6] Neuroimaging has provided essential information on the preclinical evolution of AD, regularly associated with the deposition of abeta in the brain.[7] The new insights led to the promulgation of a set of research guidelines for the diagnosis of the preclinical stages of AD[8] and for the characterization of the biology of disorders leading to dementia based in the amyloid-tau-neurodegeneration profile.[9] Here, neurodegeneration is measured by either atrophy on MRI or decreased metabolism on 18F-fluorodeoxyglucose (FDG)-PET.[9] These guidelines will probably soon permeate the thinking of clinicians and eventually become commonplace in the clinic.

Furthermore, imaging can be used to define whether experimental therapies designed to remove amyloid from the brain do reach their target and reduce brain amyloid levels.[10] Because amyloid and tau imaging are revolutionizing the management of and therapy for AD, imaging of other proteins associated with neurodegeneration is being developed. PET tracers for alpha-synuclein, key in Parkinson disease, have been the object of preliminary reports.[11] Along similar lines, active work is pursuing the development of tracers for TAR DNA-binding protein 43 (TDP-43) aggregates, characteristic of several types of FTD.[12]

VASCULAR COGNITIVE IMPAIRMENT

Cognitive impairment to the point of dementia can result from multiple bihemispheric strokes (multi-infarct dementia). Bilateral ischemic lesions in Papez circuit may present as isolated memory loss (**Fig. 1**), but the sudden onset differentiates them from AD. Successive ischemic lesions in the hemispheres may mimic one of the frontotemporal dementias, particularly primary progressive aphasia (PPA). Although ischemic lesions do not spare the primary cortices (paracentral, auditory), neurodegenerative disorders manifesting as dementia typically do (**Fig. 2**). However, autopsy studies in a general population have shown that dementia is seldom associated with large ischemic lesions: it is much more often associated with small infarcts or even microinfarcts, related to small artery disease[13] and with white matter changes on MRI (**Fig. 3**). White matter damage is more likely when the lesions are visible on T1-weighted images; enlarged perivascular spaces can give rise to marked changes on T2 images, including fluid-attenuated inversion recovery (FLAIR),[14] but have little clinical significance. Several arteriolar disorders are characterized by dementia, such as CADASIL (cerebral autosomal dominant arteriopathy with subcortical infarcts and leukoencephalopathy)[15] and cerebral amyloid angiopathy[16–18] (**Fig. 4**).

The role of vascular versus neurodegenerative factors in the genesis of cognitive impairment in older people is currently a matter of some controversy.[19] Vascular lesions are frequent in the brain of patients with neurodegenerative diseases,

CT   T2 FLAIR   MRA

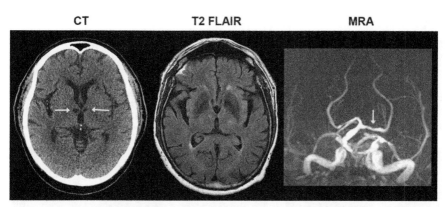

Fig. 1. Critical-location-infarct dementia. This 74-year-old man had sustained a silent infarction of the right dorsomedial-anterior nuclei of the thalamus, affecting the mammillothalamic tract of Vic-D'Azyr. He became symptomatic, with loss of episodic memory for recent events and impaired executive function, after the second infarction, almost symmetric to the first, on the left side. The chronic infarctions (*arrows*) are more apparent on computed tomography (CT) than on fluid-attenuated inversion recovery (FLAIR) imaging. Note the arteriosclerotic changes in the proximal segment of the posterior cerebral artery on magnetic resonance angiography (MRA) (*arrow*). (*From* Masdeu, J.C. and Pascual, B. Genetic and degenerative disorders primarily causing dementia. *Handb Clin Neurol* 2016;135:525-64; with permission.)

particularly in the older age groups.[20,21] These neuropathologic studies have highlighted the difficulty in attributing the cognitive impairment characteristic of dementia to either AD changes or vascular injury. Even more challenging is making a clinical differential diagnosis between vascular dementia and AD.[22,23] The presence of white matter changes or lacunar strokes on MRI or computed tomography (CT), required by the National Institute of Neurological Disorders and Stroke (NINDS)- Association Internationale pour la Recherche et l'Enseignement en Neurosciences (AIREN) diagnostic criteria for vascular dementia,[24] is of limited value, because patients with extensive changes on MRI may not be demented.[25] Some investigators have speculated that progressive vascular dementia, as associated with small-vessel disease, is simply vascular brain disease plus AD.[26] By contrast, AD has been postulated to be a vascular disorder.[27] Because both disorders increase in prevalence in patients aged 70 to 90 years, it is difficult to separate their effects in studies showing an association between cognitive impairment and vascular disease on MRI.[28] By contrast, using MRI as a marker of vascular disease and PET imaging of AD, the contribution of these two disorders can be elucidated. Patients with dementia and a large vascular load on MRI may not show the characteristic metabolic pattern of AD, but show frontal and thalamic hypometabolism on ^{18}F-FDG-PET[29] (**Fig. 5**) Likewise, vascular MRI features and amyloid deposition, the latter characteristic of AD, seem to be independent predictors of cognitive impairment[30] and of the risk of developing cognitive decline.[31] Vascular and neurodegenerative disorders are probably additive for the causation of dementia.[19,31]

ALZHEIMER DISEASE

A long time, estimated in decades, witnesses the evolution of neurobiological events leading to, but preceding, the cognitive impairment characteristic of AD.[32,33] In

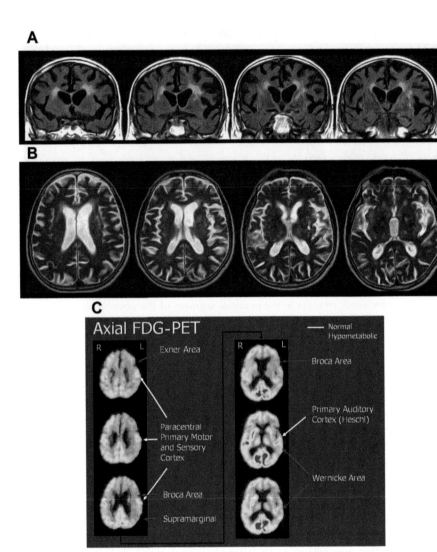

Fig. 2. Primary progressive aphasia, nonfluent type. An 80-year-old man with progressive impairment of language fluency for about 2 years before these images were obtained. Coronal FLAIR (*A*) and axial T2-weighted (*B*) MRI images showing mild to moderate leukoaraiosis of the frontal periventricular white matter and lacunar infarctions in the left putamen, globus pallidus, pulvinar, and internal and extreme capsules. Axial FDG-PET (*C*) showing hypometabolism in the perisylvian association cortex of the frontal, parietal, and temporal lobes of the left hemisphere. The primary auditory and motor-sensory cortices are spared. (*From* Masdeu, J.C. and Pascual, B. Genetic and degenerative disorders primarily causing dementia. *Handb Clin Neurol* 2016;135:525-64; with permission.)

autosomal dominant AD, in which the timing of the onset of dementia can be predicted with some accuracy, increased abeta deposition in the brain has been reported about 7 years before expected onset, decreased metabolism at the time of expected onset and decreased hippocampal volume and verbal memory about 7 years after expected onset, followed by decreased general cognition about 10 years after expected onset[34]

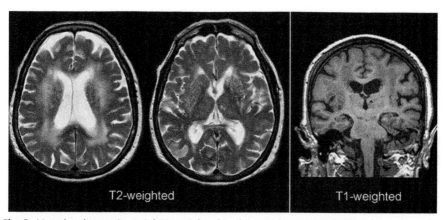

T2-weighted   **T1-weighted**

Fig. 3. Vascular dementia. Axial T2-weighted and coronal T1-weighted images from an 80-year-old woman with impairment of cognition and gait. Note the thalamic infarctions and the large areas of altered signal (increased on T2 and decreased on T1) in the centrum semiovale. (*From* Masdeu, J.C. and Pascual, B. Genetic and degenerative disorders primarily causing dementia. *Handb Clin Neurol* 2016;135:525-64; with permission.)

(**Fig. 6**). A similar sequence seems to be present with abeta deposition in sporadic, late-onset AD, although the causal mix in this more advanced age group yields more complex biomarker results.[33,35,36] Research AD diagnostic guidelines issued in 2011 distinguish a preclinical stage, characterized by abeta brain deposition and defined by the use of cerebrospinal fluid (CSF) or neuroimaging biomarkers.[8,33,37–39] Other imaging changes that could be identified at this stage, but become more prominent as the neurodegenerative process evolves, include tau deposition[4] and synaptic dysfunction, detected by impaired metabolism on ^{18}F-FDG-PET[40] and, less reliably at present, by perfusion single-photon emission computed tomography (SPECT), MRI blood oxygen level dependent (BOLD), or arterial spin labeling (ASL),[41,42] as well as medial temporal volume reduction on MRI.[34,43] Multimodal imaging, including PET and MRI biomarkers (**Table 1**),[44] is increasingly used to define the brain changes in

T2 FLAIR   Gradient Echo   T1

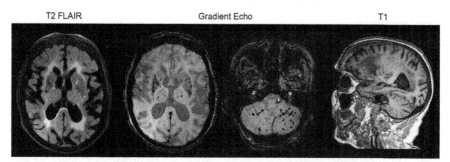

Fig. 4. Cerebral amyloid angiopathy (CAA). MRI from a 72-year-old woman with dementia and CAA. The white matter contains many abnormal areas, which appear hyperintense on the transverse FLAIR image and hypointense on the sagittal T1-weighted image. Multiple lacunar infarcts are present in the lenticular nuclei and few in the thalami. Microbleeds, best seen on the gradient-echo images, dot the lenticular nuclei, thalami, and the cerebellum. Scattered microbleeds can also be seen in the cortex or subcortical white matter. (*From* Masdeu, J.C. and Pascual, B. Genetic and degenerative disorders primarily causing dementia. *Handb Clin Neurol* 2016;135:525-64; with permission.)

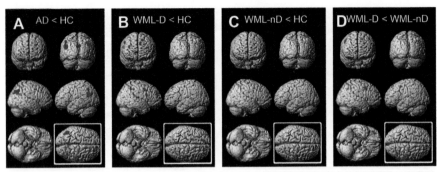

Fig. 5. Metabolism in AD and vascular dementia. (*A–D*) Shown in red are the regions of the brain with reduced metabolism in the first, compared with the second, of 2 comparison groups. (*A–C*) Each of the patient groups, AD, vascular disease, and dementia (white matter lesions–dementia [WML-D]), and vascular disease but without dementia (white matter lesions–no dementia [WML-nD]), is compared with a healthy control group (HC). (*D*) WML-D is compared with WML-nD. The height thresholds for the comparisons are as follows: (*A*) T = 4.07 (voxel-level significance, *P*<.01 false-discovery rate corrected); (*B* and *C*) T = 3.29 (voxel level *P*<.001); and (*D*) T = 2.12 (voxel level, *P*<.02). In AD (*A*), note the classic pattern of bilaterally decreased metabolism in the parietotemporal association cortex and precuneus. The pattern in vascular disease with dementia resembles more the pattern in vascular disease without dementia than the pattern in AD. In vascular disease, patients with dementia have a reduction primarily in frontal metabolism, compared with those who are not demented (*D*). Group patterns are most obvious on the superior aspect of the brain, highlighted with a frame in each panel. (*From* Pascual, B., Prieto, E., Arbizu, J. et al. Brain glucose metabolism in vascular white matter disease with dementia: differentiation from Alzheimer disease. *Stroke* 2010;41:2889-93; with permission.)

individual patients, independently of diagnosis.[9] This approach may facilitate the targeting of new therapies to specific neurobiological events, particularly at the preclinical or early clinical stages, which may be most amenable to treatment.[35]

The discovery of AD risk genes coding for proteins involved in inflammation[45–47] has rekindled the interest in neuroinflammation as a possible pathogenetic factor in AD. Inflammation is also amenable to imaging.

Abeta Deposition

Brain abeta was initially imaged with Pittsburgh compound B (^{11}C-PIB) (**Fig. 7**).[2] PIB is available bound to ^{11}C, a positron-emitting isotope with a half-life of 20.4 minutes, requiring an on-site cyclotron. However, since 2012 there are abeta-imaging compounds bound to ^{18}F, with a half-life of 109.8 min. The longer half-life allows the radiotracer to be synthesized at a facility with a cyclotron and then shipped to institutions with PET cameras, which are more widely available. Good concordance with histologically measured abeta load has been shown not only for PIB[48,49] but also for 3 ^{18}F abeta PET tracers, ^{18}F-florbetapir,[50] ^{18}F-flutemetamol,[51] and ^{18}F-florbetaben,[52] which are approved by the FDA for use in the clinical setting. In early AD, amyloid deposition is highest in frontoparietotemporal association cortex, including the precuneus, sparing the paracentral regions and primary sensory cortex. The striatum is often affected as well.

Similarly to the presence of another biomarker of AD, decreased CSF abeta 42 level,[53] abeta brain deposition begins in the preclinical stages of AD, increases during the MCI stage and, by the time of the AD diagnosis, remains relatively stable as the disease progresses.[54,55] Thus, abeta deposition is a marker of the preclinical stages

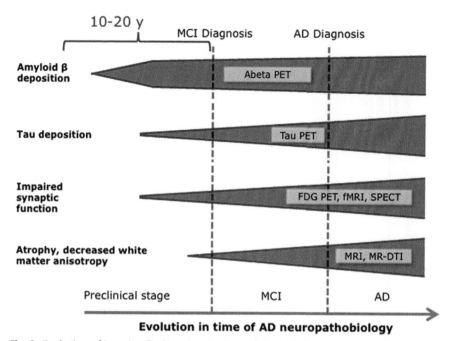

Evolution in time of AD neuropathobiology

Fig. 6. Evolution of imaging findings in AD. Neurobiological changes in the various stages in the development of AD, shown by specific neuroimaging techniques. A wider area in red indicates a greater degree of the neurobiological disorder (abeta or tau deposition, impaired synaptic function or atrophy, and decreased white matter anisotropy). Note that the sequence of tau deposition is only an estimate, because studies are still sparse. Amyloid PET, ^{11}C-Pittsburgh compound B PET; fMRI, functional MRI; MR-DTI, diffusion tensor imaging performed with fMRI; SPECT, single-photon emission CT. (*From* Masdeu, J.C. and Pascual, B. Genetic and degenerative disorders primarily causing dementia. *Handb Clin Neurol* 2016;135:525-64; with permission.)

of the disease and correlates with the degree of cognitive impairment only in the pre-clinical stages and MCI, not during AD,[55,56] although atrophy and synaptic dysfunction continue to increase and spread as clinical AD worsens and cognition deteriorates.[54]

In asymptomatic individuals of a similar age, abeta deposition has been found more often among *APOE4* carriers,[57] but this genotype may not have an effect on the risk of cognitive worsening once its effect on amyloid deposition is accounted for.[35,58] Lifetime cognitive engagement has been found to protect from preclinical abeta deposition[59] but this effect, like the protective effect of physical exercise, may be restricted to *APOE4* carriers.[60] Impaired sleep has been associated with an increased amyloid burden.[61]

Abeta deposition is the strongest and earliest neuroimaging predictor of future cognitive impairment in healthy elderly and of worsening from MCI to AD, increasing the risk between 3-fold and 7-fold.[35,36,62] The effect of abeta deposition on cognitive impairment in early stages of the AD continuum may be modulated by some common genetic variants. For instance, healthy *APOE4* carriers not only have greater abeta deposition but have worse memory and visuospatial skills for the same amount of 11C-PIB binding.[63] This finding may reflect a longer period of time with abeta deposition in the APOE4 carriers. Healthy, abeta-positive carriers of the Met genotype of the brain-derived neurotrophic factor (BDNF) *Val66Met* allele have a greater worsening on

Table 1
Clinical, imaging, and genetic findings associated with the neurodegenerative dementias

Dementia Type	Clinical Findings	Atrophy (MRI)	Decreased Metabolism (PET) Or Perfusion (SPECT, ASL)	β-Amyloid (PET)	Tau (PET)	Predisposing Gene Variants or Mutations
AD	Memory loss, language or visuospatial function impairment	Medial temporal, precuneus, lateral temporoparietal association cortex	Precuneus, lateral parietotemporal association cortex	+++	+++	APOE4, TREM2, TOMM40, APP, PS1/2
lvPPA	Impaired repetition of sentences and phrases, phonologic errors in speech	Left posterior perisylvian or parietal association cortex	Left posterior perisylvian or parietal association cortex	+>>−	+++	APOE, TREM2, TOMM40, APP, PS1/2, MAPT
nfvPPA	Nonfluent speech, agrammatism	Left posterior frontoinsular association cortex	Left posterior frontoinsular association cortex	−	+>−	MAPT, GRN
svPPA	Anomic aphasia, loss of comprehension, surface dyslexia	Left or right anterior temporal lobe	Left or right anterior temporal lobe	−>+	−>+	GRN, MAPT, C9orf72
bvFTD	Behavioral and personality changes, executive dysfunction	Symmetric to moderately right-predominant frontal or anterior temporal regions	Anterior frontal cortex and temporal association cortex	−	+ ≈ −	MAPT, GRN, C9orf72, FUS, CHMP2B
CBD	Apraxia, rigidity	Superior parietal lobule	Superior parietal lobule, premotor cortex, putamen	−	+	MAPT, GRN
PSP	Supranuclear palsy, executive function loss, parkinsonism	Midbrain	Frontal association cortex	−	+	MAPT
DLB	Memory loss, visual hallucinations, parkinsonism	Similar to AD, but less medial temporal atrophy	Posterior parieto-occipital association cortex, putamen	+	+	APOE4, GBA

Abbreviations: bvFTD, behavioral variant of FTD; CBD, corticobasal degeneration; DLB, diffuse Lewy-body; lvPPA, logopenic variant primary progressive aphasia; nfvPPA, nonfluent variant primary progressive aphasia; PSP, progressive supranuclear palsy; svPPA, semantic variant primary progressive aphasia.

¹¹C-PIB in AD

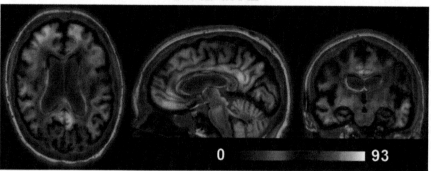

0 ▬▬▬▬▬ 93

Fig. 7. ¹¹C-PIB–positive scan in AD. In yellow, areas of the brain with abeta deposition, shown on the MRI of this 65-year-old woman. Note the distribution of amyloid binding, predominantly in the frontal and temporal lobes, as well as precuneus. There is slight binding to white matter, but not as pronounced as in the ¹⁸F-florbetapir scan (see **Fig. 8**). (*From* Masdeu, J.C. and Pascual, B. Genetic and degenerative disorders primarily causing dementia. *Handb Clin Neurol* 2016;135:525-64; with permission.)

follow-up in episodic memory, language, and executive function than the Val homozygotes despite similar abeta PET binding in both groups.[64]

Abeta imaging is also a powerful tool to separate the dementias characterized by abeta deposition, such as AD and diffuse Lewy body dementia (DLB), from the FTDs, which course without abeta deposition. Separating patient samples of AD and FTD validated clinically, areas under the receiver operating characteristic (ROC) curve for ¹¹C-PIB (0.888) and ¹⁸F-FDG (0.910) were similar.[65] ¹¹C-PIB slightly outperformed ¹⁸F-FDG in patients with known histopathology findings.[65] A confounder is the presence of abeta deposition in some older people with FTD.[66]

Patients with an AD clinical presentation may have a negative abeta PET scan. In a clinical trial of early AD, 14% had negative abeta scans among 214 with AD symptoms.[67] This proportion parallels the 14% abeta-negative results in a population sample of 154 amnesic patients with MCI and 16% of 58 patients with MCI from Alzheimer Disease Neuroimaging Initiative (ADNI)[68] and may increase to 30% when the patients studied are older than 82 years.[69] It may reflect the smaller subset of patients with dementia who do not have increased abeta or tau levels at autopsy.[70] These imaging findings could reflect the mixed pathology results in the oldest old.[71] However, even with a careful neuropathologic exclusion of other causes, clinical and neuropathologic findings are occasionally dissociated: individuals with marked abeta and neurofibrillary disorder may be cognitively intact.[70] In these individuals there is less abeta deposition in the form of fibrillar plaques and intimately related oligomeric abeta assemblies, less hyperphosphorylated soluble tau species localized in synapses, and less glial activation.[72]

Longitudinal abeta imaging allows the evaluation of the natural history of abeta deposition among at-risk genotypes,[57] and it has the potential to be a marker of effectiveness in studies performed during the preclinical stage of AD, because it has helped elucidate brain changes during AD therapy.[10,73]

Tau Deposition

In the healthy brain, the protein tau stabilizes neurotubules and is therefore essential for normal neural function (Villemagne and colleagues, 2015).[74] However, in AD and other neurodegenerative disorders, tau becomes abnormally hyperphosphorylated, dysfunctional, and misfolded, constituting the tangles observed neuropathologically in AD and other tauopathies. Recently, PET tracers have been synthesized that bind strongly to the abnormally folded tau, using the folding properties of this protein for binding. These tracers do not bind to the healthy, native form of tau, but, as has become common usage, this article refers to hyperphosphorylated tau simply as tau. The most experience exists with flortaucipir (^{18}F-AV-1451), which shows highly specific uptake in areas known neuropathologically to contain a large amount of tau in AD[3,4,75] (**Fig. 8**). It has little white matter binding but, in older individuals, even those cognitively intact, there is uptake in the lenticular nucleus; choroid plexus or its vicinity; and the region of the substantia nigra, red nucleus, and subthalamic nucleus. The reason for this uptake pattern is still unclear, but it does not seem to be related to tau deposition, except for the choroid plexus.[76] The binding to substantia nigra could be explained, at least in part, by binding of flortaucipir to melanin.[77,78] However, this would not explain the greater binding in older people, with likely less melanin in the nigra, unless they had a larger amount of extraneuronal melanin more available to the tracer, but decreased flortaucipir midbrain binding has been reported in Parkinson disease.[78]

Flortaucipir binds to tau in AD,[79] which is associated with 3-repeat (3R) and 4-repeat (4R) tau aggregates, but less with 3R or 4R tau found in most varieties of tau-related FTD, such as the behavioral variant or progressive supranuclear palsy (PSP),[77,80] although the binding pattern correlates well with the clinical syndrome.[81] The configuration of tau aggregates, which differs in various taoupathies,[82] most likely determines binding and it is only beginning to be understood. For instance, flortaucipir binds to patients harboring a p.R406W mutation in the *MAPT* gene, encoding tau.[83] This mutation results in 3R and 4R tau aggregates similar to those in AD.[83] It also binds to some extent to TDP-43 in semantic dementia,[80,84,85] probably because the abundant protein aggregates in this disease have a configuration that allows flortaucipir binding.

Tau accumulation measured with flortaucipir correlates better with the degree of cognitive impairment than amyloid accumulation,[86] a finding in agreement with prior neuropathologic studies.[87] Furthermore, there is an inverse correlation between tau accumulation and brain metabolism: regions high in tau have uniformly depressed metabolism[75] (see **Fig. 8**). This correlation is not as tight with amyloid accumulation (see **Fig. 8**). A newer tau PET tracer, ^{18}F-MK-6240, has less nonspecific binding than flortaucipir.[88]

Impaired Synaptic Function

Impaired synaptic function across the various AD stages can be gauged with techniques measuring the regional metabolism, regional perfusion, and the functional MRI (fMRI) BOLD signal. Findings are concordant, but each technique is amenable to different applications. Metabolism has been studied most extensively and has proved more helpful that the more recent use of resting state BOLD fMRI to assess functional connectivity changes and of ASL to measure regional perfusion using noninvasive MRI.

Metabolism

Regional cerebral metabolism studies with PET have used ^{18}F-FDG as a metabolic marker.[89,90] The most typical pattern found in early AD is decreased metabolism bilaterally in the parietotemporal association cortex and posterior cingulate gyrus.[91] Metabolism reflects synaptic activity and therefore is most affected early in the regions to which medial temporal neurons project,[92] and may reflect impaired connectivity even

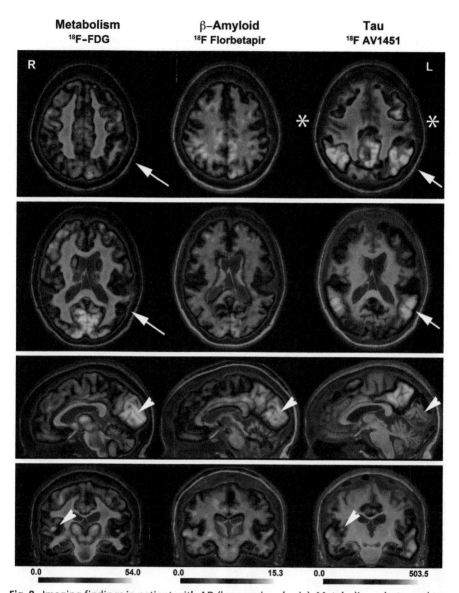

Fig. 8. Imaging findings in patient with AD (logopenic aphasia). Metabolism, abeta, and tau imaging from a 57-year-old woman with the logopenic-aphasia variety of AD. The primary sensory-motor areas (*asterisks*), as well as the primary visual (striatal cortex) and auditory (Heschl gyrus) regions (*arrowheads*) have normal metabolism and no tau deposition. By contrast, areas with high tau deposition (eg, inferior parietal lobule, *arrows*) tend to have decreased metabolism. In some areas, high amyloid deposition corresponds to low metabolism and increased tau (eg, the precuneus). However, there are areas with high amyloid load and normal metabolism, such as the medial occipital region. Uptake in the region of the substantia nigra does not correspond with tau deposition. (*From* Masdeu, J.C. and Pascual, B. Genetic and degenerative disorders primarily causing dementia. *Handb Clin Neurol* 2016;135:525-64; with permission.)

in presymptomatic individuals.[93] Large recent studies have failed to document an AD metabolic pattern in *APOE4* carriers.[1] Depending on the approach and the sample studied, the accuracy for predicting the evolution of MCI to AD varies from 0.774 to 0.983.[94]

Perfusion

In the absence of associated vascular disease,[95] perfusion is typically coupled to metabolism in neurodegenerative disorders. In current clinical practice, brain perfusion is most often studied with SPECT, using Tc-99m HMPAO (hexamethyl propylamine oxime, Ceretec), a lipid-soluble macrocyclic amine, or Tc-99m ECD (ethyl cysteinate dimer, Neurolite). However, a head-to-head comparison of perfusion SPECT with metabolism PET has shown a much better sensitivity and specificity of PET compared with SPECT in AD and diffuse Lewy body disease.[89] ASL could facilitate perfusion data at the same time that other MRI parameters are obtained but it requires further validation.[42,96]

Atrophy

Volume loss or atrophy, typically involving first the medial temporal regions, was the first reliable neuroimaging finding detected in AD (**Fig. 9**)[97] and, for a while, was thought to be the most robust, to the point of assigning the name of neurodegenerative pattern to the pattern of atrophy most often observed in AD.[98] The story may not be as simple. Although it is controverted but possible that atrophy may predate the onset of clinical findings in familial autosomal dominant AD,[34,99–101] healthy older people with the so-called neurodegeneration pattern are not at increased risk of developing cognitive impairment.[36] However, in patients with mild cognitive impairment, the presence of this pattern of atrophy predicts faster deterioration.[102]

Although atrophy can be appreciated visually (see **Fig. 9**),[103] automated methods are more precise and facilitate longitudinal follow-up. The accuracy of software that classifies clinically appropriate cases has been compared favorably with the accuracy of trained readers.[104] MRI end points compared across healthy individuals and those in various stages of the AD continuum have included hippocampal volume,

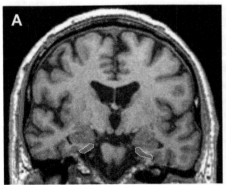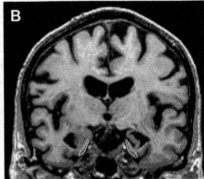

Fig. 9. Temporal atrophy in AD. Coronal MRI at the level of the mammillary bodies. The entorhinal cortex has been outlined in a normal control (*A*) and a person with mild cognitive impairment of the amnesic type (*B*). Note the dilatation of the temporal horns of the person with mild cognitive impairment corresponding with hippocampal atrophy. (*From* Masdeu, J.C. and Pascual, B. Genetic and degenerative disorders primarily causing dementia. *Handb Clin Neurol* 2016;135:525-64; with permission.)

tensor-based morphometry, and cortical thickness.[105,106] The best results are usually achieved by combining all features,[105] although temporal atrophy was associated with the shortest median dementia-free period.[107]

By correlating postmortem findings with the pattern of atrophy on MRI, 3 distinct atrophy patterns have been found in patients with typical AD neuropathology, including abeta deposition: typical AD (about 70% of cases), limbic-predominant AD (20%), and hippocampal-sparing AD (10%).[108] Particularly in patients with the early onset of the disease, posterior cortical atrophy, with prominent visual impairment, is common (**Fig. 10**).

White Matter Anisotropy Loss

White matter abnormalities in the fornix[109] or in fronto-occipital and inferior temporal fasciculi, the splenium of the corpus callosum, subcallosal white matter, and the cingulum bundle[110] were found with the use of diffusion tensor imaging (DTI) in healthy individuals at risk for AD, either with autosomal dominant mutations[109,111] or carrying the *APOE* ε4 allele.[110] In affected areas, DTI showed decreased functional anisotropy[109] or increased mean diffusivity.[111] However, the findings are not robust enough to provide reliable information on the risk in the general population.[112] In AD, higher anisotropy can be found in white matter volumes where a disrupted tract, such as the superior longitudinal fasciculus, crosses an intact one, such as the corticospinal tract, effectively increasing volume anisotropy.[113] The complexity of the changes has been addressed by means of support vector machine classifiers and multiresolution statistical analysis.[112,114] For DTI, discrimination values higher than 90% have been achieved comparing MCI with healthy controls using support vector machine classifiers.[114,115] However, these optimistic outcomes need to be validated in additional independent samples.

Inflammation

Inflammatory changes are prominent in AD: it is debated whether they are pathogenic, or simply reflect scavenging of neurons and neuronal processes, or even have a neuroprotective effect.[116–118] Animal models of tau-induced neuronal loss have shown earlier and more severe inflammation than models of increased abeta.[119] However, data in humans are essential to understand the role of inflammation in neurodegeneration. PET imaging allows in vivo quantification of neuroinflammation by measuring the density of the 18-kDa translocator protein (TSPO), which is expressed in activated, but not resting, microglia and, to a lesser extent, in astrocytes. TSPO in AD has been largely imaged with ^{11}C-PK11195, not an ideal compound because of its low affinity for the receptor[120] and a low ratio of specific to nonspecific binding.[121] However, even ^{11}C-PK11195 has shown moderately increased binding in AD[122,123] and in some patients with MCI.[120] A correlation with cognitive performance was documented in 1 study.[124] The limitations of ^{11}C-PK11195 have prompted the development of second-generation radioligands, such as ^{11}C-PBR28, which has greater signal/noise ratio than ^{11}C-PK11195 in monkey brain.[121] However, the affinity of this and other TSPO-binding compounds is strongly determined by the rs6971 polymorphism on the *TSPO* gene, leading to high-affinity and low-affinity groups, as well as an intermediate phenotype. The low-affinity group cannot be imaged with this tracer but it can be imaged with a newer TSPO tracer, ^{11}C-ER176, which also has better imaging characteristics than ^{11}C-PBR28.[125] Using a technique to determine binding in the intermediate phenotype, Kreisl and colleagues[126] have used ^{11}C-PBR28 to

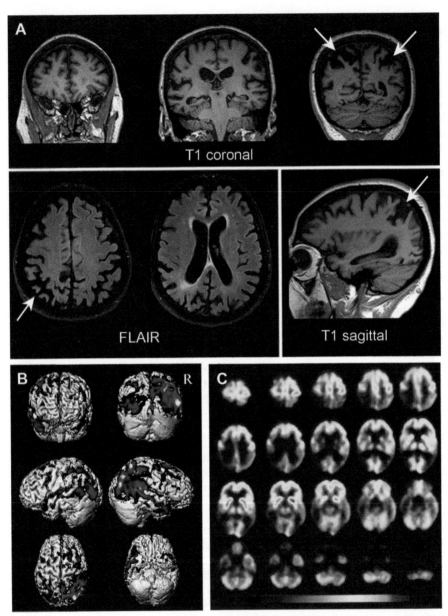

Fig. 10. Posterior cortical atrophy in AD. (A) Conventional MRI, (B) volumetric MRI on a rendered image, and (C) PET studies from a 61-year-old woman with a 3-year history of progressive reading difficulties, agraphia, and dressing apraxia. On examination she had a Balint syndrome with simultanagnosia, apraxia of eye movements, optic ataxia, and tunnel vision. Note in (A) the marked atrophy in the lateral parietal lobe, with dilatation of the intraparietal sulcus (*arrows*). There is also hippocampal atrophy, albeit less prominent. (B) Voxels with significant atrophy (compared with statistical parametric mapping to 48 controls, P<.05 uncorrected; k>20) are shown in red. Note that in (B) the right side of the brain is shown on the right side of the image, opposite to the radiologic convention on conventional MRI (A) and PET (C). Areas of decreased metabolism on PET (C) most closely match the clinical picture. (*From* Masdeu, J.C. and Pascual, B. Genetic and degenerative disorders primarily causing dementia. *Handb Clin Neurol* 2016;135:525-64; with permission.)

show increased binding in regions typically affected in AD, particularly inferior-medial temporal regions, the inferior parietal lobule, and precuneus, but only a trend for hippocampus and precuneus in MCI. There was a correlation with atrophy on MRI but not with abeta deposition. Furthermore, binding correlated with several relevant cognitive measures.[126] This study was performed using an arterial input function, but good results in AD have been obtained using a cerebellar reference region.[127] Increased astrocytosis has been detected in AD with ^{11}C-DED PET.[128]

Neuronal Loss

Atrophy on MRI correlates well with the degree of regional neuronal loss.[129] Another approach to measure neuronal loss is to quantify the regional density of neuronal receptors such as the gamma-aminobutyric acid A (GABA-A) receptor, which is abundant in neurons and widespread in the brain. Binding to GABA-A receptors by ^{11}C-flumazenil, a PET tracer, has been reported to be reduced in early AD.[130] The anatomy of reduction paralleled the distribution of neuronal loss in early AD described in neuropathologic studies (**Fig. 11**).[129]

DIFFUSE LEWY BODY DEMENTIA

Considered as the second most common neurodegenerative dementia,[131] DLB is clinically characterized by progressive, but fluctuating, cognitive impairment accompanied by visual hallucinations, parkinsonism, and in many cases rapid eye movement sleep disorder.[132] DLB is associated with Lewy body disorder not restricted to the substantia nigra and nucleus locus coeruleus, as in classic Parkinson disease, but widespread throughout the cortex. In addition to Lewy bodies, the neuropathology of DLB includes diffuse amyloid plaques,[133] rather than the rounded, circumscribed plaques of AD.[134] Both types of plaques bind ^{11}C-PIB.[133] In about half of the cases, Alzheimer-type disorder is present in the same patient, complicating the nosology

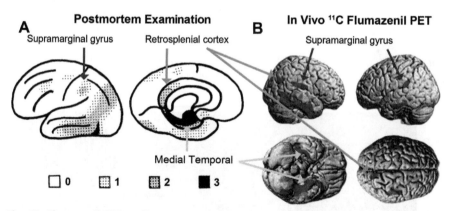

Fig. 11. Flumazenil PET to detect neuronal loss in AD. Areas showing neuronal loss in AD had a similar distribution in the flumazenil PET study[162] and in the classic histologic study of early AD by Brun and Englund[129] (1981). In a whole-brain histologic survey of neuronal loss (*A*), from 0 (no neuronal loss) to 3 (most neuronal loss), the regions most affected were the temporal lobes, particularly in their medial aspect, the retrosplenial cortex, and the supramarginal-angular gyri, which were the regions involved on flumazenil PET (*B*). (*From* Pascual, B., Prieto, E., Arbizu, J. et al. Decreased carbon-11-flumazenil binding in early Alzheimer's disease. *Brain* 2012;135:2817-25; with permission.)

of clinical DLB.[135] Many of the imaging features of AD are also present in DLB; namely, atrophy, decreased metabolism, and abeta deposition.[136] However, unlike in AD, in pure DLB there is little medial temporal atrophy.[135] Furthermore, compared with AD, DLB is associated with decreased occipital metabolism on ^{18}F-FDG-PET (**Fig. 12**) and with less total abeta deposition on ^{11}C-PIB PET, although about 80% of patients have abnormal ^{11}C-PIB PET.[133] In 1 study,[133] the combination of volumetry, metabolism, and abeta imaging effectively distinguished DLB from AD (area under the ROC = 0.98).

On studies of metabolism (^{18}F-FDG-PET) or perfusion (H_2[15]O-PET, SPECT, ASL), the posterior cingulate island sign is helpful to distinguish DLB from AD. Although the posterior cingulate gyrus, by the splenium of the corpus callosum, is uniformly hypometabolic or hypoperfused in AD, it is less so in DLB[131,137] (**Fig. 13**). Dopaminergic markers, such as ^{18}F-fluorodopa (FDOPA) PET or 2beta-carbomethoxy-3beta-(4-iodophenyl)tropane (^{123}I-beta-CIT) SPECT, are likely to show decreased striatal uptake in DLB disease (see **Fig. 13**), but not in AD.[138] Characteristically, the decrease is greatest at the tail of the putamen and less pronounced in anterior putamen and caudate[137] (**Fig. 14**).

Frontotemporal Dementia

FTD or frontotemporal lobar degeneration is a group of diseases accounting for about 10% to 20% of all dementias worldwide. It affects a younger age group than AD: FTD occurs in about 3 to 15 per 100,000 individuals aged between 55 years and 65 years.[139] Atrophy and white matter abnormalities on MRI, decreased metabolism on FDG-PET, and decreased perfusion on SPECT or ASL tend to be regional and correspond well to the area preferentially affected by the disorder (see **Table 1**).[140–144] Except for rare cases with motor neuron involvement, FTD, like AD, tends to affect association cortex, rather than primary motor or sensory cortices (see **Figs. 5** and **18**). Unlike AD, which tends to affect posterior brain regions, FDT tends to affect the anterior portion of the brain.[90] Hippocampal volume alone differentiates AD from FTD poorly; hippocampal sclerosis associated with FTD could explain the overlap.[145] Frontotemporal abnormalities on FDG-PET/SPECT may antedate the atrophy that eventually becomes obvious on MRI (**Fig. 15**).[146,147] For this reason, PET has been approved for FTD diagnosis by the US Centers for Medicare & Medicaid Services (CMS). Amyloid imaging is

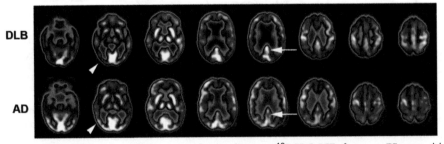

Fig. 12. Metabolism in diffuse Lewy body disease. ^{18}F-FDG-PET from a 75-year-old man with DLB showing decreased metabolism in the lateral aspect of the occipital lobes (*arrowheads*) and greater metabolism than the patient with AD in the posterior cingulate region (*arrows*). (*From* Masdeu, J.C. and Pascual, B. Genetic and degenerative disorders primarily causing dementia. *Handb Clin Neurol* 2016;135:525-64; with permission.)

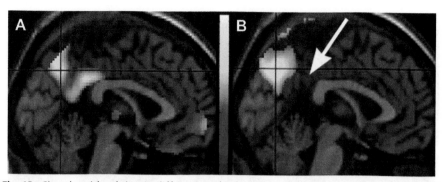

Fig. 13. Cingulate island sign in diffuse Lewy body disease. On MRI templates of the medial aspect of the brain, areas of decreased metabolism (^{18}F-FDG-PET) in AD (*A*) and decreased perfusion ($H_2{}^{15}O$-PET) in DLB (*B*). Metabolism and perfusion are coupled in AD and DLB. Note involvement of the posterior cingulate gyrus in AD, but sparing of this region (*arrow*) in DLB. (*Adapted from* Goker-Alpan, O., Masdeu, J.C., Kohn, P.D. et al. The neurobiology of glucocerebrosidase-associated parkinsonism: a positron emission tomography study of dopamine synthesis and regional cerebral blood flow. *Brain* 2012;135:2440-8; with permission.)

generally negative in the FTDs.[136] Tau imaging using flortaucipir shows considerably lower uptake in FTD than in AD.[80] However, ^{18}F-AV-1451 uptake correlated well with quantitatively measured 4R tau burden, as determined postmortem in the brain of a patient presenting with nonfluent variant PPA (nfvPPA).[148]

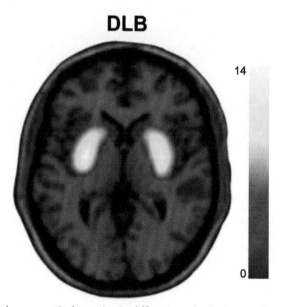

Fig. 14. Decreased presynaptic dopamine in diffuse Lewy body disease. On an axial MRI template, areas of decreased presynaptic dopamine (^{18}F-FDOPA-PET) in a sample of patients with DLB. (*From* Goker-Alpan, O., Masdeu, J.C., Kohn, P.D. et al. The neurobiology of glucocerebrosidase-associated parkinsonism: a positron emission tomography study of dopamine synthesis and regional cerebral blood flow. *Brain* 2012;135:2440-8; with permission.)

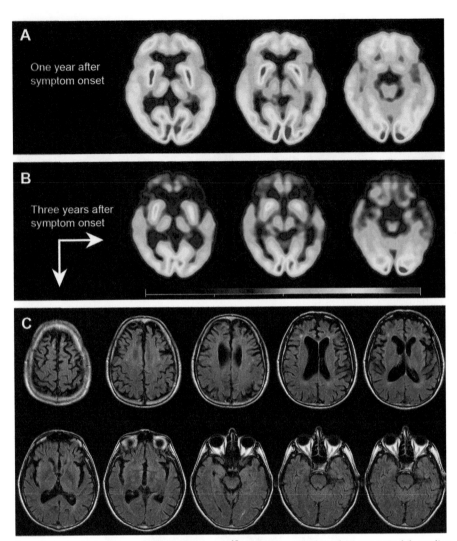

Fig. 15. Behavioral form of FTD. Shown are ^{18}F-FDG-PET (*A, B*) and FLAIR MRI (*C*) studies from a 51-year-old man with progressive speech apraxia and impaired planning, to the point of mutism and complete dependency for activities of daily living when studies (*B*) and (*C*) were obtained, on the same day. Metabolism was already decreased on the initial PET study, particularly on the frontal opercula and temporal tips, but it is much more obvious on the follow-up study, showing extensive frontotemporal hypometabolism. Note that the frontotemporal abnormality is much more obvious on the PET study (*A, B*) than on the MRI study (*C*), which shows frontal atrophy. (*From* Masdeu, J.C. and Pascual, B. Genetic and degenerative disorders primarily causing dementia. *Handb Clin Neurol* 2016;135:525-64; with permission.)

Furthermore, unlike other tau PET tracers, ^{18}F-AV-1451 is not appreciably blocked by monoamine oxidase B (MAO-B) inhibitors,[149] ruling out the possibility that the increased ^{18}F-AV-1451 signal may simply correspond with an increase in MAO-B induced by the pathologic process.[150] In FTD, small but detectable and accurate ^{18}F-AV-1451 binding has been found in most studies[80,148] and its regional distribution corresponds well to the clinical syndromes.[81] The lower ^{18}F-AV-1451 signal in FTD compared with AD could be related to lower ^{18}F-AV-1451 binding to FTD tau but also reflects the lower tau load in FTD, which is about 10% of that in AD.[151]

Clinically, anatomically, neuropathologically, and genetically, FTD comprises a heterogeneous set of disorders[152] (see **Table 1**). The clinical presentation depends on the region of the brain earliest and most affected by the disease.[141–144] It can present with a frontal lobe syndrome, characterized by impulsivity and disinhibition, the so-called behavioral variant of FTD (classic Pick disease, affecting the frontotemporal poles; see **Fig. 15**)[153,154]; with an aphasic syndrome, named PPA (with left hemispheric involvement)[155]; or with progressive prosopagnosia, when the anterior portion of the right temporal lobe is affected.[156] PPA can be either semantic (involving predominantly the left temporal tip; **Fig. 16**) or nfvPPA (involving the left anterior perisylvian area; see **Fig. 2**). There is a third PPA variant, termed logopenic aphasia (involving the left posterior perisylvian area; see **Fig. 8**),[157] which is most often associated with AD, rather than FTD, pathology.[158] FTD can also co-occur with motor neuron disease, and atypical parkinsonian disorders, such as corticobasal degeneration (CBD) and PSP. These 2 disorders are associated with tau disorder, and their clinical and pathologic features overlap: the clinical syndrome of PSP can be associated with CBD pathology and vice versa.[159,160] The clinical syndromes correspond with well-defined neuroimaging. At stages beyond the initial gait impairment, PSP is easy to diagnose clinically by the characteristic parkinsonism associated with markedly impaired postural reflexes and downward-gaze palsy; frank dementia, of a frontal-lobe type, only supervenes as the disease advances. MRI shows minimal frontal atrophy[141] but remarkable midbrain atrophy (hummingbird sign; **Fig. 17**) such that a decreased midbrain/pons area ratio on sagittal images distinguishes this disorder well.[161] Corticobasal degeneration is characterized by progressive apraxia, accompanied by apractic agraphia when the left hemisphere is affected. Typically, both atrophy and decreased metabolism affect the superior parietal lobule (**Fig. 18**). This region is the area of representation of the hand. Thus, CBD causes apraxia, whereas PPA, involving the perisylvian cortex, which subserves the mouth region of the motor strip (see **Fig. 2**), is associated with aphasia.

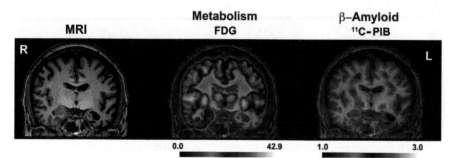

Fig. 16. Semantic dementia. Metabolism (^{18}F-FDG) and abeta (^{11}C-PIB) PET data superimposed on the MRI of a 65-year-old man with marked anomia, but preserved repetition. Note the marked left anterior temporal atrophy. Metabolism is markedly decreased on the left but also, to a lesser degree, on the right temporal tip. (*From* Masdeu, J.C. and Pascual, B. Genetic and degenerative disorders primarily causing dementia. *Handb Clin Neurol* 2016;135:525-64; with permission.)

Control   ## PSP

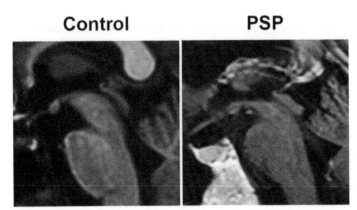

Fig. 17. Midbrain atrophy in PSP. Sagittal T1-weighted MRI from a 79-year-old woman with PSP shows marked atrophy of the midbrain, which has the appearance of a hummingbird (hummingbird sign). Compare with the morphology of the midbrain at the same level in a healthy individual of a similar age. (*From* Masdeu, J.C. and Pascual, B. Genetic and degenerative disorders primarily causing dementia. *Handb Clin Neurol* 2016;135:525-64; with permission.)

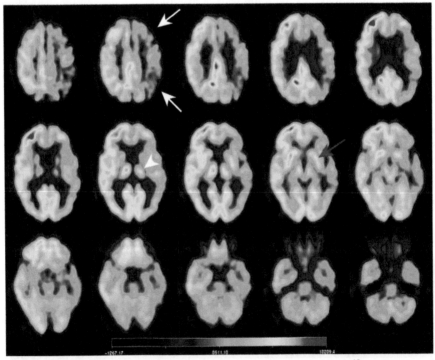

Fig. 18. Metabolism in corticobasal degeneration. Axial sections of an ^{18}F-FDG-PET study from a 47-year-old man with progressive agraphia and apraxia, as well as right-sided parkinsonism. Metabolism in the association cortex of the frontal and parietal lobe is decreased (*white arrows*), as well as in the ipsilateral thalamus (*arrowhead*) and lenticular nucleus (*red arrow*). Note that the greatest decrease in metabolism is in the higher sections, corresponding with the area of representation of the hand in the motor strip. (*From* Masdeu, J.C. and Pascual, B. Genetic and degenerative disorders primarily causing dementia. *Handb Clin Neurol* 2016;135:525-64; with permission.)

SUMMARY

Although MRI is being used to rule out rare causes of dementia, such as tumors or prion disorders, and more frequent ones, such as vascular disease, it can also be used advantageously to support the clinical impression in neurodegenerative dementias, particularly with the aid of automated measurement of cortical thickness and the volume of the amygdala and hippocampus, structures that are critical for episodic memory processing. PET allows the quantification of regional cerebral metabolism, characteristically altered in AD, diffuse Lewy body disease, and the FTDs. PET is also used to determine the abnormal brain deposition of β-amyloid and tau, as well as brain inflammation. These instruments allow quantification in vivo and the longitudinal follow-up of key neurobiological events in neurodegeneration. For instance, amyloid imaging is being used not only to determine who has excess amyloid in the brain but also to investigate whether removing it may slow the deposition of tau and delay cognitive impairment in AD. Tau imaging provides an important outcome measure for ongoing clinical trials targeting not only amyloid but tau as well. Neuroimaging, already critical for the diagnosis and follow-up of diseases that cause dementia, will increasingly apply in the clinic and in research.

REFERENCES

1. Knopman DS, Jack CR Jr, Wiste HJ, et al. Age and neurodegeneration imaging biomarkers in persons with Alzheimer disease dementia. Neurology 2016;87: 691–8.
2. Klunk WE, Koeppe RA, Price JC, et al. The Centiloid Project: standardizing quantitative amyloid plaque estimation by PET. Alzheimers Dement 2015;11:1–15.e1-4.
3. Scholl M, Lockhart SN, Schonhaut DR, et al. PET imaging of tau deposition in the aging human brain. Neuron 2016;89:971–82.
4. Johnson KA, Schultz A, Betensky RA, et al. Tau positron emission tomographic imaging in aging and early Alzheimer disease. Ann Neurol 2016;79:110–9.
5. Sanchez-Juan P, Ghosh PM, Hagen J, et al. Practical utility of amyloid and FDG-PET in an academic dementia center. Neurology 2014;82:230–8.
6. Sperling RA, Rentz DM, Johnson KA, et al. The A4 study: stopping AD before symptoms begin? Sci Transl Med 2014;6:228fs13.
7. Mungas D, Tractenberg R, Schneider JA, et al. A 2-process model for neuropathology of Alzheimer's disease. Neurobiol Aging 2014;35:301–8.
8. Sperling RA, Aisen PS, Beckett LA, et al. Toward defining the preclinical stages of Alzheimer's disease: recommendations from the National Institute on Aging-Alzheimer's Association workgroups on diagnostic guidelines for Alzheimer's disease. Alzheimers Dement 2011;7:280–92.
9. Jack CR Jr, Bennett DA, Blennow K, et al. NIA-AA research framework: toward a biological definition of Alzheimer's disease. Alzheimers Dement 2018;14: 535–62.
10. Sevigny J, Chiao P, Bussiere T, et al. The antibody aducanumab reduces abeta plaques in Alzheimer's disease. Nature 2016;537:50–6.
11. Zhang X, Jin H, Padakanti PK, et al. Radiosynthesis and in vivo evaluation of two PET radioligands for imaging alpha-synuclein. Appl Sci (Basel) 2014;4:66–78.
12. ALS Association. ALS find a cure 2016. Available at: http://www.alsa.org/news/media/press-releases/grand-challenge-generation-020816.html. Accessed September 8, 2016.

13. Esiri MM, Wilcock GK, Morris JH. Neuropathological assessment of the lesions of significance in vascular dementia. J Neurol Neurosurg Psychiatry 1997;63: 749–53.
14. Kirkpatrick J, Hayman L. White-matter lesions on MR imaging of clinically healthy brains of elderly subjects: possible pathologic basis. Radiology 1987;162: 509–11.
15. Viswanathan A, Gschwendtner A, Guichard JP, et al. Lacunar lesions are independently associated with disability and cognitive impairment in CADASIL. Neurology 2007;69:172–9.
16. Reijmer YD, van Veluw SJ, Greenberg SM. Ischemic brain injury in cerebral amyloid angiopathy. J Cereb Blood Flow Metab 2016;36(1):40–54.
17. Johnson KA, Gregas M, Becker JA, et al. Imaging of amyloid burden and distribution in cerebral amyloid angiopathy. Ann Neurol 2007;62:229–34.
18. Gurol ME, Viswanathan A, Gidicsin C, et al. Cerebral amyloid angiopathy burden associated with leukoaraiosis: a positron emission tomography/magnetic resonance imaging study. Ann Neurol 2013;73:529–36.
19. Chui HC, Ramirez-Gomez L. Clinical and imaging features of mixed Alzheimer and vascular pathologies. Alzheimers Res Ther 2015;7:21.
20. Savva GM, Wharton SB, Ince PG, et al. Age, neuropathology, and dementia. N Engl J Med 2009;360:2302–9.
21. Schneider JA, Arvanitakis Z, Bang W, et al. Mixed brain pathologies account for most dementia cases in community-dwelling older persons. Neurology 2008; 70(10):816.
22. Ballard CG, Burton EJ, Barber R, et al. NINDS AIREN neuroimaging criteria do not distinguish stroke patients with and without dementia. Neurology 2004;63: 983–8.
23. Knopman DS, DeKosky ST, Cummings JL, et al. Practice parameter: diagnosis of dementia (an evidence-based review). Report of the Quality Standards Subcommittee of the American Academy of Neurology. Neurology 2001;56: 1143–53.
24. Roman GC, Tatemichi TK, Erkinjuntti T, et al. Vascular dementia: diagnostic criteria for research studies. Report of the NINDS-AIREN International Workshop. Neurology 1993;43:250–60.
25. de Leeuw FE, de Groot JC, Achten E, et al. Prevalence of cerebral white matter lesions in elderly people: a population based magnetic resonance imaging study. The Rotterdam Scan Study. J Neurol Neurosurg Psychiatry 2001;70:9–14.
26. Nolan KA, Lino MM, Seligmann AW, et al. Absence of vascular dementia in an autopsy series from a dementia clinic. J Am Geriatr Soc 1998;46:597–604.
27. de la Torre JC. Alzheimer disease as a vascular disorder: nosological evidence. Stroke 2002;33:1152–62.
28. van der Flier WM, van Straaten EC, Barkhof F, et al. Small vessel disease and general cognitive function in nondisabled elderly: the LADIS study. Stroke 2005;36:2116–20.
29. Pascual B, Prieto E, Arbizu J, et al. Brain glucose metabolism in vascular white matter disease with dementia: differentiation from Alzheimer disease. Stroke 2010;41:2889–93.
30. Marchant NL, Reed BR, Sanossian N, et al. The aging brain and cognition: contribution of vascular injury and abeta to mild cognitive dysfunction. JAMA Neurol 2013;70:488–95.

31. Vemuri P, Lesnick TG, Przybelski SA, et al. Vascular and amyloid pathologies are independent predictors of cognitive decline in normal elderly. Brain 2015;138: 761–71.
32. Jack CR Jr, Knopman DS, Jagust WJ, et al. Tracking pathophysiological processes in Alzheimer's disease: an updated hypothetical model of dynamic biomarkers. Lancet Neurol 2013;12:207–16.
33. Villemagne VL, Burnham S, Bourgeat P, et al. Amyloid beta deposition, neurodegeneration, and cognitive decline in sporadic Alzheimer's disease: a prospective cohort study. Lancet Neurol 2013;12:357–67.
34. Yau WY, Tudorascu DL, McDade EM, et al. Longitudinal assessment of neuroimaging and clinical markers in autosomal dominant Alzheimer's disease: a prospective cohort study. Lancet Neurol 2015;14:804–13.
35. Petersen RC, Wiste HJ, Weigand SD, et al. Association of elevated amyloid levels with cognition and biomarkers in cognitively normal people from the community. JAMA Neurol 2016;73:85–92.
36. Burnham SC, Bourgeat P, Dore V, et al. Clinical and cognitive trajectories in cognitively healthy elderly individuals with suspected non-Alzheimer's disease pathophysiology (SNAP) or Alzheimer's disease pathology: a longitudinal study. Lancet Neurol 2016;15:1044–53.
37. Jack CR Jr, Bennett DA, Blennow K, et al. A/T/N: an unbiased descriptive classification scheme for Alzheimer disease biomarkers. Neurology 2016;87: 539–47.
38. Vos SJ, Xiong C, Visser PJ, et al. Preclinical Alzheimer's disease and its outcome: a longitudinal cohort study. Lancet Neurol 2013;12:957–65.
39. Su Y, Blazey TM, Owen CJ, et al. Quantitative amyloid imaging in autosomal dominant Alzheimer's disease: results from the DIAN study group. PLoS One 2016;11:e0152082.
40. Mosconi L, Rinne JO, Tsui WH, et al. Amyloid and metabolic positron emission tomography imaging of cognitively normal adults with Alzheimer's parents. Neurobiol Aging 2013;34:22–34.
41. Orban P, Madjar C, Savard M, et al. Test-retest resting-state fMRI in healthy elderly persons with a family history of Alzheimer's disease. Sci Data 2015;2:150043.
42. Bron EE, Steketee RM, Houston GC, et al. Diagnostic classification of arterial spin labeling and structural MRI in presenile early stage dementia. Hum Brain Mapp 2014;35:4916–31.
43. Andrews KA, Frost C, Modat M, et al. Acceleration of hippocampal atrophy rates in asymptomatic amyloidosis. Neurobiol Aging 2016;39:99–107.
44. Masdeu JC, Pascual B. Genetic and degenerative disorders primarily causing dementia. Handb Clin Neurol 2016;135:525–64.
45. Lambert JC, Ibrahim-Verbaas CA, Harold D, et al. Meta-analysis of 74,046 individuals identifies 11 new susceptibility loci for Alzheimer's disease. Nat Genet 2013;45:1452–8.
46. Guerreiro R, Wojtas A, Bras J, et al. TREM2 variants in Alzheimer's disease. N Engl J Med 2013;368:117–27.
47. Bradshaw EM, Chibnik LB, Keenan BT, et al. CD33 Alzheimer's disease locus: altered monocyte function and amyloid biology. Nat Neurosci 2013;16:848–50.
48. Villeneuve S, Rabinovici GD, Cohn-Sheehy BI, et al. Existing Pittsburgh Compound-B positron emission tomography thresholds are too high: statistical and pathological evaluation. Brain 2015;138:2020–33.

49. Murray ME, Lowe VJ, Graff-Radford NR, et al. Clinicopathologic and 11C-Pitts-burgh compound B implications of Thal amyloid phase across the Alzheimer's disease spectrum. Brain 2015;138:1370–81.

50. Choi SR, Schneider JA, Bennett DA, et al. Correlation of amyloid PET ligand flor-betapir F 18 binding with abeta aggregation and neuritic plaque deposition in postmortem brain tissue. Alzheimer Dis Assoc Disord 2012;26:8–16.

51. Wolk DA, Grachev ID, Buckley C, et al. Association between in vivo fluorine 18-labeled flutemetamol amyloid positron emission tomography imaging and in vivo cerebral cortical histopathology. Arch Neurol 2011;68:1398–403.

52. Sabri O, Sabbagh MN, Seibyl J, et al. Florbetaben PET imaging to detect amy-loid beta plaques in Alzheimer's disease: phase 3 study. Alzheimers Dement 2015;11:964–74.

53. Palmqvist S, Zetterberg H, Mattsson N, et al. Detailed comparison of amyloid PET and CSF biomarkers for identifying early Alzheimer disease. Neurology 2015;85:1240–9.

54. Jack CR Jr, Lowe VJ, Senjem ML, et al. 11C PiB and structural MRI provide com-plementary information in imaging of Alzheimer's disease and amnestic mild cognitive impairment. Brain 2008;131:665–80.

55. Villemagne VL, Pike KE, Chetelat G, et al. Longitudinal assessment of Abeta and cognition in aging and Alzheimer disease. Ann Neurol 2011;69:181–92.

56. Chetelat G, Villemagne VL, Pike KE, et al. Relationship between memory perfor-mance and beta-amyloid deposition at different stages of Alzheimer's disease. Neurodegener Dis 2012;10:141–4.

57. Vlassenko AG, Mintun MA, Xiong C, et al. Amyloid-beta plaque growth in cogni-tively normal adults: longitudinal [11C]Pittsburgh compound B data. Ann Neurol 2011;70:857–61.

58. Lim YY, Laws SM, Villemagne VL, et al. Abeta-related memory decline in APOE epsilon4 noncarriers: implications for Alzheimer disease. Neurology 2016;86: 1635–42.

59. Landau SM, Marks SM, Mormino EC, et al. Association of lifetime cognitive engagement and low beta-amyloid deposition. Arch Neurol 2012;69:623–9.

60. Vemuri P, Lesnick TG, Przybelski SA, et al. Effect of intellectual enrichment on AD biomarker trajectories: longitudinal imaging study. Neurology 2016;86: 1128–35.

61. Brown BM, Rainey-Smith SR, Villemagne VL, et al. The relationship between sleep quality and brain amyloid burden. Sleep 2016;39:1063–8.

62. Schreiber S, Landau SM, Fero A, et al. Comparison of visual and quantitative florbetapir F 18 positron emission tomography analysis in predicting mild cogni-tive impairment outcomes. JAMA Neurol 2015;72:1183–90.

63. Kantarci K, Lowe V, Przybelski SA, et al. APOE modifies the association between Abeta load and cognition in cognitively normal older adults. Neurology 2012;78: 232–40.

64. Lim YY, Villemagne VL, Laws SM, et al. BDNF Val66Met, Abeta amyloid, and cognitive decline in preclinical Alzheimer's disease. Neurobiol Aging 2013;34: 2457–64.

65. Rabinovici GD, Rosen HJ, Alkalay A, et al. Amyloid vs FDG-PET in the differen-tial diagnosis of AD and FTLD. Neurology 2011;77:2034–42.

66. Serrano GE, Sabbagh MN, Sue LI, et al. Positive florbetapir PET amyloid imag-ing in a subject with frequent cortical neuritic plaques and frontotemporal lobar degeneration with TDP43-positive inclusions. J Alzheimers Dis 2014;42:813–21.

67. Vellas B, Carrillo MC, Sampaio C, et al. Designing drug trials for Alzheimer's disease: what we have learned from the release of the phase III antibody trials: a report from the EU/US/CTAD Task Force. Alzheimers Dement 2013;9:438–44.
68. Petersen RC, Aisen P, Boeve BF, et al. Mild cognitive impairment due to Alzheimer disease in the community. Ann Neurol 2013;74:199–208.
69. Mathis CA, Kuller LH, Klunk WE, et al. In vivo assessment of amyloid-beta deposition in nondemented very elderly subjects. Ann Neurol 2013;73:751–61.
70. Monsell SE, Mock C, Roe CM, et al. Comparison of symptomatic and asymptomatic persons with Alzheimer disease neuropathology. Neurology 2013;80: 2121–9.
71. Nelson PT, Head E, Schmitt FA, et al. Alzheimer's disease is not "brain aging": neuropathological, genetic, and epidemiological human studies. Acta Neuropathol 2011;121:571–87.
72. Perez-Nievas BG, Stein TD, Tai HC, et al. Dissecting phenotypic traits linked to human resilience to Alzheimer's pathology. Brain 2013;136:2510–26.
73. Sperling R, Salloway S, Brooks DJ, et al. Amyloid-related imaging abnormalities in patients with Alzheimer's disease treated with bapineuzumab: a retrospective analysis. Lancet Neurol 2012;11:241–9.
74. Villemagne VL, Fodero-Tavoletti MT, Masters CL, et al. Tau imaging: early progress and future directions. Lancet Neurol 2015;14:114–24.
75. Pascual B, Masdeu JC. Tau, amyloid, and hypometabolism in the logopenic variant of primary progressive aphasia. Neurology 2016;86:487–8.
76. Ikonomovic MD, Abrahamson EE, Price JC, et al. [F-18]AV-1451 positron emission tomography retention in choroid plexus: more than "off-target" binding. Ann Neurol 2016;80:307–8.
77. Marquie M, Normandin MD, Vanderburg CR, et al. Validating novel tau positron emission tomography tracer [F-18]-AV-1451 (T807) on postmortem brain tissue. Ann Neurol 2015;78:787–800.
78. Hansen AK, Knudsen K, Lillethorup TP, et al. In vivo imaging of neuromelanin in Parkinson's disease using 18F-AV-1451 PET. Brain 2016;139:2039–49.
79. Ossenkoppele R, Schonhaut DR, Scholl M, et al. Tau PET patterns mirror clinical and neuroanatomical variability in Alzheimer's disease. Brain 2016;139: 1551–67.
80. Lowe VJ, Curran G, Fang P, et al. An autoradiographic evaluation of AV-1451 Tau PET in dementia. Acta Neuropathol Commun 2016;4:58.
81. Josephs KA, Martin PR, Botha H, et al. [(18) F]AV-1451 tau-PET and primary progressive aphasia. Ann Neurol 2018;83:599–611.
82. Taniguchi-Watanabe S, Arai T, Kametani F, et al. Biochemical classification of tauopathies by immunoblot, protein sequence and mass spectrometric analyses of sarkosyl-insoluble and trypsin-resistant tau. Acta Neuropathol 2016; 131:267–80.
83. Smith R, Puschmann A, Scholl M, et al. 18F-AV-1451 tau PET imaging correlates strongly with tau neuropathology in MAPT mutation carriers. Brain 2016;139: 2372–9.
84. Makaretz SJ, Quimby M, Collins J, et al. Flortaucipir tau PET imaging in semantic variant primary progressive aphasia. J Neurol Neurosurg Psychiatry 2018;89: 1024–31.
85. Bevan-Jones WR, Cope TE, Jones PS, et al. [(18)F]AV-1451 binding in vivo mirrors the expected distribution of TDP-43 pathology in the semantic variant of primary progressive aphasia. J Neurol Neurosurg Psychiatry 2018;89:1032–7.

86. Wang L, Benzinger TL, Su Y, et al. Evaluation of tau imaging in staging Alzheimer disease and revealing interactions between beta-amyloid and tauopathy. JAMA Neurol 2016;73:1070–7.

87. Nelson PT, Alafuzoff I, Bigio EH, et al. Correlation of Alzheimer disease neuropathologic changes with cognitive status: a review of the literature. J Neuropathol Exp Neurol 2012;71:362–81.

88. Lohith TG, Bennacef I, Vandenberghe R, et al. Brain imaging of Alzheimer dementia patients and elderly controls with (18)F-MK-6240, a PET tracer targeting neurofibrillary tangles. J Nucl Med 2019;60:107–14.

89. O'Brien JT, Firbank MJ, Davison C, et al. 18F-FDG PET and perfusion SPECT in the diagnosis of Alzheimer and Lewy body dementias. J Nucl Med 2014;55: 1959–65.

90. Herholz K. Guidance for reading FDG PET scans in dementia patients. Q J Nucl Med Mol Imaging 2014;58:332–43.

91. Chen K, Ayutyanont N, Langbaum JB, et al. Characterizing Alzheimer's disease using a hypometabolic convergence index. Neuroimage 2011;56:52–60.

92. Bozoki AC, Korolev IO, Davis NC, et al. Disruption of limbic white matter pathways in mild cognitive impairment and Alzheimer's disease: a DTI/FDG-PET Study. Hum Brain Mapp 2012;33(8):1792–802.

93. Drzezga A, Becker JA, Van Dijk KR, et al. Neuronal dysfunction and disconnection of cortical hubs in non-demented subjects with elevated amyloid burden. Brain 2011;134:1635–46.

94. Caroli A, Prestia A, Chen K, et al. Summary metrics to assess Alzheimer disease-related hypometabolic pattern with 18F-FDG PET: head-to-head comparison. J Nucl Med 2012;53:592–600.

95. Wong CY, Thie J, Gaskill M, et al. A statistical investigation of normal regional intra-subject heterogeneity of brain metabolism and perfusion by F-18 FDG and O-15 H2O PET imaging. BMC Nucl Med 2006;6:4.

96. Chen Y, Wolk DA, Reddin JS, et al. Voxel-level comparison of arterial spin-labeled perfusion MRI and FDG-PET in Alzheimer disease. Neurology 2011; 77:1977–85.

97. Masdeu J, Aronson M. CT findings in early dementia. Gerontologist 1985;25:82.

98. Jack CR Jr, Knopman DS, Chetelat G, et al. Suspected non-Alzheimer disease pathophysiology–concept and controversy. Nat Rev Neurol 2016;12:117–24.

99. Bateman RJ, Xiong C, Benzinger TL, et al. Clinical and biomarker changes in dominantly inherited Alzheimer's disease. N Engl J Med 2012;367:795–804.

100. Reiman EM, Quiroz YT, Fleisher AS, et al. Brain imaging and fluid biomarker analysis in young adults at genetic risk for autosomal dominant Alzheimer's disease in the presenilin 1 E280A kindred: a case-control study. Lancet Neurol 2012;11:1048–56.

101. Apostolova LG, Hwang KS, Medina LD, et al. Cortical and hippocampal atrophy in patients with autosomal dominant familial Alzheimer's disease. Dement Geriatr Cogn Disord 2011;32:118–25.

102. Caroli A, Prestia A, Galluzzi S, et al. Mild cognitive impairment with suspected nonamyloid pathology (SNAP): prediction of progression. Neurology 2015;84: 508–15.

103. Scheltens P, Fox N, Barkhof F, et al. Structural magnetic resonance imaging in the practical assessment of dementia: beyond exclusion. Lancet Neurol 2002; 1:13–21.

104. Kloppel S, Stonnington CM, Barnes J, et al. Accuracy of dementia diagnosis: a direct comparison between radiologists and a computerized method. Brain 2008;131:2969–74.
105. Wolz R, Julkunen V, Koikkalainen J, et al. Multi-method analysis of MRI images in early diagnostics of Alzheimer's disease. PLoS One 2011;6:e25446.
106. Hua X, Leow AD, Parikshak N, et al. Tensor-based morphometry as a neuroimaging biomarker for Alzheimer's disease: an MRI study of 676 AD, MCI, and normal subjects. Neuroimage 2008;43:458–69.
107. Heister D, Brewer JB, Magda S, et al. Predicting MCI outcome with clinically available MRI and CSF biomarkers. Neurology 2011;77:1619–28.
108. Whitwell JL, Dickson DW, Murray ME, et al. Neuroimaging correlates of pathologically defined subtypes of Alzheimer's disease: a case-control study. Lancet Neurol 2012;11:868–77.
109. Ringman JM, O'Neill J, Geschwind D, et al. Diffusion tensor imaging in preclinical and presymptomatic carriers of familial Alzheimer's disease mutations. Brain 2007;130:1767–76.
110. Smith CD, Chebrolu H, Andersen AH, et al. White matter diffusion alterations in normal women at risk of Alzheimer's disease. Neurobiol Aging 2010;31:1122–31.
111. Fortea J, Sala-Llonch R, Bartres-Faz D, et al. Increased cortical thickness and caudate volume precede atrophy in PSEN1 mutation carriers. J Alzheimers Dis 2010;22:909–22.
112. Kim WH, Adluru N, Chung MK, et al. Multi-resolution statistical analysis of brain connectivity graphs in preclinical Alzheimer's disease. Neuroimage 2015;118:103–17.
113. Douaud G, Jbabdi S, Behrens TE, et al. DTI measures in crossing-fibre areas: increased diffusion anisotropy reveals early white matter alteration in MCI and mild Alzheimer's disease. Neuroimage 2011;55:880–90.
114. Wee CY, Yap PT, Zhang D, et al. Identification of MCI individuals using structural and functional connectivity networks. Neuroimage 2012;59:2045–56.
115. O'Dwyer L, Lamberton F, Bokde AL, et al. Using support vector machines with multiple indices of diffusion for automated classification of mild cognitive impairment. PLoS One 2012;7:e32441.
116. Ferretti MT, Cuello AC. Does a pro-Inflammatory process precede Alzheimer's disease and mild cognitive impairment? Curr Alzheimer Res 2011;8:164–74.
117. Serrano-Pozo A, Mielke ML, Gomez-Isla T, et al. Reactive glia not only associates with plaques but also parallels tangles in Alzheimer's disease. Am J Pathol 2011;179:1373–84.
118. Hoozemans JJ, Rozemuller AJ, van Haastert ES, et al. Neuroinflammation in Alzheimer's disease wanes with age. J Neuroinflammation 2011;8:171.
119. Maeda J, Zhang MR, Okauchi T, et al. In vivo positron emission tomographic imaging of glial responses to amyloid-beta and tau pathologies in mouse models of Alzheimer's disease and related disorders. J Neurosci 2011;31:4720–30.
120. Okello A, Edison P, Archer HA, et al. Microglial activation and amyloid deposition in mild cognitive impairment: a PET study. Neurology 2009;72:56–62.
121. Kreisl WC, Fujita M, Fujimura Y, et al. Comparison of [(11)C]-(R)-PK 11195 and [(11)C]PBR28, two radioligands for translocator protein (18 kDa) in human and monkey: implications for positron emission tomographic imaging of this inflammation biomarker. Neuroimage 2010;49:2924–32.
122. Cagnin A, Brooks DJ, Kennedy AM, et al. In-vivo measurement of activated microglia in dementia. Lancet 2001;358:461–7.

123. Schuitemaker A, Kropholler MA, Boellaard R, et al. Microglial activation in Alzheimer's disease: an (R)-[(1)(1)C]PK11195 positron emission tomography study. Neurobiol Aging 2013;34:128–36.
124. Edison P, Archer HA, Gerhard A, et al. Microglia, amyloid, and cognition in Alzheimer's disease: an 11C (R)PK11195-PET and 11C PIB-PET study. Neurobiol Dis 2008;32:412–9.
125. Zanotti-Fregonara P, Pascual B, Veronese M, et al. Head-to-head comparison of 11C-PBR28 and 11C-ER176 for quantification of the translocator protein in the human brain. Eur J Nucl Med Mol Imaging 2019;46(9):1822–9.
126. Kreisl WC, Lyoo CH, McGwier M, et al. In vivo radioligand binding to translocator protein correlates with severity of Alzheimer's disease. Brain 2013;136: 2228–38.
127. Lyoo CH, Ikawa M, Liow JS, et al. Cerebellum can serve as a pseudo-reference region in Alzheimer disease to detect neuroinflammation measured with PET radioligand binding to translocator protein. J Nucl Med 2015;56:701–6.
128. Carter SF, Scholl M, Almkvist O, et al. Evidence for astrocytosis in prodromal Alzheimer disease provided by 11C-deuterium-L-deprenyl: a multitracer PET paradigm combining 11C-Pittsburgh compound B and 18F-FDG. J Nucl Med 2012; 53:37–46.
129. Brun A, Englund E. Regional pattern of degeneration in Alzheimer's disease: neuronal loss and histopathological grading. Histopathology 1981;5:549–64.
130. Pascual B, Prieto E, Arbizu J, et al. Decreased carbon-11-flumazenil binding in early Alzheimer's disease. Brain 2012;135:2817–25.
131. Graff-Radford J, Murray ME, Lowe VJ, et al. Dementia with Lewy bodies: basis of cingulate island sign. Neurology 2014;83:801–9.
132. McKeith IG, Dickson DW, Lowe J, et al. Diagnosis and management of dementia with Lewy bodies: third report of the DLB Consortium. Neurology 2005;65: 1863–72.
133. Kantarci K, Lowe VJ, Boeve BF, et al. Multimodality imaging characteristics of dementia with Lewy bodies. Neurobiol Aging 2012;33:2091–105.
134. Montine TJ, Phelps CH, Beach TG, et al. National Institute on Aging-Alzheimer's Association guidelines for the neuropathologic assessment of Alzheimer's disease: a practical approach. Acta Neuropathol 2012;123:1–11.
135. Nedelska Z, Ferman TJ, Boeve BF, et al. Pattern of brain atrophy rates in autopsy-confirmed dementia with Lewy bodies. Neurobiol Aging 2015;36: 452–61.
136. Rowe CC, Ng S, Ackermann U, et al. Imaging beta-amyloid burden in aging and dementia. Neurology 2007;68:1718–25.
137. Goker-Alpan O, Masdeu JC, Kohn PD, et al. The neurobiology of glucocerebrosidase-associated parkinsonism: a positron emission tomography study of dopamine synthesis and regional cerebral blood flow. Brain 2012;135: 2440–8.
138. Lim SM, Katsifis A, Villemagne VL, et al. The 18F-FDG PET cingulate island sign and comparison to 123I-beta-CIT SPECT for diagnosis of dementia with Lewy bodies. J Nucl Med 2009;50:1638–45.
139. Ferrari R, Hernandez DG, Nalls MA, et al. Frontotemporal dementia and its subtypes: a genome-wide association study. Lancet Neurol 2014;13:686–99.
140. Kerklaan BJ, van Berckel BN, Herholz K, et al. The added value of 18-fluorodeoxyglucose-positron emission tomography in the diagnosis of the behavioral variant of frontotemporal dementia. Am J Alzheimers Dis Other Demen 2014;29: 607–13.

141. Agosta F, Galantucci S, Magnani G, et al. MRI signatures of the frontotemporal lobar degeneration continuum. Hum Brain Mapp 2015;36(7):2602–14.

142. Zhang Y, Tartaglia MC, Schuff N, et al. MRI signatures of brain macrostructural atrophy and microstructural degradation in frontotemporal lobar degeneration subtypes. J Alzheimers Dis 2013;33:431–44.

143. Kirshner HS. Primary progressive aphasia and Alzheimer's disease: brief history, recent evidence. Curr Neurol Neurosci Rep 2012;12:709–14.

144. Sapolsky D, Bakkour A, Negreira A, et al. Cortical neuroanatomic correlates of symptom severity in primary progressive aphasia. Neurology 2010;75:358–66.

145. de Souza LC, Chupin M, Bertoux M, et al. Is hippocampal volume a good marker to differentiate Alzheimer's disease from frontotemporal dementia? J Alzheimers Dis 2013;36:57–66.

146. Mendez MF, Shapira JS, McMurtray A, et al. Accuracy of the clinical evaluation for frontotemporal dementia. Arch Neurol 2007;64:830–5.

147. Foster NL, Heidebrink JL, Clark CM, et al. FDG-PET improves accuracy in distinguishing frontotemporal dementia and Alzheimer's disease. Brain 2007;130: 2616–35.

148. Josephs KA, Whitwell JL, Tacik P, et al. [18F]AV-1451 tau-PET uptake does correlate with quantitatively measured 4R-tau burden in autopsy-confirmed corticobasal degeneration. Acta Neuropathol 2016;132:931–3.

149. Hansen AK, Brooks DJ, Borghammer P. MAO-B Inhibitors do not block in vivo Flortaucipir([(18)F]-AV-1451) binding. Mol Imaging Biol 2018;20:356–60.

150. Olsen M, Aguilar X, Sehlin D, et al. Astroglial responses to amyloid-beta progression in a mouse model of Alzheimer's disease. Mol Imaging Biol 2018;20: 605–14.

151. Shiarli AM, Jennings R, Shi J, et al. Comparison of extent of tau pathology in patients with frontotemporal dementia with Parkinsonism linked to chromosome 17 (FTDP-17), frontotemporal lobar degeneration with Pick bodies and early onset Alzheimer's disease. Neuropathol Appl Neurobiol 2006;32: 374–87.

152. Rascovsky K, Hodges JR, Knopman D, et al. Sensitivity of revised diagnostic criteria for the behavioural variant of frontotemporal dementia. Brain 2011;134: 2456–77.

153. Liscic RM, Storandt M, Cairns NJ, et al. Clinical and psychometric distinction of frontotemporal and Alzheimer dementias. Arch Neurol 2007;64:535–40.

154. Whitwell JL, Przybelski SA, Weigand SD, et al. Distinct anatomical subtypes of the behavioural variant of frontotemporal dementia: a cluster analysis study. Brain 2009;132:2932–46.

155. Gorno-Tempini ML, Hillis AE, Weintraub S, et al. Classification of primary progressive aphasia and its variants. Neurology 2011;76:1006–14.

156. Josephs KA, Whitwell JL, Knopman DS, et al. Two distinct subtypes of right temporal variant frontotemporal dementia. Neurology 2009;73:1443–50.

157. Gorno-Tempini ML, Dronkers NF, Rankin KP, et al. Cognition and anatomy in three variants of primary progressive aphasia. Ann Neurol 2004;55:335–46.

158. Mesulam MM, Weintraub S, Rogalski EJ, et al. Asymmetry and heterogeneity of Alzheimer's and frontotemporal pathology in primary progressive aphasia. Brain 2014;137:1176–92.

159. Whitwell JL, Jack CR Jr, Parisi JE, et al. Midbrain atrophy is not a biomarker of progressive supranuclear palsy pathology. Eur J Neurol 2013;20:1417–22.

160. Josephs KA, Hodges JR, Snowden JS, et al. Neuropathological background of phenotypical variability in frontotemporal dementia. Acta Neuropathol 2011;122: 137–53.
161. Massey LA, Jager HR, Paviour DC, et al. The midbrain to pons ratio: a simple and specific MRI sign of progressive supranuclear palsy. Neurology 2013;80: 1856–61.
162. Pascual B, Prieto E, Marti-Climent J, et al. Decreased 11C-flumazenil binding in early Alzheimer disease. J Neuroimaging 2012;22:106.

Imaging of Central Nervous System Tumors Based on the 2016 World Health Organization Classification

K. Ina Ly, MD[a], Patrick Y. Wen, MD[b],
Raymond Y. Huang, MD, PhD[c],*

KEYWORDS

- Gliomas • Medulloblastomas • MRI • IDH • 1p/19q codeletion • MGMT
- Machine learning • Radiogenomics

KEY POINTS

- The 2016 World Health Organization Classification of Tumors of the Central Nervous System added a novel classification system for gliomas and medulloblastomas based on phenotypic and molecular characteristics, with the goal to create more homogeneous diagnostic groups to improve patient risk stratification and guide management decisions.
- Specific radiographic features on anatomic and physiologic MRI have been shown to correlate with certain molecular subgroups in gliomas and medulloblastomas and represent a promising means to noninvasively assess tumor genotype.
- Radiomics and machine learning techniques extract a large set of quantitative imaging features from whole-tumor regions of interest and may add significant value to traditional imaging approaches.

Disclosures: Dr K.I. Ly has nothing to disclose. Dr P.Y. Wen has received research support from Agios, Astra Zeneca Beigene, Eli Lilly, Genentech/Roche, Karyopharm, Kazia, MediciNova, Merck, Novartis, Oncoceutics, Sanofi-Aventis, and VBI Vaccines. He has served on the advisory board for Abbvie, Agios, Astra Zeneca, Blue Earth Diagnostics, Eli Lilly, Genentech/Roche, Immunomic Therapeutics, Karyopharm, Kiyatec, Puma, Vascular Biogenics, Taiho, Deciphera, VBI Vaccines, and Tocagen; as a speaker for Merck and Prime Oncology; and as an Editor for UpToDate and Elsevier. Dr R.Y. Huang has nothing to disclose.

[a] Stephen E. and Catherine Pappas Center for Neuro-Oncology, Yawkey 9E, Massachusetts General Hospital, 55 Fruit Street, Boston, MA 02114, USA; [b] Center for Neuro-Oncology, Dana-Farber Cancer Institute, 450 Brookline Avenue, Boston, MA 02215, USA; [c] Department of Radiology, Brigham and Women's Hospital, 75 Francis Street, Boston, MA 02215, USA
* Corresponding author.
E-mail address: ryhuang@bwh.harvard.edu

Neurol Clin 38 (2020) 95–113
https://doi.org/10.1016/j.ncl.2019.08.004

INTRODUCTION
Updates to the World Health Organization Classification of Tumors of the Central Nervous System

The classification of central nervous system (CNS) tumors has historically been based on phenotypic characteristics seen on light microscopy, such as histologic features on hematoxylin-eosin–stained sections and immunohistochemical staining of lineage-associated proteins, as well as assessment of ultrastructural features on electron microscopy.[1] The 2016 World Health Organization (WHO) Classification of Tumors of the Central Nervous System introduced a major paradigm shift by adding a classification system based on genotypic alterations known to underlie the tumorigenesis of CNS tumors. The goal of this integrated phenotypic and genotypic classification system is to generate more homogenous diagnostic groups to improve correlations with [1] prognosis, guide the use of therapies, and aid in the prediction of treatment response. As a result, the 2016 classification system has led to a significant restructuring of certain tumor categories, most notably the diffuse gliomas and medulloblastomas.[1] Diffuse gliomas are now classified according to a 3-tiered system that requires a histologic diagnosis of glioma as well as assessment of the mutation status of the isocitrate dehydrogenase (IDH) gene and, in some cases, co-deletion status of the chromosomal arms of 1p and 19q (**Fig. 1**). Similar to gliomas, medulloblastomas were also

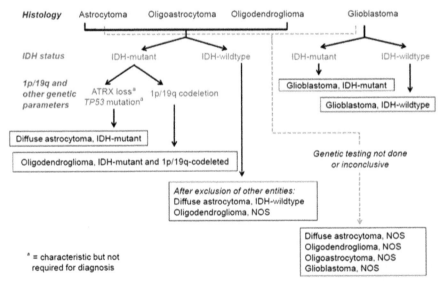

Fig. 1. Algorithm for classification of grade II and III diffuse gliomas based on histologic and genetic characteristics (IDH mutation and 1p/19q-codeletion status). Diffuse gliomas can be classified histologically into astrocytomas, oligodendrogliomas, and oligoastrocytomas (although this is a rare entity based on the 2016 WHO classification) and genetically into IDH-mutant and IDH-wild-type tumors. IDH-mutant tumors can further be categorized by 1p/19q-codeletion status (1p/19q codeleted vs 1p/19q intact). By definition, gliomas that carry the IDH mutation and 1p/19q codeletion are oligodendrogliomas. IDH-mutant gliomas that do not demonstrate 1p/19q codeletion are categorized as diffuse astrocytomas. If genetic testing cannot be performed or is inconclusive, the tumor is classified as not otherwise specified (NOS). (From Louis DN, Perry A, Reifenberger G, et al. The 2016 World Health Organization Classification of Tumors of the Central Nervous System: a summary. Acta Neuropathol. 2016;131(6):803-820; with permission.)

historically classified by histologic variants. With the 2016 WHO classification, four distinct molecular subgroups were introduced, with each subgroup defined by characteristic histologic features, genetic alterations, demographic groups, and prognoses value (**Table 1**).

The Role of MRI and Radiogenomics in Neuro-Oncology

MRI plays a vital role in the diagnosis and management of patients with brain tumors (**Box 1**). Given the importance of tumor molecular features for patient risk stratification and guiding treatment decisions, there has been increasing emphasis on correlating imaging features derived from anatomic and physiologic MRI modalities with molecular markers to characterize imaging phenotypes of brain tumors (collectively referred to as radiogenomics). **Table 2** provides an overview of common MRI modalities and their biological correlates.[2]

Anatomic MRI sequences such as T1-weighted (T1W) post-contrast and T2-weighted (T2W) fluid-attenuated inversion recovery (FLAIR) sequences provide excellent tissue contrast and are routinely acquired in clinical practice, whereas physiologic MRI techniques capture functional or metabolic properties of tumors.

Diffusion-weighted imaging (DWI) measures the diffusivity of water molecules in tissue, which varies depending on the geometry and structure of the microenvironment of tissue. The apparent diffusion coefficient (ADC), a quantitative measure of water diffusion derived from DWI, can provide valuable information on tissue properties, including cellularity, necrosis, and cytotoxic edema.[3]

Several perfusion-weighted imaging (PWI) techniques permit evaluation of tumor vascular properties and are available for most modern clinical MRI scanners. Dynamic

Table 1
Clinical and histologic characteristics of the four molecular subgroups (WNT, SHH, Group 3, Group 4) of medulloblastoma

	WNT (~10%)	SHH (~30%)	Group 3 (~25%)	Group 4 (~35%)
Histologic correlate	Classic; rarely LCA	Classic> desmoplastic/ nodular>LCA> MBEN	Classic>LCA	Classic; rarely LCA
Affected age group	Children, adults; rarely infants	Infants, adults; rarely children	Pediatric patients; rarely adults	Children>infants, adults
Metastasis at diagnosis	~5%–10%	~15%–20%	~40%–45%	~35%–40%
5-y overall survival	>95%	~75%	~50%	~75%
Prognosis	Best	Intermediate	Worst	Intermediate in children but worse in adults

Each molecular subgroup has one or more histologic correlates, is associated with characteristic genetic alterations and demographic factors, and has distinct prognostic implications.

Abbreviations: LCA, large cell/anaplastic; MBEN, medulloblastoma with extensive nodularity; SHH, sonig hedgehog; WNT, wingless.

Adapted from Northcott PA, Jones DT, Kool M, et al. Medulloblastomics: the end of the beginning. *Nat Rev Cancer.* 2012;12(12):818-834; with permission.

Box 1
Utility of MRI and radiogenomics in the care of patients with brain tumors

Defining anatomic boundaries of tumors (T1W post-contrast and T2/FLAIR sequences)

Characterizing physiologic and metabolic properties of tumors (DWI, PWI, MRS)

Targeting specific tumor areas during surgery/biopsy; for example, contrast-enhancing areas (reflective of most aggressive part of tumor) to increase diagnostic accuracy

Longitudinal monitoring of tumor behavior, including response to treatment and signs of recurrence

Noninvasive global assessment of tumor spatial heterogeneity

Abbreviations: DWI, diffusion-weighted imaging; FLAIR, fluid-attenuated inversion recovery; MRS, magnetic resonance spectroscopy; PWI, perfusion-weighted imaging; T1W, T1-weighted.

---

contrast enhancement (DCE) imaging is a T1W-based technique that quantifies changes in signal intensity as intravascular contrast agent permeates through a leaky vasculature into the interstitium.[3] High K^{trans}, a transfer constant coefficient that measures vascular permeability, is typically associated with high-grade tumors because of the presence of increased capillary permeability in malignant lesions.[4,5] Unlike DCE imaging, dynamic susceptibility contrast (DSC) imaging is acquired based on T2W or T2*-weighted sequences.[3] The most commonly used parameter derived from DSC imaging is relative cerebral blood volume (rCBV; normalized to contralateral brain). Among diffuse gliomas, increased rCBV is associated with higher tumor grade because of a greater degree of angiogenesis.[6]

Proton magnetic resonance spectroscopy (MRS) measures metabolite concentrations in tissue. Examples of the most commonly measured metabolites for the evaluation of CNS tumors are listed in **Table 2**.

Radiomics and machine learning techniques, including deep learning, constitute high-throughput computational approaches that extract and synthesize a large number of quantitative imaging features, with the goal to identify diagnostic or predictive models that correlate with tumor genotype or behavior. In contrast to traditional qualitative or quantitative approaches that typically focus on one or a few imaging characteristics or regional measurements and that are subject to intrarater and interrater variability, radiomics and machine learning extract imaging features from whole-tumor regions of interest. Commonly extracted features in radiomics include tumor shape, tumor location, and tumor signal intensity and texture from different MRI sequences and modalities (see **Table 2**). Supervised learning approaches involve inputting extracted imaging features from a predefined set of patients (training set) into machine learning algorithms to construct multivariable models that are associated with a specific clinical correlate or outcome (eg, absence vs presence of malignancy or overall survival). In a separate validation set of a comparable patient population, the trained models can then be tested for their ability to predict the same set of outcomes. This approach can reduce overinflation of model performance caused by the combined use of a large number of imaging features.

In this article, we review the MRI features associated with various genetic subgroups of gliomas and medulloblastomas as defined by the 2016 WHO classification (**Table 3**). We also provide a summary of the imaging characteristics of *MGMT* promoter-methylated gliomas (**Table 3**), given the importance of this genetic alteration for predicting patient treatment response and prognosis.

Table 2
Overview of common MRI modalities, commonly measured parameters, and biological correlates

Imaging Modality	Parameter	Biological Correlate/Significance
T1W post-contrast sequences	Enhancement	• Reflects areas of blood-brain barrier breakdown • Typically associated with high-grade tumors
T2W FLAIR sequences	Hyperintensity	• Reflects areas of edema or gliosis
DWI	ADC	• Low ADC typically seen in highly cellular tumors, cytotoxic edema, and necrosis • High ADC typically seen in vasogenic edema
PWI: DCE	K^{trans}, v_e, v_p	• High K^{trans} typically seen in high-grade tumors • v_e: reflects volume fraction in extracellular extravascular space • v_p: reflects volume fraction in intravascular space
PWI: DSC	rCBV, rCBF, MTT	• High rCBV typically seen in high-grade tumors, may be accompanied by high rCBF
MRS	NAA, choline, creatine, lactate, 2HG	• NAA: marker of neuronal integrity • Choline: marker of cell membrane turnover • Creatine: marker of energy metabolism • Lactate: marker of nonoxidative glycolysis, necrosis, and hypoxia • 2HG: oncometabolite in *IDH*-mutant gliomas • Increased choline/NAA and choline/creatine ratios typically seen in high-grade tumors
Radiomics	Tumor intensity, shape, texture, and wavelet features	• Intensity features: derived from histogram distribution of signal intensity • Texture features: measure of tissue heterogeneity or spatial variation of tumor intensity • Wavelet features: reflect transformed domain representations of intensity and texture features

Abbreviations: 2HG, 2-hydroxyglutarate; ADC, apparent diffusion coefficient; DCE, dynamic contrast enhancement; DSC, dynamic susceptibility contrast; DWI, diffusion-weighted imaging; FLAIR, fluid-attenuated inversion recovery; MRS, magnetic resonance spectroscopy; MTT, mean transit time; NAA, *N*-acetylaspartate; PWI, perfusion-weighted imaging; rCBF, relative cerebral blood flow; rCBV, relative cerebral blood volume; T1W, T1 weighted; T2W, T2 weighted.

Adapted from Ly KI, Gerstner ER. The Role of Advanced Brain Tumor Imaging in the Care of Patients with Central Nervous System Malignancies. *Curr Treat Options Oncol.* 2018;19(8):40; with permission.

GLIOMAS
IDH Mutation

Significance
The isocitrate dehydrogenase (IDH) enzymes constitute a group of metabolic enzymes that catalyze the oxidative decarboxylation of isocitrate to α-ketoglutarate in normal

Table 3
Summary of characteristic imaging features of *IDH*-mutant, 1p/19q-codeleted, and *MGMT* promoter-methylated gliomas, compared with their *IDH*-wild-type, 1p/19q-intact, and *MGMT* promoter-unmethylated counterparts, respectively

Imaging Modality	*IDH* Mutation	1p/19q Codeletion	*MGMT* Promoter Methylation
Anatomic MRI	• Single lobe (especially frontal) • Less enhancement • Sharp tumor margins • Homogeneous signal intensity • Cystic changes	• No difference in contrast enhancement • Unclear whether there are differences in signal intensity or tumor margins • Increased susceptibility artifacts (calcifications, hemorrhage) • T2/FLAIR mismatch sign	• Unclear whether there are differences in location and signal intensity
DWI	• Higher ADC values	• Unclear whether there are differences in ADC values	• Higher ADC values
PWI	• No clear difference in rCBV	• Possibly mildly increased rCBV	• Unclear whether there are differences in rCBV • Possibly increased K^{trans}
MRS	• 2HG spectroscopic peak	• No difference (but based on single-voxel MRS)	—
Radiomics/deep learning	• Classification accuracy 80%–89% when including patient age and imaging features	• Classification accuracy 78%–88% • Lower homogeneity based on texture analysis	• Classification accuracy 71%–83%

cells. Mutations in the *IDH* gene, as seen in a subgroup of diffuse gliomas and glioblastomas (GBMs), result in conversion of isocitrate to D-2-hydroxyglutarate (D-2HG),[7] which, in turn, leads to epigenetic alterations and changes in global genomic methylation patterns that are thought to promote tumorigenesis.[8] Approximately 80% of grade II and grade III gliomas and 5% of GBMs harbor *IDH* mutations.[9,10] *IDH* mutations are key prognostic drivers: patients to *IDH*-mutant (mut) gliomas demonstrate significantly longer survival times compared with those with *IDH*-wild-type (wt) tumors of the same histologic type and grade.[11,12] Furthermore, *IDH* mutations are a defining feature of tumors of oligodendroglial lineage, in addition to codeletion of chromosomes 1p and 19q (1p/19q codeletion).[13,14] In contrast, gliomas with intact chromosomes 1p and 19q are classified as astrocytomas.[1] Knowledge about a patient's *IDH* status has important implications for patient management and prognostic assessment. For instance, depending on individual patient factors, some clinicians may treat a grade II *IDH*-wt astrocytoma the same as a GBM with concurrent chemoradiation and adjuvant temozolomide, but consider a more conservative treatment approach in a grade II *IDH*-mut astrocytoma, such as observation or radiation and chemotherapy.

Anatomic MRI

IDH-mut gliomas show a predilection for involvement of a single cerebral lobe, particularly the frontal lobe.[15–18] By contrast, *IDH*-wt tumors tend to involve multiple lobes and have a more central and infratentorial location (**Fig. 2**).[18–20] This includes a higher proportion of *IDH*-wt tumors in the brainstem, which may reflect the presence of undiagnosed histone H3K27M-mutated tumors, a group of predominantly pediatric and highly aggressive tumors that, by definition, are exclusively *IDH*-wt.[19] On T1W post-contrast sequences, *IDH*-mut tumors, including *IDH*-mut GBMs, typically demonstrate less enhancement,[16,18,21] which is likely driven by decreased levels of angiogenesis and vascular endothelial growth factor in mutant tumors.[22]

In addition, *IDH*-mut gliomas typically display sharper tumor margins,[17] more homogeneous signal intensity,[18] and latter (defined as circumscribed nonenhancing T2-hyperintense foci).[19] The latter may be explained by the strong association between cystic changes and oligodendrogliomas,[23] which, by definition, always harbor an *IDH* mutation (see **Fig. 1**).

Diffusion-weighted and perfusion-weighted imaging

With respect to DWI, the minimum ADC value measured within a tumor volume of interest (ADC_{min}) may be a more useful marker of cellularity than the mean ADC value (ADC_{mean}), given that the latter may not accurately reflect the spatial heterogeneity of gliomas. Multiple retrospective studies have shown that the ADC_{min} is lower in grade II and III *IDH*-wt gliomas compared to *IDH*-mut counterparts of the same grade,[17,19] which likely reflects higher tumor cellularity and increased tumor aggressiveness of *IDH*-wt tumors. In one study, an ADC_{min} threshold of $\leq$ 0.9×10^{-3} mm²/s showed the greatest sensitivity (91%) to predict *IDH* status in grade II gliomas.[19] These findings were confirmed in a large study of 131 *IDH*-wt and 72 *IDH*-mut gliomas from The Cancer Genome Atlas, which found lower median ADC_{mean}, ADC_{min}, and ADC_{max} values (normalized to contralateral normal-appearing white matter) in *IDH*-wt tumors, with a relative ADC_{mean} cutoff value of 1.2×10^{-3} mm²/s generating the highest sensitivity (82%), specificity (75%), and area under the curve (AUC) (0.79).[24]

Contrary to the general assumption that biologically more aggressive tumors show higher rCBV because of increased angiogenesis, mean or maximum rCBV does not seem to differentiate between *IDH*-wt and *IDH*-mut grade II gliomas.[19] Notably, oligodendrogliomas are known to display higher rCBV compared with astrocytomas,[25] and their inclusion in the *IDH*-mut category may at least partly explain this observation.

Magnetic resonance spectroscopy

The presence of D-2HG (the oncometabolite produced as a result of the *IDH* mutation) in *IDH*-mut gliomas has proved to be a valuable imaging biomarker. D-2HG is virtually absent in *IDH*-wt tumors but can reach high concentrations between 5 and 30 mM in *IDH*-mut cells, thus providing a high contrast/noise ratio between mutant cells and background.[26] The ability of MRS to detect D-2HG depends on the density of *IDH*-mut tumor cells, efficiency of cellular D-2HG production, and technical considerations such as spectral resolution and presence of artifacts.[8] While early studies focused on demonstrating the feasibility of 2HG MRS with single-voxel MRS,[27–29] the field has advanced to the implementation of three-dimensional MRS imaging techniques for complete spatial coverage of tumors. A recent prospective study[30] of 24 patients compared the sensitivity and specificity of 2 MRS methods (edited MRS using

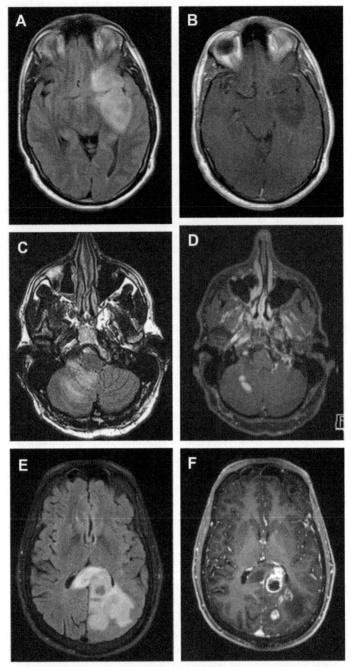

Fig. 2. FLAIR and T1W post-contrast images from a patient with a grade III *IDH*-mutant (*A, B*) and grade III *IDH*-wild-type astrocytoma (*C, D*) as well as an *IDH*-wild-type GBM (*E, F*). The *IDH*-mutant astrocytoma shows characteristic involvement of the frontotemporal lobe, homogeneous signal intensity, and well-demarcated tumor borders on FLAIR sequences (*A*) as well as lack of contrast enhancement on T1W post-contrast sequences (*B*). By contrast, the *IDH*-wild-type astrocytoma is located infratentorially (right cerebellar hemisphere) and shows more diffuse astrocytoma margins (*C*) and contrast enhancement (*D*). Note that gliomas are not usually located in the cerebellum; a more typical appearance is periventricular location, involvement of the corpus callosum, presence of ring enhancement, and necrosis (*E, F*).

Mescher-Garwood point-resolved spectroscopy [MEGA-PRESS] sequence vs PRESS sequence) for preoperative 2HG detection and found that edited MRS (which removes the spectral signal from other metabolites (e.g. glutamate, glutamine, and N-acetylaspartate) in the same range of frequencies) showed superior sensitivity and specificity (both 100%).

In the clinical setting, D-2HG may be useful to diagnose *IDH*-mut gliomas inaccessible for biopsies and potentially guide neurosurgical planning, as complete resection of *IDH*-mut tumors in young patients is associated with an improved prognosis.[31] D-2HG levels decrease after treatment with radiation and/or chemotherapy[32,33] and increase in the setting of tumor progression.[33] In addition, D-2HG levels were shown to decrease by 70% after 1 week of treatment with an *IDH* inhibitor in a phase I clinical trial (**Fig. 3**).[34] These data make D-2HG a potentially useful biomarker of response, although further validation in prospective studies will be required.

Machine learning

Multiple studies suggest that *IDH*-mut and *IDH*-wt tumors can be differentiated based on quantitative MRI features, with accuracies ranging from 80% to 89%.[35–37] In one study, a model that combined patient age, enhancement intensity, tumor volume/edema ratio, and multiple texture features predicted *IDH* status with an accuracy of up to 89%.[35] Another study found that textural features alone on T1W post-contrast, T2W, and FLAIR sequences could predict *IDH* status in GBMs and low-grade gliomas with an accuracy of > 88%, sensitivity > 85%, and specificity of 93% to 100% in the training and validation cohort, supporting the notion that spatial variations of tumor intensity may vary significantly between *IDH*-mut and *IDH*-wt tumors.[37]

Deep learning methods have shown a similar performance. Using a residual convolutional neural network on a multi-institutional dataset of 496 cases, Chang and colleagues[38] achieved prediction accuracies for *IDH* status of up to 86%, which increased to 89% when patient age was added to the model. In another study using a single neural network architecture, *IDH* status could be predicted with a mean

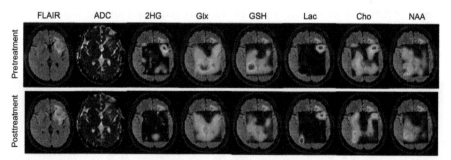

Fig. 3. Metabolic maps from MRS in a patient with an *IDH*-mutant glioma before and after treatment with an *IDH* inhibitor. Pretreatment, there are increased levels of 2HG in the area of FLAIR hyperintensity in the left frontal lobe. There are also corresponding areas of high lactate (Lac) and choline (Cho) and low N-acetylaspartate (NAA) levels, which is typical for neoplasms. One week after treatment, there is reduction of 2HG levels, suggesting a potential role for 2HG as a marker of response. (*Adapted from* Andronesi OC, Arrillaga-Romany IC, Ly KI, et al. Pharmacodynamics of mutant-IDH1 inhibitors in glioma patients probed by in vivo 3D MRS imaging of 2-hydroxyglutarate. *Nat Commun.* 2018;9(1):1474; with permission.)

accuracy of 94% based on absent or minimal areas of enhancement, central areas of cystlike necrosis, and well-defined tumor margins.[39]

Chromosomal 1p/19q Codeletion

Significance

Whole-arm deletion of 1p and 19q occurs as a result of an unbalanced translocation between chromosomes 1p and 19q and is invariably associated with an *IDH* mutation (see **Fig. 1**).[40] It is a defining feature of oligodendrogliomas and a strong predictor of a favorable treatment response to chemotherapy and survival.[41]

Anatomic MRI

Unlike *IDH* status, the differences between 1p/19q-codeleted and 1p/19q-intact tumors on anatomic MRI are less clear. Codeleted tumors are commonly found in the frontal, parietal, and occipital lobes, whereas intact gliomas tend to be located in the temporal, insular, or temporoinsular regions.[42,43] Existing studies have found no group differences in contrast enhancement[43,44] and conflicting results on differences in the degree of heterogeneity on T1W or T2W sequences.[43,45] Similarly, there is conflicting evidence on whether tumor margins have any predictive value,[45,46] which may be explained by the difficulty of objectively assessing tumor margins and the high degree of interrater variability. In general, codeleted tumors display susceptibility artifacts on MRI,[45–47] reflecting areas of calcification and hemorrhage typical of oligodendrogliomas (**Fig. 4**).[1]

A recent study of *IDH*-mut low-grade gliomas showed that the presence of the T2-FLAIR mismatch sign (defined as complete or near-complete hyperintense signal on T2W sequences and relatively hypointense signal on FLAIR sequences except for a hyperintense rim) had a positive predictive value of 100% for 1p/19q-intact cases (**Fig. 5**).[47] However, the negative predictive value was only 44%; that is, the absence of the T2-FLAIR mismatch sign did not rule out a 1p/19q-intact tumor. For these cases, applying a model that combines tumor homogeneity, age, T2* susceptibility blooming, location, and hydrocephalus had 79% to 81% predictive accuracy.[47]

Diffusion-weighted imaging, perfusion-weighted imaging, and magnetic resonance spectroscopy

A study of *IDH*-mut tumors (of which 54 were 1p/19q-intact and 48 were 1p/19q-codeleted) found that the presence of mixed restricted diffusion (defined as a mixed pattern of high and intermediate ADC values) was associated with 1p/19q

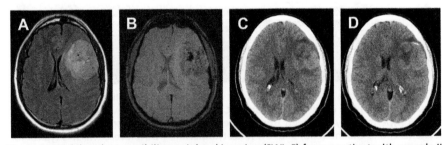

Fig. 4. FLAIR (*A*) and susceptibility-weighted imaging (SWI; *B*) from a patient with a grade III left frontal *IDH*-mutant and 1p/19q-codeleted oligodendroglioma. SWI shows areas of increased susceptibility within the tumor, reflecting underlying calcification. Computed tomography of the head confirms the absence of hemorrhage and shows areas of peripheral calcification (*C, D*).

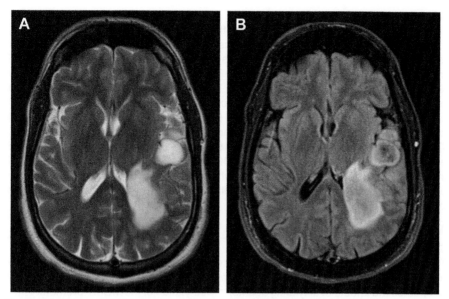

Fig. 5. T2W (*A*) and FLAIR sequences (*B*) showing the T2/FLAIR mismatch sign in a patient with an *IDH*-mutant, 1p/19q-intact glioma. Note the near-complete hyperintense signal on T2W sequences (*A*) and relatively hypointense signal on FLAIR sequences (*B*) with a hyperintense rim.

codeletion.[21] Others did not find an association between ADC_{min} and 1p/19q status[48,49] but reported higher ADC_{max} in 1p/19-intact tumors, possibly reflecting differences in vasogenic and/or cytotoxic edema.[49] Overall, it is difficult to draw clear conclusions from these studies, given the differences in the type of measured ADC parameter as well as how patient groups were stratified. For instance, in the latter studies,[48,49] *IDH* mutation status was not assessed and it is possible that some *IDH*-wt tumors were included.

Similar conflicting results have been found on PWI. Fellah and colleagues[48] reported no group differences between rCBV, rCBF, and rKF2 (relative permeability index) in a cohort of grade II and III tumors, although rCBV and rCBF were higher in the codeleted group among those with grade II tumors. By contrast, others found that a rCBV > 1.59 predicted 1p/19q codeletion with a sensitivity of 92% and specificity of 76%.[50] Biologically, increased rCBV may be explained by areas of microvascular proliferation even in low-grade oligodendrogliomas. Multiple factors may contribute to the discrepant results between studies, including the small sample size (37–50 patients), inclusion of recurrent tumors,[50] and differences in image acquisition and postprocessing techniques. Notably, the combination of conventional and physiologic imaging resulted only in modest improvement of the misclassification error (from 48% to 40%) and sensitivity (from 70% to 79%) compared with conventional imaging alone.[48] Future investigations should focus on the inclusion of a homogeneous patient population with available genotyping for both *IDH* mutations and 1p/19q codeletion and standardized imaging acquisition and postprocessing methods.

Lastly, metabolite ratios on single-voxel MRS did not seem to differ between codeleted and intact tumors, although the investigators acknowledged the limitation of single-voxel MRS in capturing tumor spatial heterogeneity.[48]

Machine learning

One way to assess texture is by analyzing the local spatial frequency content: strong lower frequencies appear as homogeneous smooth regions, whereas strong higher frequencies are reflected as heterogeneous detailed regions.[51] In one study, spectral frequencies in the intermediate range on T2W sequences had superior sensitivity (93%) and specificity (96%) for codeletion status compared with assessment by an expert reader (sensitivity 70% and specificity 63%).[51] Another study[52] showed that codeleted tumors had lower homogeneity (potentially explained by the presence of calcifications and susceptibility artifact) and less distinct borders on FLAIR images. The reported accuracy of texture features to distinguish between 1p/19q-codeleted and 1p/19q-intact gliomas ranges from 78% to 88%.[37,53] The performance appeared improved with a deep learning algorithm, which achieved a mean predictive accuracy of 92% based on left frontal lobe location, ill-defined tumor margins, and larger areas of enhancement.[39]

MGMT Promoter Methylation

Significance

The *MGMT* gene encodes the DNA repair enzyme O-6-methylguanine DNA methyltransferase, which removes alkyl groups from the O6 position of guanine and thereby attenuates the effects of alkylating agents.[54] Methylation of the *MGMT* promoter inactivates the enzyme and sensitizes gliomas to alkylating chemotherapy, and is a cardinal predictor of treatment response and survival. Although the 2016 WHO classification does not stratify gliomas by their *MGMT* promoter methylation status, knowledge thereof significantly influences patient risk stratification and treatment decision.

Anatomic MRI

Studies of up to approximately 200 patients did not observe a difference in tumor location between methylated and unmethylated tumors,[16,55] whereas a large study of 358 patients by Ellingson and colleagues[56] found a preferential distribution of methylated tumors in the left hemisphere and unmethylated tumors in the right hemisphere. Biologically, this may be explained by anatomic differences in the expression of genes involved in cell proliferation and tumorigenesis. However, others have reported an association between methylated tumors and the right hemisphere[57] and a predilection for the parietal and occipital lobes.[58] These discrepancies may partly be explained by the inclusion of different patient populations (primary[56] vs secondary[57] GBMs) and significant differences in sample size.

Similarly, there is conflicting evidence whether there are group differences on FLAIR and contrast-enhanced sequences. Some investigators have observed an association between ring enhancement and unmethylated tumors[55] and between mixed-nodular enhancement and methylated tumors,[58] but the sample sizes in each group were very small ($\leq$8 cases). In the study by Ellingson and colleagues,[56] FLAIR volume was smaller in methylated tumors, which was corroborated in a meta-analysis that included more than 2000 patients.[59] Overall, it seems that there is insufficient evidence to unequivocally distinguish between methylated and unmethylated tumors based on conventional MRI features alone; in one series, imaging characteristics had a predictive accuracy of only 66%.[16]

Diffusion-weighted and perfusion-weighted MRI

Methylated GBMs appear to show higher ADC[60,61] and ADC_{min} values[62,63] than unmethylated GBMs, consistent with the notion that lower ADC reflects increased tumor cellularity and aggressiveness. The utility of rCBV to distinguish between the

2 molecular groups is unclear: although some investigators have shown lower rCBV in methylated GBMs (mean 5.4 vs 9.5),[64] others did not find such a difference.[61] One study reported increased K^{trans} on preoperative MRI of methylated tumors, but the AUC was only 0.756, with a sensitivity of 56% and specificity of 85%.[65] It is interesting to note, however, that this increased permeability may facilitate drug delivery and blood flow to reverse the immunosuppressive and tumor-promoting microenvironment and contribute to the improved survival seen in patients with methylated tumors.

Machine learning
Compared to its ability to classify tumors by *IDH*-mutation and 1p/19q-codeletion status, the performance of machine learning seems to be lower for classification of *MGMT* promoter methylation status. For instance, the classification accuracy of textural features on T2W sequences to distinguish between methylated and unmethylated GBMs was only 71%.[55] Similarly, using the same convolutional neural network architecture to predict *IDH*-mutation, 1p19q-codeletion, and *MGMT* promoter methylation status, the accuracy was lowest for methylation status (mean 83%, compared to >90% for the other 2 groups).[39] The most predictive features for methylated tumors were mixed, nodular enhancement; presence of an eccentric cyst or area of necrosis; more masslike edema with cortical involvement; and slight frontal and superficial temporal predominance.[39]

MEDULLOBLASTOMAS
Molecular Subgroups of Medulloblastomas

In addition to retaining the existing histopathologic classification into classic, large cell/anaplastic, desmoplastic/nodular, and extensive nodularity tumors, the 2016 WHO classification distills medulloblastomas into 4 molecular groups: wingless (WNT)-activated, sonic hedgehog (SHH)-activated group 3, and group 4 tumors (see **Table 1**).[66] Notably, each molecular group has distinct prognostic value. Because molecular analyses may not be routinely available at some centers, identification of MRI features that can distinguish between different molecular subgroups may be particularly helpful for risk stratification and management.

Anatomic MRI

In a retrospective study of 99 patients, tumor location was predictive of underlying molecular subtype: tumors along the cerebellar peduncle and cerebellopontine angle were associated with the WNT subgroup, whereas cerebellar hemispheric location was predictive of SHH tumors (**Fig. 6**). Group 3 and 4 tumors were typically found along the midline and along the fourth ventricle.[67] These anatomic differences may be explained by different developmental origins of tumor cells.[68] Minimal or lack of enhancement was typically seen in midline group 4 tumors. Including tumor location and enhancement pattern in a regression model resulted in $\geq$ 65% of medulloblastomas being correctly classified by molecular subgroup.[67] Notably, other studies found that a large proportion of WNT-subtype tumors have a midline location.[69,70] These discrepancies may relate to the small number of WNT-subtype tumors included in each study (because they constitute the least common molecular group) and the difficulty in clearly distinguishing between tumors originating from the midline and the cerebellar peduncles. Quantitative MR analysis using machine learning in a large cohort may help shed light on the predictive value of structural MRI features.

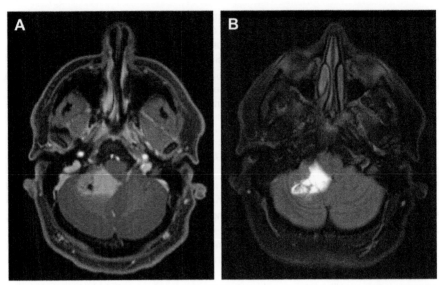

Fig. 6. T1-weighted post-contrast (*A*) and FLAIR MRI sequences (*B*) from a patient with a medulloblastoma (SHH-activated, TP53 wild-type), showing a large cystic mass with nodular enhancement in the right cerebellar hemisphere.

Magnetic Resonance Spectroscopy

A study of 30 medulloblastomas showed that in vivo ^{1}H MRS may help differentiate between the four different molecular subgroups. SHH medulloblastomas are characterized by high levels of choline and lipids and low levels of creatine and taurine.[71] By contrast, group 3 and 4 medulloblastomas typically show high levels of taurine and lower lipid and creatine levels.[71] In addition, application of a 5-metabolite model (creatine, myoinositol, taurine, aspartate, and lipid 13a) differentiated between group 3/4 and SHH tumors with very good accuracy (AUC 0.88). In another study, high levels of glutamate on ^{1}H MRS were associated with improved survival in patients with medulloblastoma.[72]

Machine Learning

In a multi-institutional study of 109 tumors, radiomic features extracted from T1W and T2W images resulted in good to very good predictive performance for SHH, group 3 and group 4 tumors (AUCs 0.7–0.83).[73] Specifically, tumor-edge sharpness was most predictive of SHH and group 4 tumors. The model performance was less robust in predicting WNT and group 3 tumors, possibly because of the smaller sample size in these groups and higher molecular heterogeneity across group 3 tumors.[73]

SUMMARY

Imaging features on anatomic and physiologic MRI can help distinguish between certain molecular subgroups of diffuse gliomas and medulloblastomas, particularly *IDH*-mut and *IDH*-wt gliomas. Radiomics and machine learning–based approaches may augment the ability to distinguish between genetic subgroups by identifying quantitative features from whole-tumor regions of interest. Future studies should focus on prospective validation of these imaging markers in larger and more homogenous patient populations.

REFERENCES

1. Louis DN, Ohgaki H, Wiestler OD, et al. WHO classification of tumours of the central nervous system. 4th edition. Lyon: International Agency for Research on Cancer; 2016.

2. Ly KI, Gerstner ER. The role of advanced brain tumor imaging in the care of patients with central nervous system malignancies. Curr Treat Options Oncol 2018; 19(8):40.

3. Kalpathy-Cramer J, Gerstner ER, Emblem KE, et al. Advanced magnetic resonance imaging of the physical processes in human glioblastoma. Cancer Res 2014;74(17):4622–37.

4. Roberts HC, Roberts TP, Bollen AW, et al. Correlation of microvascular permeability derived from dynamic contrast-enhanced MR imaging with histologic grade and tumor labeling index: a study in human brain tumors. Acad Radiol 2001;8(5):384–91.

5. Roberts HC, Roberts TP, Brasch RC, et al. Quantitative measurement of microvascular permeability in human brain tumors achieved using dynamic contrast-enhanced MR imaging: correlation with histologic grade. AJNR Am J Neuroradiol 2000;21(5):891–9.

6. Rollin N, Guyotat J, Streichenberger N, et al. Clinical relevance of diffusion and perfusion magnetic resonance imaging in assessing intra-axial brain tumors. Neuroradiology 2006;48(3):150–9.

7. Dang L, White DW, Gross S, et al. Cancer-associated IDH1 mutations produce 2-hydroxyglutarate. Nature 2009;462(7274):739–44.

8. Miller JJ, Shih HA, Andronesi OC, et al. Isocitrate dehydrogenase-mutant glioma: evolving clinical and therapeutic implications. Cancer 2017;123(23):4535–46.

9. Yan H, Parsons DW, Jin G, et al. IDH1 and IDH2 mutations in gliomas. N Engl J Med 2009;360(8):765–73.

10. Parsons DW, Jones S, Zhang X, et al. An integrated genomic analysis of human glioblastoma multiforme. Science 2008;321(5897):1807–12.

11. Hartmann C, Hentschel B, Wick W, et al. Patients with IDH1 wild type anaplastic astrocytomas exhibit worse prognosis than IDH1-mutated glioblastomas, and IDH1 mutation status accounts for the unfavorable prognostic effect of higher age: implications for classification of gliomas. Acta Neuropathol 2010;120(6): 707–18.

12. Olar A, Wani KM, Alfaro-Munoz KD, et al. IDH mutation status and role of WHO grade and mitotic index in overall survival in grade II-III diffuse gliomas. Acta Neuropathol 2015;129(4):585–96.

13. Kraus JA, Koopmann J, Kaskel P, et al. Shared allelic losses on chromosomes 1p and 19q suggest a common origin of oligodendroglioma and oligoastrocytoma. J Neuropathol Exp Neurol 1995;54(1):91–5.

14. von Deimling A, Louis DN, von Ammon K, et al. Evidence for a tumor suppressor gene on chromosome 19q associated with human astrocytomas, oligodendrogliomas, and mixed gliomas. Cancer Res 1992;52(15):4277–9.

15. Wang Y, Zhang T, Li S, et al. Anatomical localization of isocitrate dehydrogenase 1 mutation: a voxel-based radiographic study of 146 low-grade gliomas. Eur J Neurol 2015;22(2):348–54.

16. Carrillo JA, Lai A, Nghiemphu PL, et al. Relationship between tumor enhancement, edema, IDH1 mutational status, MGMT promoter methylation, and survival in glioblastoma. AJNR Am J Neuroradiol 2012;33(7):1349–55.

17. Xing Z, Yang X, She D, et al. Noninvasive assessment of IDH mutational status in World Health Organization grade II and III astrocytomas using DWI and DSC-PWI combined with conventional MR imaging. AJNR Am J Neuroradiol 2017;38(6):1138–44.

18. Qi S, Yu L, Li H, et al. Isocitrate dehydrogenase mutation is associated with tumor location and magnetic resonance imaging characteristics in astrocytic neoplasms. Oncol Lett 2014;7(6):1895–902.

19. Villanueva-Meyer JE, Wood MD, Choi BS, et al. MRI features and IDH mutational status of grade II diffuse gliomas: impact on diagnosis and prognosis. AJR Am J Roentgenol 2018;210(3):621–8.

20. Metellus P, Coulibaly B, Colin C, et al. Absence of IDH mutation identifies a novel radiologic and molecular subtype of WHO grade II gliomas with dismal prognosis. Acta Neuropathol 2010;120(6):719–29.

21. Park YW, Han K, Ahn SS, et al. Prediction of IDH1-mutation and 1p/19q-codeletion status using preoperative MR imaging phenotypes in lower grade gliomas. AJNR Am J Neuroradiol 2018;39(1):37–42.

22. Lacerda S, Law M. Magnetic resonance perfusion and permeability imaging in brain tumors. Neuroimaging Clin N Am 2009;19(4):527–57.

23. Koeller KK, Rushing EJ. From the archives of the AFIP: oligodendroglioma and its variants: radiologic-pathologic correlation. Radiographics 2005;25(6):1669–88.

24. Wu CC, Jain R, Radmanesh A, et al. Predicting genotype and survival in glioma using standard clinical MR imaging apparent diffusion coefficient images: a pilot study from the cancer genome atlas. AJNR Am J Neuroradiol 2018;39(10):1814–20.

25. Cha S, Tihan T, Crawford F, et al. Differentiation of low-grade oligodendrogliomas from low-grade astrocytomas by using quantitative blood-volume measurements derived from dynamic susceptibility contrast-enhanced MR imaging. AJNR Am J Neuroradiol 2005;26(2):266–73.

26. Andronesi OC. Precision oncology in the era of radiogenomics: the case of D-2HG as an imaging biomarker for mutant IDH gliomas. Neuro Oncol 2018;20(7):865–7.

27. Andronesi OC, Kim GS, Gerstner E, et al. Detection of 2-hydroxyglutarate in IDH-mutated glioma patients by in vivo spectral-editing and 2D correlation magnetic resonance spectroscopy. Sci Transl Med 2012;4(116):116ra114.

28. Choi C, Ganji SK, DeBerardinis RJ, et al. 2-hydroxyglutarate detection by magnetic resonance spectroscopy in IDH-mutated patients with gliomas. Nat Med 2012;18(4):624–9.

29. Pope WB, Prins RM, Albert Thomas M, et al. Non-invasive detection of 2-hydroxyglutarate and other metabolites in IDH1 mutant glioma patients using magnetic resonance spectroscopy. J Neurooncol 2012;107(1):197–205.

30. Branzoli F, Di Stefano AL, Capelle L, et al. Highly specific determination of IDH status using edited in vivo magnetic resonance spectroscopy. Neuro Oncol 2018;20(7):907–16.

31. Buckner J, Giannini C, Eckel-Passow J, et al. Management of diffuse low-grade gliomas in adults - use of molecular diagnostics. Nat Rev Neurol 2017;13(6):340–51.

32. Andronesi OC, Loebel F, Bogner W, et al. Treatment response assessment in IDH-mutant glioma patients by noninvasive 3D functional spectroscopic mapping of 2-hydroxyglutarate. Clin Cancer Res 2016;22(7):1632–41.

33. Choi C, Raisanen JM, Ganji SK, et al. Prospective longitudinal analysis of 2-hydroxyglutarate magnetic resonance spectroscopy identifies broad clinical utility

for the management of patients with IDH-mutant glioma. J Clin Oncol 2016; 34(33):4030–9.

34. Andronesi OC, Arrillaga-Romany IC, Ly KI, et al. Pharmacodynamics of mutant-IDH1 inhibitors in glioma patients probed by in vivo 3D MRS imaging of 2-hydroxyglutarate. Nat Commun 2018;9(1):1474.

35. Zhang B, Chang K, Ramkissoon S, et al. Multimodal MRI features predict isocitrate dehydrogenase genotype in high-grade gliomas. Neuro Oncol 2017;19(1): 109–17.

36. Yu J, Shi Z, Lian Y, et al. Noninvasive IDH1 mutation estimation based on a quantitative radiomics approach for grade II glioma. Eur Radiol 2017;27(8):3509–22.

37. Lu CF, Hsu FT, Hsieh KL, et al. Machine learning-based radiomics for molecular subtyping of gliomas. Clin Cancer Res 2018;24(18):4429–36.

38. Chang K, Bai HX, Zhou H, et al. Residual convolutional neural network for the determination of IDH status in low- and high-grade gliomas from MR imaging. Clin Cancer Res 2018;24(5):1073–81.

39. Chang P, Grinband J, Weinberg BD, et al. Deep-learning convolutional neural networks accurately classify genetic mutations in gliomas. AJNR Am J Neuroradiol 2018;39(7):1201–7.

40. Louis DN, Perry A, Reifenberger G, et al. The 2016 World Health Organization classification of tumors of the central nervous system: a summary. Acta Neuropathol 2016;131(6):803–20.

41. Cairncross JG, Ueki K, Zlatescu MC, et al. Specific genetic predictors of chemotherapeutic response and survival in patients with anaplastic oligodendrogliomas. J Natl Cancer Inst 1998;90(19):1473–9.

42. Kim JW, Park CK, Park SH, et al. Relationship between radiological characteristics and combined 1p and 19q deletion in World Health Organization grade III oligodendroglial tumours. J Neurol Neurosurg Psychiatry 2011;82(2):224–7.

43. Sherman JH, Prevedello DM, Shah L, et al. MR imaging characteristics of oligodendroglial tumors with assessment of 1p/19q deletion status. Acta Neurochir (Wien) 2010;152(11):1827–34.

44. Chawla S, Krejza J, Vossough A, et al. Differentiation between oligodendroglioma genotypes using dynamic susceptibility contrast perfusion-weighted imaging and proton MR spectroscopy. AJNR Am J Neuroradiol 2013;34(8):1542–9.

45. Megyesi JF, Kachur E, Lee DH, et al. Imaging correlates of molecular signatures in oligodendrogliomas. Clin Cancer Res 2004;10(13):4303–6.

46. Jenkinson MD, du Plessis DG, Smith TS, et al. Histological growth patterns and genotype in oligodendroglial tumours: correlation with MRI features. Brain 2006;129(Pt 7):1884–91.

47. Batchala PP, Muttikkal TJE, Donahue JH, et al. Neuroimaging-based classification algorithm for predicting 1p/19q-codeletion status in IDH-mutant lower grade gliomas. AJNR Am J Neuroradiol 2019;40(3):426–32.

48. Fellah S, Caudal D, De Paula AM, et al. Multimodal MR imaging (diffusion, perfusion, and spectroscopy): is it possible to distinguish oligodendroglial tumor grade and 1p/19q codeletion in the pretherapeutic diagnosis? AJNR Am J Neuroradiol 2013;34(7):1326–33.

49. Jenkinson MD, Smith TS, Brodbelt AR, et al. Apparent diffusion coefficients in oligodendroglial tumors characterized by genotype. J Magn Reson Imaging 2007;26(6):1405–12.

50. Jenkinson MD, Smith TS, Joyce KA, et al. Cerebral blood volume, genotype and chemosensitivity in oligodendroglial tumours. Neuroradiology 2006;48(10): 703–13.

51. Brown R, Zlatescu M, Sijben A, et al. The use of magnetic resonance imaging to noninvasively detect genetic signatures in oligodendroglioma. Clin Cancer Res 2008;14(8):2357–62.

52. Bahrami N, Hartman SJ, Chang YH, et al. Molecular classification of patients with grade II/III glioma using quantitative MRI characteristics. J Neurooncol 2018; 139(3):633–42.

53. Zhou H, Chang K, Bai HX, et al. Machine learning reveals multimodal MRI patterns predictive of isocitrate dehydrogenase and 1p/19q status in diffuse low- and high-grade gliomas. J Neurooncol 2019;142(2):299–307.

54. Gerson SL. MGMT: its role in cancer aetiology and cancer therapeutics. Nat Rev Cancer 2004;4(4):296–307.

55. Drabycz S, Roldan G, de Robles P, et al. An analysis of image texture, tumor location, and MGMT promoter methylation in glioblastoma using magnetic resonance imaging. Neuroimage 2010;49(2):1398–405.

56. Ellingson BM, Cloughesy TF, Pope WB, et al. Anatomic localization of O6-methylguanine DNA methyltransferase (MGMT) promoter methylated and unmethylated tumors: a radiographic study in 358 de novo human glioblastomas. Neuroimage 2012;59(2):908–16.

57. Wang Y, Fan X, Zhang C, et al. Anatomical specificity of O6-methylguanine DNA methyltransferase protein expression in glioblastomas. J Neurooncol 2014; 120(2):331–7.

58. Eoli M, Menghi F, Bruzzone MG, et al. Methylation of O6-methylguanine DNA methyltransferase and loss of heterozygosity on 19q and/or 17p are overlapping features of secondary glioblastomas with prolonged survival. Clin Cancer Res 2007;13(9):2606–13.

59. Suh CH, Kim HS, Jung SC, et al. Clinically relevant imaging features for MGMT promoter methylation in multiple glioblastoma studies: a systematic review and meta-analysis. AJNR Am J Neuroradiol 2018;39(8):1439–45.

60. Han Y, Yan LF, Wang XB, et al. Structural and advanced imaging in predicting MGMT promoter methylation of primary glioblastoma: a region of interest based analysis. BMC Cancer 2018;18(1):215.

61. Moon WJ, Choi JW, Roh HG, et al. Imaging parameters of high grade gliomas in relation to the MGMT promoter methylation status: the CT, diffusion tensor imaging, and perfusion MR imaging. Neuroradiology 2012;54(6):555–63.

62. Romano A, Calabria LF, Tavanti F, et al. Apparent diffusion coefficient obtained by magnetic resonance imaging as a prognostic marker in glioblastomas: correlation with MGMT promoter methylation status. Eur Radiol 2013;23(2):513–20.

63. Rundle-Thiele D, Day B, Stringer B, et al. Using the apparent diffusion coefficient to identifying MGMT promoter methylation status early in glioblastoma: importance of analytical method. J Med Radiat Sci 2015;62(2):92–8.

64. Ryoo I, Choi SH, Kim JH, et al. Cerebral blood volume calculated by dynamic susceptibility contrast-enhanced perfusion MR imaging: preliminary correlation study with glioblastoma genetic profiles. PLoS One 2013;8(8):e71704.

65. Ahn SS, Shin NY, Chang JH, et al. Prediction of methylguanine methyltransferase promoter methylation in glioblastoma using dynamic contrast-enhanced magnetic resonance and diffusion tensor imaging. J Neurosurg 2014;121(2):367–73.

66. Northcott PA, Jones DT, Kool M, et al. Medulloblastomics: the end of the beginning. Nat Rev Cancer 2012;12(12):818–34.

67. Perreault S, Ramaswamy V, Achrol AS, et al. MRI surrogates for molecular subgroups of medulloblastoma. AJNR Am J Neuroradiol 2014;35(7):1263–9.

68. Gibson P, Tong Y, Robinson G, et al. Subtypes of medulloblastoma have distinct developmental origins. Nature 2010;468(7327):1095–9.
69. Patay Z, DeSain LA, Hwang SN, et al. MR imaging characteristics of wingless-type-subgroup pediatric medulloblastoma. AJNR Am J Neuroradiol 2015; 36(12):2386–93.
70. Teo WY, Shen J, Su JM, et al. Implications of tumor location on subtypes of medulloblastoma. Pediatr Blood Cancer 2013;60(9):1408–10.
71. Bluml S, Margol AS, Sposto R, et al. Molecular subgroups of medulloblastoma identification using noninvasive magnetic resonance spectroscopy. Neuro Oncol 2016;18(1):126–31.
72. Wilson M, Gill SK, MacPherson L, et al. Noninvasive detection of glutamate predicts survival in pediatric medulloblastoma. Clin Cancer Res 2014;20(17): 4532–9.
73. Iv M, Zhou M, Shpanskaya K, et al. MR imaging-based radiomic signatures of distinct molecular subgroups of medulloblastoma. AJNR Am J Neuroradiol 2019;40(1):154–61.

Cranial Nerve Imaging and Pathology

Zoltan Klimaj, MD[a], Joshua P. Klein, MD, PhD[b], Gabriella Szatmary, MD, PhD[c,d,*]

KEYWORDS

- Cranial nerve imaging • MRI of cranial nerves • Neuroimaging • Neuroradiology
- Neuro-ophthalmology • Cranial neuropathies • Diplopia • Visual loss

KEY POINTS

- Describe common and less common adult, and some pediatric, neuroimaging findings in the differential diagnosis of cranial neuropathies.
- Provide a framework for clinically driven neuroimaging-based differentiation among intra- and extracranial causes of cranial neuropathies and other causes masquerading as cranial nerve palsy.
- Take home points: neuroimaging is the most frequently ordered ancillary test today in neurology. The neurologist must have the expertise to interpret patient-related neuroimaging studies in order to translate the significance of often nonspecific imaging findings to the bedside.

INTRODUCTION

Dysfunction of the cranial nerves (CNs) is a common neurologic scenario that might exist in isolation or in association with other symptoms or signs. Localization of lesions along the central and peripheral segments of the CNs and confirming a diagnosis very often necessitates the acquisition of specific MR sequences and less frequently computed tomography (CT). The purpose of this review is to provide an approach to neuroimaging of the CNs, correlating anatomic and pathophysiologic abnormalities to neuroimaging findings. Some of the latest technical improvements in neuroimaging of the CNs are highlighted as well.

This review follows a localization-based approach, beginning with the extra-axial (extracranial, cavernous sinus, cisternal) segments of the CNs and ending with the intra-axial (parenchymal, nuclear, internuclear) segments of the CNs.

[a] MR Research Center, Semmelweis University, Balassa utca 6, Budapest 1083, Hungary; [b] Clinical Affairs, Department of Neurology, Brigham and Women's Hospital, Harvard Medical School, Room BB-334, 75 Francis Street, Boston, MA 02116, USA; [c] Neuroimaging Hattiesburg Clinic, PA, 415 South 28th Avenue, Hattiesburg, MS 39401, USA; [d] University of Mississippi Medical Center, Jackson, MS, USA
* Corresponding author. 415 South 28th Avenue, Hattiesburg, MS 39401.
E-mail address: gabriella.szatmary@hattiesburgclinic.com

Neuroimaging is the best tool to differentiate cranial neuropathies from other disorders masquerading as such. Therefore, even a negative imaging study is helpful by excluding a potentially life-threatening structural lesion. This role of neuroimaging can be summarized by the aphorism "MRI never shows everything but always shows something."

IMAGING OF THE CRANIAL NERVES

Foraminal and orbital segments of CNs are well depicted on native T1-weighted fluid-attenuated inversion recovery (FLAIR) high-resolution images against the sharp contrast of orbital fat and on contrast-enhanced (CE) 3-dimensional constructive interference in steady state (3D-CISS) fast gradient echo sequences.

Contrast administration and use of mixed weighting steady-state free precession (SSFP) is a useful technique for visualization of CNs in the cavernous sinus. CE magnetic resonance angiography (MRA) is another option for imaging CNs within the cavernous sinus, although it requires 15% to 20% more time than CE-SSFP.[1]

Imaging of cisternal segments of CNs primarily depends on negative contrast with a heavily T2-weighted image (T2WI) appearance of CSF, and 3D acquisition is preferable over 2D. CISS, fast imaging using steady-state acquisition or driven equilibrium (DRIVE) sequences are best for depicting this contrast.[1,2] Segmentation and fusion of different modalities, such as high-resolution computed angiography, time-of-flight MRA, and T2W 3D DRIVE, are especially helpful in presurgical planning by 3D modeling relationship of CNs to adjacent vasculature and brain parenchyma (**Fig. 1**, Video 1 [see https://drive.google.com/file/d/11yER3IMFarMw0DtygBu7Ct1GVZjqQ9fh/view?usp=sharing]).

T2WI allows direct identification of several CN nuclei in fetal and neonatal brains because the nuclei and proximal fibers myelinate earlier than the surrounding mesencephalic and rhombencephalic white matter tracts. In adults, the location of CN nuclei is possible only by using anatomic landmarks.[2]

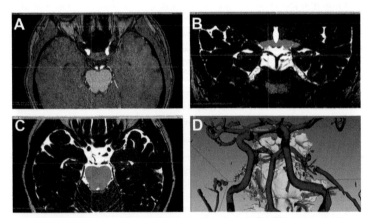

Fig. 1. 3D visualization of segmented objects in the skull base (see Video 1). The segmentation was made by Slicer software based on TOF MRA (*A*) and heavily T2W 3D DRIVE sequences (*B, C*). The oculomotor nerves (*dark blue*) arise between the posterior cerebral and superior cerebellar arteries shown on surface-rendered image (*D*). Optic chiasm (*green*), oculomotor nerves (*dark blue*, pointed by *blue arrow*), trigeminal nerve (*light blue*), abducens nerve (*purple*), vestibular and facial nerves (*brown*), and arteries (*orange*).

Although the parenchymal fascicular segments of CNs are poorly delineated, identification is possible in research settings with multishot diffusion-weighted imaging (DWI) with periodically rotated overlapping parallel lines with enhanced reconstruction sequence. For depicting lesions in the brainstem, multiple sequences including DWI, T2-FLAIR, T2WI, T1-weighted imaging (T1WI) with and without contrast, as well as T2* or susceptibility-weighted imaging sequences to evaluate for blood products, are often required. Axial image resolution of approximately 0.5 × 0.5 mm and 0.7 mm of section thickness might be sufficient to identify most CNs by 2D sequences, except for CN4 that can be imaged with higher spatial resolution that requires 0.3 mm isovolumetric 3D imaging, and this requires the use of at least a 3T magnet.[2] High-resolution and CE T1WI is needed for full characterization of most pathologic processes, especially inflammatory and mass lesions, as many of these conditions manifest by abnormal enhancement of the nerves.

CRANIAL NERVE ANATOMY, PATHOLOGY, AND DIFFERENTIAL DIAGNOSIS

The olfactory nerve, CN I, can be considered an intracranial brain extension, similar to the optic nerve and the neuroretina. The optic nerve, CN II, is composed of axons of the ganglion cells of the entire retina. These axons are myelinated by oligodendrocytes after they pass through the lamina cribrosa, unlike CN I that is myelinated by olfactory ensheathing cells, and CNs III–XII that are myelinated by Schwann cells. This distinction explains why diseases affecting Schwann cells do not affect the optic nerve, and diseases involving the central nervous system may also affect the optic nerve.[3]

The clinical examination is most important in identifying functional abnormalities of the CNs, and the clinical history is most important in establishing a specific cause. In addition, the presence of aberrant regeneration of a CN, such as synkinesis, confirms both an extra-axial location of nerve damage and chronicity of disease.

The most common pathologies affecting any CN are vascular, inflammatory (noninfectious and infectious), compressive-infiltrative, and degenerative. Less common causes include trauma, inherited diseases, and paraneoplastic processes. Although there are a limited number of pathologies affecting the CNs, due to their long intra- and extracranial courses, disorders mimicking cranial neuropathies are extensive. Coverage of detailed anatomy and all diseases affecting CNs is beyond the scope of this article, and for such the reader is referred to several CN-specific reviews.[1,4–8]

In order to avoid repetition of the same cause affecting the CNs, typical imaging characteristics of common lesions affecting any CN will be described in order of first appearance. On neuroimaging studies, in the acute setting, end-organ edema and, in the chronic setting, atrophy help to confirm CN involvement, but findings are often nonspecific on traditional sequences, as most lesions are hypo-to-isointense on T1WI and hyperintense on T2WI. DWI can be helpful in the differential diagnosis when diffusion restriction or facilitation is demonstrated.

Anterior Cranial Fossa

The most common causes of olfactory neuropathy are trauma (**Fig. 2**) and neurodegenerative disorders and, less frequently, infections, tumors, and congenital disorders. Injury of the afferent fibers of the olfactory bulb may result in bulb atrophy months after the event, similar to optic atrophy. Olfactory dysfunction with decreased olfactory bulb volume is one of the initial symptoms and imaging signs appearing years before motor and cognitive symptoms in several neurodegenerative diseases (eg, Parkinson and Alzheimer disease) and may be used as a biomarker of disease progression.

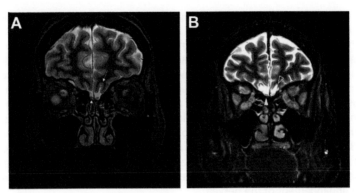

Fig. 2. Olfactory neuropathy. A 55-year-old patient with history of pseudotumor cerebri syndrome diagnosed 18 years ago with low-lying olfactory bulbs that are within the superior ethmoid air cells symmetrically likely secondary to cribriform plate defect at the olfactory recess due to raised intracranial pressure, but olfactory bulb (*arrow*) and olfactory sulcus (*dashed arrow*) are intact on coronal STIR sequence (*A*). It is assumed that the development of an olfactory recess defect spontaneously decompresses increased intracranial pressure (ICP). Therefore, patching of the bony defect, when the underlying cause is not recognized, may worsen elevated ICP-related symptoms and signs, including papilledema. A 69-year-old patient evaluated for thyroid eye disease and incidentally noted to have atrophy of the olfactory bulb (*filled arrow head*) and olfactory sulcus (*empty arrow head*) from remote head trauma on coronal STIR sequence (*B*).

A compressive cranial neuropathy affecting any CN, including CN I, is most commonly from tumors that are either extra-axial (eg, benign tumors such as meningioma or malignant tumors such as tumors with perineural spread, lymphoma, leukemia, leptomeningeal carcinomatosis (LMC), or lymphomatosis) or intra-axial such as nerve sheath tumors. Olfactory groove meningioma has the same imaging appearance as meningiomas occurring elsewhere in the central nervous system (CNS), that is, hypo-to-isointensity on T1WI and hyperintensity on T2WI, with variable calcification inside the tumor (**Fig. 3**), avid and homogenous contrast enhancement, and very often a dural tail. Malignant tumors that cause olfactory dysfunction not originating from the olfactory nerve include ethmoid carcinoma (**Fig. 4**) and leptomeningeal cancer (LMC).[9] Olfactory ensheathing cell tumor is exceedingly rare. Esthesioneuroblastoma is a rare malignant neuroendocrine tumor originating either from the olfactory neuroepithelium or the intracranial olfactory tract. This tumor typically invades the nasal fossa and the skull base (**Fig. 5**).

Congenital anosmia may be associated with Kallmann syndrome. The common imaging findings in Kallmann syndrome include absent olfactory sulci and bulb. Kallmann syndrome has been encountered in patients with congenital fibrosis of extraocular muscles subtype 1, a group of disorders that result from the dysinnervation of oculomotor and/or trochlear nerves and secondary atrophy of their target muscles.[10]

Extracranial Orbital Pathologies

The optic nerve: cranial nerve II

In an adult, the most common causes of an optic neuropathy include glaucoma, ischemic optic neuropathy, papilledema (PE), and optic neuritis (ON). Less frequent types of optic neuropathy are compressive-infiltrative, nutritional-toxic-metabolic, hereditary, traumatic, and paraneoplastic. For a comprehensive list of optic neuropathies with Web links to a large clinical, neuro- and ophthalmic imaging database, the reader

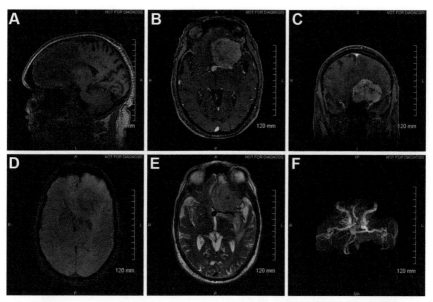

Fig. 3. Olfactory groove meningioma. An 85-year-old patient with history of syncope, headaches for approximately 6 months, and convulsions. Left frontal lobe partially necrotic heterogeneously enhancing olfactory groove meningioma causing significant perilesional edema and subfalcine herniation is shown on sagittal T1-weighted sequence as a hypointense mass (*A*). Pronounced contrast enhancement by the meningioma is depicted on axial and coronal T1WI after contrast administration (*B, C*). Microbleeds or calcification is not visible on axial SWAN sequence (*D*). Axial T2-weighted sequence (*E*) demonstrates an anterior communicating artery aneurysm just dorsal to the mass lesion as a flow void, which is clearly visible on axial T1WI with contrast sequence as well (*B, arrow*). MIP image of 3D TOF MRA shows the aneurysm (*F, arrow*). MIP, maximum intensity projection.

is referred to the neuro-ophthalmology curriculum and the Neuro-Ophthalmology Virtual Educational Library.[11]

The most frequent cause of an acute optic neuropathy in patients older than 50 years is ischemic optic neuropathy (ION), with the nonarteritic variant more common than the arteritic. The diagnosis of ION is clinical and in typical cases neuroimaging is not needed. When obtained, it is usually normal but diffusion restriction of the optic disc or part of the optic nerve may be seen.

PE is defined as optic disc swelling secondary to elevated intracranial pressure (ICP). PE must be differentiated from pseudo-PE resulting from optic disc drusen (**Fig. 6**). The most frequent cause of PE is idiopathic intracranial hypertension, also known as pseudotumor cerebri. The primary role of imaging is to rule out an intracranial tumor or a dural venous sinus thrombosis (DVST).[4] It is recommended to obtain a brain MRI with gadolinium for typical patients, with the addition of magnetic resonance venography for atypical patients (eg, men, children, thin or postmenopausal women) and for patients with risk factors for DVST (**Fig. 7**). In patients with the typical phenotype, MR venography often shows bilateral distal transverse sinus stenosis. In children, Down syndrome, craniosynostosis (**Fig. 8**), and DVST secondary to otomastoiditis are the more common conditions associated with PE.

Inflammatory ON can be categorized by noninfectious and infectious causes. There are a growing number of causes of autoimmune ON. The most frequent autoimmune

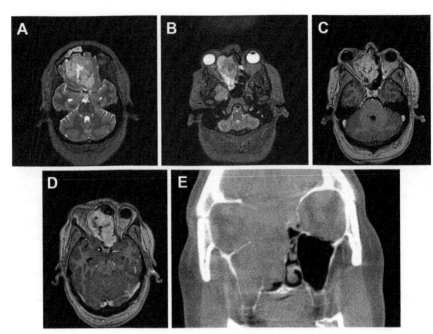

Fig. 4. Large adenoid cystic carcinoma of right nasal cavity. Large heterogeneous mass, protruding preseptally and invades the right maxillary and bilaterally the ethmoid, sphenoid and frontal sinuses, and nasopharynx are shown on axial T2WI (*A*, *B*). Contrast enhancement of the lesion is shown in axial T1-weighted sequences after contrast administration on 3D MPRAGE sequences (*C,D*). Note bony erosions on coronal CT slice (*E*).

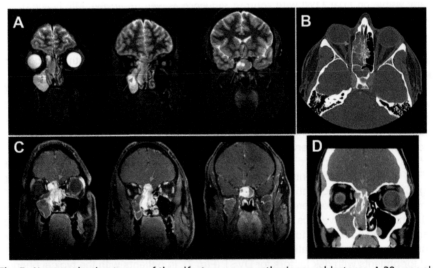

Fig. 5. Neuroendocrine tumor of the olfactory nerve: esthesioneuroblastoma. A 29-year-old man developed right-sided nasal congestion, anosmia, and had an episode of epistaxis. STIR (*A, arrow*) and T1-weighted fat-suppressed contrast-enhanced (*C, arrow*) images are shown in the first and second rows, respectively). Esthesioneuroblastoma is hyperintense on STIR sequence containing cysts and have polypoid appearance; it shows enhancement after contrast administration and bone destruction on CT scans (*B, D, arrows*).

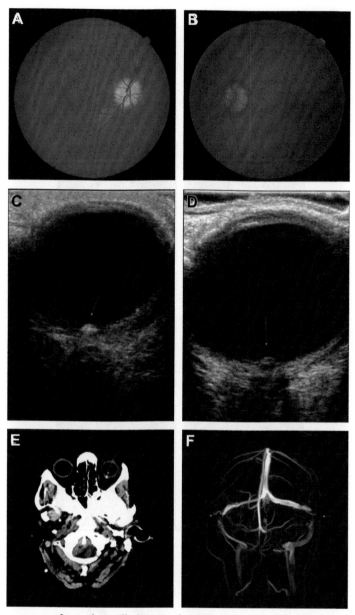

Fig. 6. Appearance of pseudopapilledema and papilledema. Pseudopapilledema due to optic disc drusen on fundus photo (*A, arrow*), B-scan ultrasound (*C, arrow*), head CT (*E, arrow*). Papilledema due to idiopathic intracranial hypertension on fundus photo (*B, arrow*), B-scan ultrasound (*D, arrow*). Blurred optic disc margins with irregular (*A*) and elevated (*B*) disc margins. Protrusion of the optic disc into posterior globe with (*C*) and without (*D*) an echogenic focus is depicted. Calcified drusen is visible on axial head CT with brain window (*E*). MR venogram (*F, arrow*) of the head without contrast demonstrates bilateral distal transverse sinus stenosis that has been described in association with idiopathic intracranial hypertension.

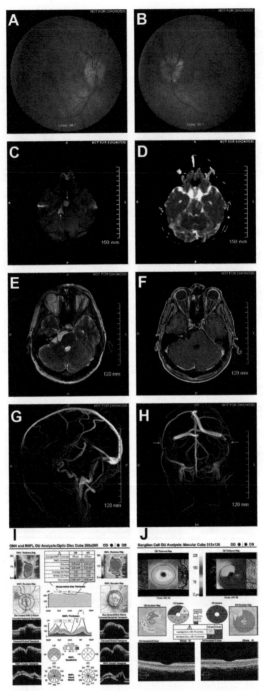

Fig. 7. Prepontine epidermoid cyst with secondary pseudotumor cerebri syndrome. A 47-year-old patient with swollen optic nerves, new onset of headaches and right facial pain. Right (*A*) and left (*B*) fundus photographs show chronic optic disc swelling (more pronounced in the left eye). Large extra-axial right infratentorial mass from the prepontine

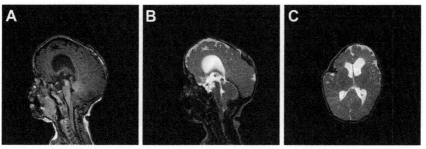

Fig. 8. Craniosynostosis in Pfeiffer syndrome with secondary pseudotumor cerebri syndrome. A 7-week-old infant with Pfeiffer syndrome with multiple developmental anomalies. Arnold-Chiari malformation and turribrachycephaly is pronounced on sagittal T1-weighted (*A*) and T2-weighted (*B*) sequences. The severely deformed skull is visible on axial T2-weighted sequence (*C*). Enlarged ventricles indicate communicating hydrocephalus. (*Courtesy of* György Várallyay, MD from MR Research Center at Semmelweis University. Budapest, Hungary.)

optic neuropathy is acute demyelinating ON.[12] The diagnosis is clinical, although orbital MRI can confirm the diagnosis and brain MRI delivers prognostic information about the risk of future demyelinating events and the diagnosis of multiple sclerosis (MS). Imaging findings in ON are nonspecific and include hyperintensity and swelling of the involved segment of the optic nerve, best seen on sequences such as T2WI, short tau inversion recovery (STIR), spectral attenuated inversion recovery, and DWI secondary to T2-shine-through, and associated contrast enhancement on fat-suppressed T1WI.[12] Increased apparent diffusion coefficient values of lesions in the optic nerve might be spots for locations of axonal disruption. Neuromyelitis optica spectrum disorder (NMOSD) is another autoimmune process that affects the optic nerve and spinal cord and, in most of the patients, is caused by a pathogenic autoantibody against aquaporin-4 (AQP4) water channel (**Fig. 9**). The transverse myelitis in NMOSD is longitudinally extensive, spanning at least 3 spinal cord segments. The area postrema (**Fig. 10**) is often a selective target of the disease process due to higher levels of expression of AQP4 at this location. Myelin oligodendrocyte glycoprotein (MOG)-immunoglobulin G (IgG) is a nonpathogenic antibody typically associated with bilateral optic neuritis that is distinct from the optic neuritis seen in AQP4-IgG seropositive patients or in patients with MS (**Fig. 11**). Typical MRI findings include confinement of the lesion to the orbit (as opposed to AQP4-IgG optic neuritis where posterior optic pathway involvement even beyond the optic chiasm is more frequent) (see **Fig. 9**), DWI restriction, perineural enhancement, elongated optic nerve-sheath complex enlargement with T2 hyperintense signal and enhancement, and diencephalon and periventricular lesions adjacent to the third and fourth ventricles.[13]

---

to the interpeduncular cistern demonstrating DWI and ADC hyperintensity corresponding to T2-shine-through effect [DWI (*C*), ADC map (*D*)], multilobed cyst laterally displacing the right CN V [hyperintense on T2WI (*E*) and does not show contrast enhancement (*F*)], consistent with an epidermoid. Severe right and mild to moderate left distal transverse sinus stenosis is shown on sagittal and coronal maximum intensity projections of MR venograms (*G*, *H*). OCT with thickening of the peripapillary nerve fiber layer OU (*I*) and superior thinning OD and circumferential of ganglion cell–inner plexiform layers (*J*). ADC, apparent diffusion coefficient; OCT, optical coherence tomography.

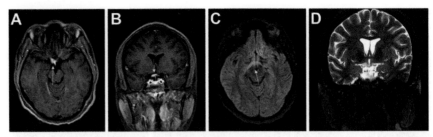

Fig. 9. Optic neuritis and chiasmitis in neuromyelitis optica. A 26-year-old African American woman with history of neuromyelitis optica and myasthenia gravis complained of acute visual loss with improvement following methylprednisolone infusion and eye pain, bilaterally. Edema and enhancement are seen on the right aspect of the optic chiasm and prechiasmal optic nerve on axial and coronal CE fat-suppressed T1-weighted sequences (*A, B* marked by *yellow arrow*) and T2-weighted hyperintense signal on axial T2 FLAIR (*C, arrow*) and coronal T2-weighted (*D*) images.

Neurosarcoidosis may be confined to CN II and behave either as an inflammatory (**Fig. 12**) or as an infiltrative optic neuropathy (**Fig. 13**), often posing diagnostic difficulty and sometimes requiring lesion biopsy. The MRI signs of sarcoidosis-related ON include nonspecific hyperintensity on T2WI and STIR images and longitudinal avid enhancement of the optic pathway from the globe to the chiasm. Thickening of the frontobasal meninges and/or enlargement of the lacrimal glands on MRI renders the diagnosis of optic nerve sarcoidosis more likely.[14]

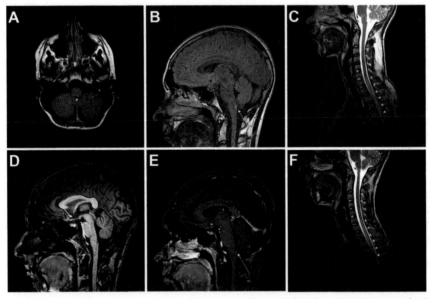

Fig. 10. Neuromyelitis optica spectrum disorder. A 13-year-old male patient presented with hiccup for 2 weeks, paresthesia, and later paraplegia in the legs. A hyperintense focus can be observed on axial and sagittal T2 FLAIR sequences (*A, B*) in the area postrema, hypointense on T1-weighted (*D*), and shows contrast enhancement on CE T1-weighted sequences (*E*). Longitudinally extensive hyperintensity of the cervical and thoracic spine can be seen on sagittal T2 and T2 SPAIR sequences (*C, F*). These findings confirmed NMO. (*Courtesy of* Anna Szőcs, MD from MR Research Center at Semmelweis University, Budapest Hungary.)

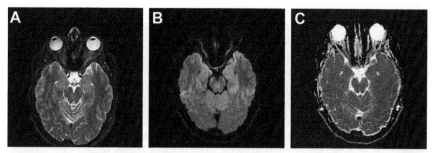

Fig. 11. Inflammatory-demyelinating optic neuritis related to MOG antibody disease. A 33-year-old 33-week pregnant Caucasian woman presented with headaches and subacute simultaneous visual loss. On examination, moderate optic disc edema (not shown) and opening pressure of 23 cm of water on lumbar puncture were noted. Therefore, she was diagnosed with probable idiopathic intracranial hypertension. Because of visual field loss in the left greater than right eye, she underwent optic nerve sheath fenestration on the left side but continued with visual loss. She responded to methylprednisolone IV but relapsed couple of weeks later off corticosteroids. Serum was positive for myelin oligodendrocyte glycoprotein antibody. Axial T2-weighted fat-saturated slice (*A*) show elongated optic nerve-sheath complex enlargement with T2 hyperintense signal of the entire intraorbital segments bilaterally; no diffusion restriction is visible on axial DWI (*B*) and ADC (*C*) map (likely T2-shine-through). IV, intravenous.

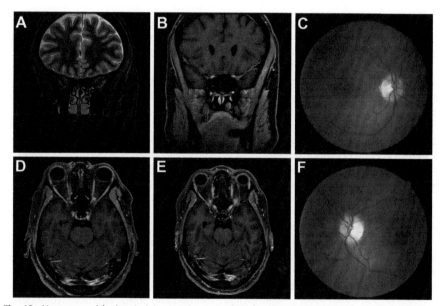

Fig. 12. Neurosarcoidosis mimicking optic nerve sheath meningioma. A 49-year-old Caucasian woman with history of bilateral gradual visual loss. There is enlargement on coronal T2WI (*A*) and peripheral intense enhancement of the optic nerves (left greater than right) within the posterior orbit, orbital apex, and intracranial segment but not extending to the optic chiasm on coronal (*B*) and axial (*D*) CE fat-suppressed T1WI with tram tracking (*arrows*) bilaterally and progressing to more solid enhancement 1 year later (*E*). Fundus photographs demonstrate temporal OU [right (*C*), left (*F*)]. These findings mimic optic nerve sheath meningioma, but biopsy proved neurosarcoidosis.

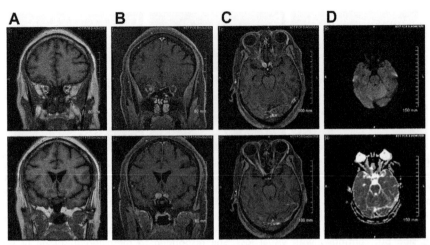

Fig. 13. Infiltrative type sarcoid optic neuropathy. A 46-year-old patient with optic atrophy and visual loss in the right eye. MRI manifestations of neuro-ophthalmic sarcoidosis involving the optic nerves are shown. Coronal T1WI (*A*), T1WI fat-suppressed postcontrast (*B*), and axial T1WI demonstrate right swollen enhancing intraorbital, intracanalicular, and intracranial optic nerve and less severe enhancement of the left intracranial optic nerve (*C*). DWI sequences with corresponding ADC map show restricted diffusion in the right optic nerve (*D*) (upper: DWI, lower: ADC).

Systemic lupus erythematosus and periarteritis nodosa can cause optic neuropathy by inflammatory and/or ischemic mechanisms. Granulomatosis with polyangiitis and eosinophilic granuloma may cause noninfectious ON. A rare form of autoimmune optic neuropathy has been described in chronic ataxic neuropathy with ophthalmoplegia, monoclonal gammopathy, cold agglutinins, and disialosyl antibodies syndrome, although the disease is most typically associated with ophthalmoplegia.

Optic perineuritis (OPN) affects the optic nerve sheath and is typically not associated with optic nerve dysfunction, but it may be associated with perineural inflammatory changes and posterior scleritis, best evaluated by orbital B-scan ultrasonography and MRI. Other findings on MRI include enhancement of the optic nerve sheath and adjacent perineural fat.

A variety of infectious agents can cause ON (and/or OPN) occasionally associated with neuroretinitis, including *Bartonella henselae*, *Borrelia burgdorferi*, cytomegalovirus, herpes zoster ophthalmicus, syphilis, tuberculosis, and West Nile virus.

The causes of compressive and infiltrative optic neuropathies include optic pathway gliomas (OPG), optic nerve sheath and diaphragma sellae meningiomas, orbital tumors, infiltrative and inflammatory processes, mucoceles, fibrous dysplasia, aneurysms, pituitary macroadenomas (**Fig. 14**), and craniopharyngiomas. The most common orbital tumor in an adult is orbital cavernous angioma. Rhabdomyosarcoma is the most common primary malignancy of the orbit in children, appearing as a mass adjacent to or attached to one of the orbital muscles. OPG is the most common primary neoplasm of the optic nerve. OPGs can be subdivided into a low-grade form (typically in children) (**Figs. 15** and**16**) and a more aggressive high-grade form (typically in adults (**Fig. 17**).[15] The low-grade form is frequently associated with neurofibromatosis type 1 (NF1). Histologically, benign optic nerve gliomas are World Health Organization (WHO) grade 1 pilocytic astrocytomas, whereas more aggressive gliomas are

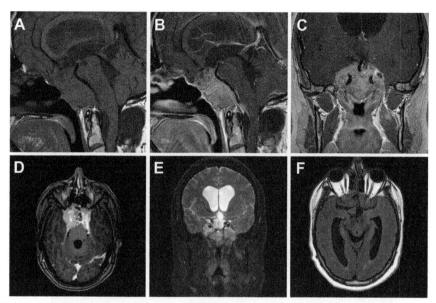

Fig. 14. Atypical ACTH-producing pituitary adenoma. A 33-year-old male patient with atypical ACTH-producing pituitary adenoma presented with visual loss in the right eye and headaches years before the examination, several surgical procedures aimed to decrease the volume of the slowly growing macroadenoma over the years. Total resection of the tumor was not possible. Sagittal native (*A*) and CE T1W spin echo images about the sella show the large heterogeneous enhancing tumor ventral to the brainstem (*B, C*); axial extension of the tumor is depicted on T1W CE gradient echo sequence (*D*). Hydrocephalus is due to the obstructing effect of the tumor ventral to the brainstem that exerts slight compression onto the basilar artery. The tumor is hyperintense with cystic parts on coronal T2WI (*E*) and appears isointense to gray matter on T2 FLAIR sequence (*F*).

either anaplastic astrocytomas (WHO III) or glioblastomas (WHO IV).[4] Gliomas are hypointense to isointense on T1WI and slightly hyperintense on T2WI with a variable enhancement pattern roughly correlated to the grade of the tumor.

Optic nerve sheath meningioma (ONSM) constitutes about 2% of all orbital tumors. Primary ONSM originates from the intraorbital or intracanalicular segments of the optic nerve (**Fig. 18**), whereas secondary ONSM are intraorbital extensions of intracranial neoplasms (**Fig. 19**). Histologically, both arise from the cap cells of the arachnoid sheath.[16] ONSM can extend through the optic canal along the planum sphenoidale to the contralateral optic nerve.[4] Thin-slice CT and gradient echo sequences may show calcification and hyperostosis of adjacent bone, features that are less common in glioma. Peripheral calcification and contrast enhancement may be observed around the nerve as a "tram-track" sign on axial images but even this finding is nonspecific and may be encountered in cases of sarcoidosis (see **Fig. 12**), metastases, or lymphoma. Molecular imaging could aid in diagnosing meningioma in view of relatively high levels of somatostatin receptor expression by these tumors.[17]

Secondary tumors of CN II are more common than primary tumors and may arise from direct invasion from intraocular, intraorbital, or intracranial primary malignancies, from hematopoietic malignancy, from LMC, or from distant primary tumors (**Fig. 20**).[18] Breast and lung cancer and melanoma are the most frequent causes of LMC among

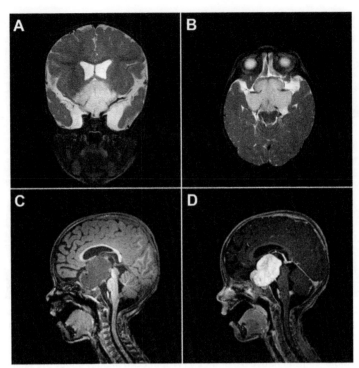

Fig. 15. Pilocytic astrocytoma.Optic pathway glioma, a WHO grade 1 pilocytic astrocytoma in a 16-month-old female child is shown as a homogeneous hyperintense large mass on T2-weighted coronal and axial slices (*A, B*). The tumor is hypointense on T1-weighted (*C*) and demonstrates intense gadolinium contrast enhancement (*D*).

solid tumors in adults. Brain MRI should include axial native T1WI images, FLAIR, DWI sequences, and 3D T1WI sequences following contrast administration. CE-T1WI and FLAIR sequences are the most sensitive to detect LMC. The most frequent MRI findings are subarachnoid and parenchymal enhancing nodules (10%–35%), diffuse or focal pial enhancement (10%–20%), and spinal nerve root enhancement.[9] Typically, on DWI, persistent restricted diffusion can be seen, unlike ischemic stroke-related restriction that is transient.

Thyroid orbitopathy may be complicated by compressive optic neuropathy from enlarged extraocular muscles (EOMs), typically in the orbital apex in the active stage of the disease, or from severe proptosis with stretching of the optic nerves from proliferation of the orbital fat in the chronic stage. CT and MRI typically show increased size of the EOMs bilaterally (although may be asymmetrical) with the inferior and medial recti most commonly involved followed by the superior and lateral recti and the superior oblique muscles[19] (**Fig. 21**). In case of optic nerve compression, abnormal signal intensity of the nerve on T2WI is often observed.

The ocular motor nerves: cranial nerves III, IV, and VI
The extracranial orbital segment of the ocular motor nerves (OMNs) can be affected by infectious/inflammatory disease, tumors, Tolosa–Hunt syndrome, or trauma with fracture involving the superior orbital fissure.

Orbital inflammation may extend intracranially through the superior orbital fissure and/or optic canal and into the cavernous sinus leading to CN dysfunction, typically

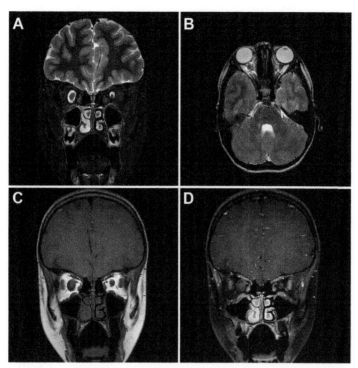

Fig. 16. Optic nerve glioma in neurofibromatosis type 1. A 10-year-old male patient with bilateral optic nerve glioma in Recklinghausen syndrome. Right greater than left enlarged isointense optic nerves on coronal STIR (*A*) and axial T2-weighted (*B*) with widened optic canals; native T1WI and fat suppressed T1-weighted contrast-enhanced spin echo (*C, D*) images show isointense signal and no contrast enhancement. (*Courtesy of* Péter Barsi, MD, PhD from MR Research Center at Semmelweis University, Budapest, Hungary.)

external ophthalmoplegia. Noninfectious orbital inflammation can further be divided into idiopathic and syndromic. Idiopathic orbital inflammation is characterized by orbital pain, diplopia, swelling, and hyperemia of the eyelid. Imaging findings may include myositis, dacryoadenitis, and perineuritis with and without associated infiltrations. In rare cases, orbital inflammation can be associated with systemic disorders such as the histioproliferative Erdheim-Chester and Rosai-Dorfman diseases and systemic inflammatory process due to IgG4-related disease (IgG4-RD). Imaging findings are nonspecific and include infiltrative intraconal tumefactive masses, or diffuse ill-defined processes, that are hyperintense on T2WI, enhance after gadolinium administration, and have no DWI restriction.[20] Orbital IgG4-RD may be distinguished by associated enlargement of the infraorbital nerve.

Orbital infections may have a dental or paranasal sinus origin. MRI or CT imaging is necessary to assess extraocular spread of infection and for differentiation of preseptal periorbital versus postseptal orbital cellulitis. MRI can be used to help visualize early inflammatory changes within the postseptal orbit and to detect intracranial extension and thrombosis of the cavernous sinus. DWI is helpful in assessing for optic nerve ischemia or infarction, which can occur secondarily from orbital infection.[21] Immuno-compromised patients are at increased risk of developing fungal cellulitis (often mucormycosis or aspergillosis) that can lead to severe secondary complications

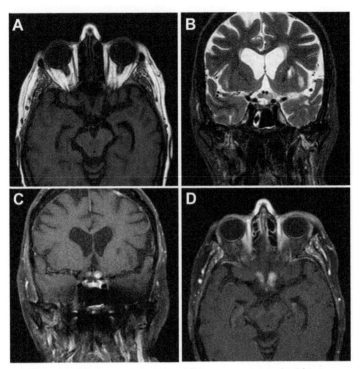

Fig. 17. Optic nerve glioblastoma. A 75-year-old woman presented with severe progressive sequential painless visual loss, first in the left and 2 months later in the right eye. In 4 months, visual acuity declined to no light perception in the left eye and hand motion in the right eye. MRI showed T1 iso- and T2 hyperintense signal (*A*, *B*) (with small central cystic changes in the latter stage of the disease, not shown) and progressive enlargement and intense contrast enhancement of the orbital, intracanalicular, and intracranial segments extending to the optic chiasm in coronal (*C*) and axial (*D*) CE fat-suppressed T1WI. Biopsy of the blind left eye revealed WHO grade IV glioblastoma. Brain metastasis developed in 4 months and patient expired in 6 months from symptom onset.WHO, World Health Organization.

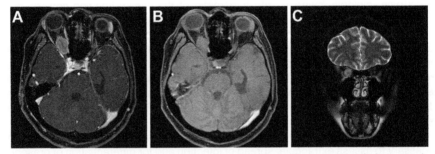

Fig. 18. Optic nerve sheath meningioma. A 49-year-old woman complained about gradual visual loss and weekly headaches for half a year, she had right periorbital crawling sensation. Optic nerve sheath meningioma is seen in the right orbital apex and shows contrast enhancement on axial T1-weighted CE fat-suppressed image (*A*). The lesion is isointense with brain tissue on T1-weighted CE SPIR (*B*) and slightly hyperintense on coronal T2-weighted fat-suppressed images (*C*). (*Courtesy of* György Várallyay, MD from MR Research Center at Semmelweis University, Budapest, Hungary.)

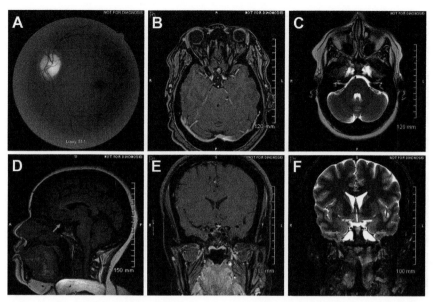

Fig. 19. Small tuberculum sellae meningioma causing compressive optic neuropathy on the left in a patient with idiopathic intracranial hypertension. A 48-year-old patient with headaches and blurred vision, elevated ICP but optic atrophy OS on fundus photograph (*A*). Small left paracentral intensely and fairly homogeneously enhancing meningioma centered at the tuberculum sellae is shown on CE and fat-suppressed axial 3D T1 VIBE (*B, arrow*) and coronal T1WI (*E, arrowhead*) and isointense lesion on sagittal native T1WI (*D*, marked by *blue arrow*). Symmetric enlargement of Meckel caves is visible on axial and coronal T2WI (*C, F* marked by *blue arrow*) in association with increased intracranial pressure.

including thrombosis, CN II-VI palsies, meningoencephalitis, or brain abscess. Imaging findings may be subtle, thus specific assessment of the sphenoid sinus is needed and may be best seen on MRI with focal enhancement of the mucosal lining. On CT, a focal hypodense area is suspicious for an abscess, and bone erosion may be seen as well.[22]

Extracranial Peripheral Segments

The trigeminal nerve: cranial nerve V
The extracranial peripheral segment of a CN is most commonly involved in perineural tumor spread of head and neck malignancies that most frequently involves the V2 (maxillary) branch and CN VII (**Fig. 22**). MRI may show obliteration of the juxtaforaminal fat pads on T1WI with or without associated foraminal enlargement and when chronic, atrophy of denervated muscle. Primary tumors of the peripheral branches of CN V include nerve sheath tumors, comprising only 5% of all schwannomas. The V1 (ophthalmic) branch is the most commonly affected, and about 25% are associated with NF1.

Trauma is a significant cause of distal peripheral branch neuropathy. Neural compression at the bony foramina due to fibro-osseous conditions such as fibrous dysplasia and Paget disease can cause peripheral trigeminal neuropathy.

Cavernous Sinus

Lesions affecting the cavernous sinus often produce multiple CN palsies (CNs III–VI). Among vascular lesions, cavernous carotid aneurysms (CCAs) account for 2% to 9%

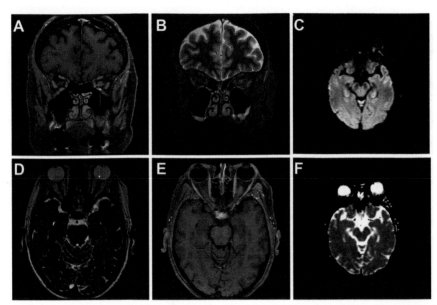

Fig. 20. Intraorbital optic nerve infiltration in chronic lymphocytic leukemia. A 62-year-old patient with history of chronic lymphocytic leukemia presented with sudden severe visual loss in the left eye and eye pain. Enlargement and enhancement of the left intraorbital and intracanalicular segments of the optic nerve is depicted on coronal [arrow on image (*A*)] and axial (*E*) contrast-enhanced fat-saturated T1-weighted sequence. The lesion is hyperintense on coronal STIR (*B*) and does not show restricted diffusion on DWI and ADC (*C, F*). Protrusion of the optic nerve head into the vitreous, consistent with left optic disc edema on axial heavily T2-weighted image [*dashed arrow* on image (*D*)].

of all intracranial aneurysms. CCAs cause CN palsies when a critical size is reached, and most commonly affect CN VI (**Fig. 23**). CTA and MRA are usually diagnostic of this entity. Carotid-cavernous fistula (CCF) is an abnormal communication between the cavernous segment of the internal carotid artery and the venous blood in the cavernous sinus itself. Patients with CCF may present with decreased vision secondary to glaucoma and external ophthalmoplegia (**Fig. 24**). When the arterialized blood is shunted anteriorly, imaging may show an enlarged superior ophthalmic vein (SOV), thickened extraocular muscles, and an enlarged cavernous sinus with abnormal convexity of the lateral wall; when shunted posteriorly enlarged cortical veins may be observed. MRA images of the head, even without contrast, frequently demonstrate abnormal flow signal not readily seen by other techniques. Lemierre syndrome is associated with cavernous sinus thrombosis secondary to peripheral infection like a retropharyngeal abscess. The syndrome may be bilateral and may cause SOV thrombosis. The differential diagnosis of SOV thrombosis principally includes infection and CCF. Characteristically, enhancement of the thrombus on T1WI and absence of normal flow void on T2WI images is seen. Meningiomas involve the cavernous sinus in 5% to 10% of cases and can cause OMN palsy (**Fig. 25**).[5]

Noninfectious inflammatory entities affecting the cavernous sinus include entities affecting the orbits, some previously described, and sarcoidosis, granulomatosis with polyangiitis, periarteritis nodosa, and Tolosa-Hunt syndrome. These entities are characterized by a T1 and T2 hypointense soft tissue mass and associated with abnormal thickening and enhancement of the dura and may extend into the orbital

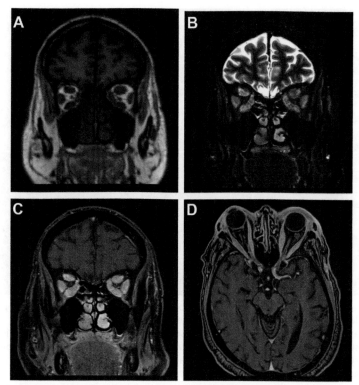

Fig. 21. Thyroid eye disease. A 69-year-old man presented with diplopia followed by visual loss in the left eye. Severe bilateral (left greater than right) enlargement of all the extraocular muscles with heterogeneous T2 signal and severe crowding in the orbital apex with compression of the left optic nerve is seen on coronal T1-weighted, STIR, T1-weighted TSE fat-saturated CE, and axial 3D T1-weighted VIBE fat-saturated CE sequences (*A, B, C, D*, respectively).

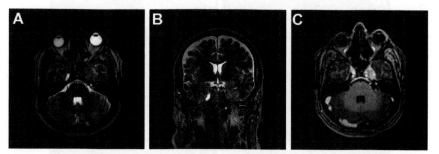

Fig. 22. Intracranial extension by perineural spread of large B-cell lymphoma. A 49-year-old man presented with left-sided visual loss, ophthalmoplegia, CN VII palsy, and trigeminal neuralgia due to intracavernous manifestation of large B-cell lymphoma. Expansion of the left cavernous sinus on axial and coronal T2-weighted slices (*A, B*) that is conspicuous on axial contrast-enhanced T1-weighted sequence (*C*). Perineural tumor spread is visible along branches of CN V through the foramen ovale into the pterygopalatine fossa. (*Courtesy of* Péter Barsi, MD, PhD from MR Research Center at Semmelweis University, Budapest, Hungary.)

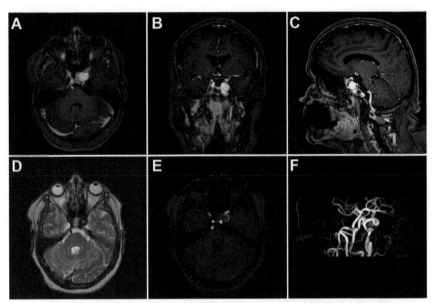

Fig. 23. Cavernous sinus aneurysm. A 68-year-old patient presented with left CN VI palsy. MR examination revealed an aneurysm within the left cavernous sinus and is shown on axial, coronal, and sagittal T1-weighted spin echo sequences after contrast administration (*A, B,* and *C,* respectively). The aneurysm shows flow void on axial T2WI (*D*) and slow flow within the aneurysm is likely based on TOF MRA examination (*E, F*). (*Courtesy of* István Gyuricza, MD, Budapest, Hungary.)

apex. Tolosa-Hunt syndrome is a diagnosis of exclusion that seems as an enhancing ill-defined process in the orbital apex, cavernous sinus, or both, with possible extension along the optic nerve and, therefore, must be differentiated from neoplasm. It is commonly unilateral and presents with painful ophthalmoplegia and often decreased vision.

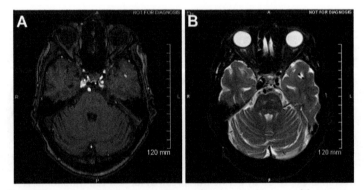

Fig. 24. Carotid-cavernous dural arteriovenous fistula. An 81-year-old woman presented with complete bilateral CN VI palsy secondary dural arteriovenous fistula that could be seen in the right parasellar region arising from the right internal carotid artery on axial slices of TOF MRA (*A, red arrow*) and on T2-weighted sequences as flow voids (*B, red arrow*). Diagnostic cerebral angiogram showed complex dAVF with outflow via veins exiting the left parasellar venous plexus with extensive cortical venous reflux. Following surgery, no recovery of CN VI paresis.

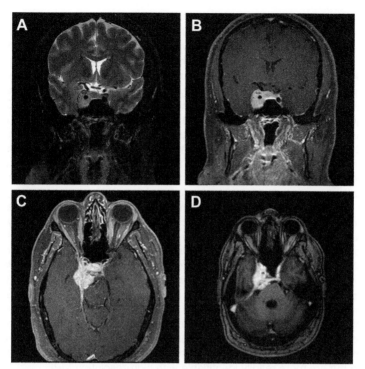

Fig. 25. Cavernous sinus meningioma. A 38-year-old man presented with diplopia due to right CN VI palsy. Head MR shows expanded cavernous sinus by a markedly homogeneously enhancing mass at the right orbital apex, right prepontine cistern, and encasing CNs III, V, and VI as seen on coronal T2WI fat-suppressed (*A*), coronal and axial T1-weighted spin echo sequences (*B, C*). Dural tail sign can be observed on axial slices. Note the difference between spin echo and gradient echo sequences: tissues that are not part of the brain are better assessable on spin echo sequences (*C*), and brain is better assessable on gradient echo sequence (*D*). (*Courtesy of* György Várallyay, MD from MR Research Center at Semmelweis University, Budapest, Hungary.)

Cisternal

A sellar lesion when extending into the *suprasellar cistern* can give rise to a compressive optic neuropathy or chiasmopathy, but when extending laterally into the cavernous sinus it typically causes OMN dysfunction. When evaluating a sellar, lesion note should always be made of whether the lesion extends to the lateral cavernous sinus or not, as that has significance regarding management. Pituitary adenomas are the most common sellar region tumors. Macroadenomas (>1 cm) with suprasellar extension are typically associated with bitemporal hemianopia and have areas of cystic degeneration (see **Fig. 14**). High-resolution T2WI and CE-FS T1WI delineate the tumor and its relationship to adjacent visual pathway structures. Previous craniotomy and sellar surgery are risk factors for aspergillosis. On MRI, variable T1 and hypointense T2 signal is due to associated necrosis, melanin, and iron content of the fungi.

Pituitary apoplexy is caused by acute hemorrhage or infarction of a pituitary adenoma or in rare cases, may occur in postpartum hypovolemic shock (Sheehan syndrome). The acute hemorrhage within the adenoma seems hyperintense on T1WI, hypointense on T2WI, and hyperdense on unenhanced CT.[4]

Abrupt onset of a complete pupil-sparing CN III palsy in a patient older than 50 years is most likely from microvascular ischemia involving the cisternal segment of the nerve. It is a clinical diagnosis and in typical cases, especially when improving, does not necessitate imaging, although this is a presently debated statement. An incomplete CN III palsy, with or without pupil sparing, is more worrisome for an externally compressive lesion (aneurysm, tumor), and neuroimaging should be obtained urgently with MRI with contrast and a vascular imaging study, either MRA and CTA. The most frequent cause of an isolated pupil-involved CN III palsy is a posterior communicating artery aneurysm (**Fig. 26**).[23] A meta-analysis showed MRA to be comparable but slightly less sensitive than CTA in diagnosing of small intracranial aneurysms, but the most important factor in diagnosing an aneurysm was found to be the interpreter, not the technique itself.[24] If MRA or CTA is normal but suspicion of aneurysm is high, then digital subtraction angiography should be obtained. Aneurysms rarely account for CN III palsies in children. Children with tuberous sclerosis are at increased risk of cerebral aneurysms. Other causes of cisternal compressive OMN palsy include those caused by a basilar artery aneurysm (**Fig. 27**, Video 2 [see https://drive. google.com/open?id=1ZYalBZIISLCuCUCmR7J7S-Oau7SXTRiU]) or normal or tortuous vessels. Downward displacement of the brainstem in trauma, intracranial hypertension, or in spontaneous intracranial hypotension can induce isolated CN III or CN IV palsies (**Fig. 28**), either secondary to cisternal, or when herniation occurs, brain parenchymal involvement.

Inflammatory causes of CN III palsies have been described, most commonly from bacterial or viral meningitis (**Fig. 29**).[25] Other inflammatory causes include sarcoidosis and Miller-Fisher syndrome. Oculomotor nerve schwannomas may be small and difficult to see but are more readily identifiable with high-resolution MRI.

Ophthalmoplegic migraine is a diagnosis of exclusion and is considered a neuralgia. CN III is most commonly affected, followed by the CN VI and CN IV. A complete CN III palsy with pupil involvement is most common. MRI studies have shown enlargement and enhancement of the perimesencephalic oculomotor nerve during an attack. After the attack, MRI shows reduced enhancement with residual enlargement of the oculomotor nerve, although complete resolution with normal MRI has been described.

Pathologies of the cisternal segment of CN V typically manifest as trigeminal neuralgia (TN) reflecting compression of the nerve at the root entry zone (REZ) (see **Fig. 7**). The secondary form of TN is most commonly induced by neurovascular conflict (NVC)

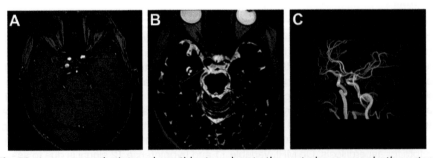

Fig. 26. Aneurysm at the internal carotid artery close to the posterior communicating artery junction laterally displacing the right CN III. A 61-year-old woman presented with right trigeminal neuralgia but no complaint of diplopia; therefore, the aneurysm was incidentaloma. The aneurysm is recognizable on TOF MRA [*red arrow* on axial slice (*A*) and on maximal intensity projection image from TOF MRA– (*C*)], and the right CN III could be seen on axial heavily T2-weighted sequence (*B*).

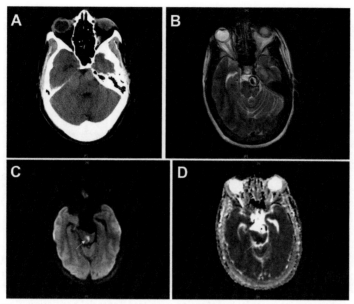

Fig. 27. CN VI palsy due to fusiform basilar artery aneurysm (see Video 2). A 39-year-old woman presents with progressive binocular horizontal diplopia from complete abduction deficit in left eye secondary to compression of the cisternal segment of CN VI by very large fusiform basilar artery aneurysm on axial CT (*A*). Axial T2WI (*B*) shows partial thrombosis (hyperintense part of the vessel) of a large basilar artery aneurysm (black area is flow void consistent with patent vessel). Subsequently, patient developed an acute brainstem infarction. Axial DWI (*C*) shows midline dorsal mesencephalon hyperintensity and corresponding ADC (*D*) hypointensity consistent with water restriction secondary to acute cerebral infarction.

at the trigeminal ganglion, sensory root, or REZ at the pons. The diagnosis is confirmed by imaging and requires the demonstration of an artery perpendicular to the long axis of the cisternal segment of the nerve, which is deviated or indented at the REZ by the vessel. The most frequently implicated vessels are vascular loops of the superior and anterior inferior cerebellar arteries, pontine branches of the basilar artery, and infrequently aberrant veins. Vascular lesions such as aneurysms, dural arteriovenous fistulas, and tortuous and ectatic vessels can also impinge on the cisternal segment of CNs V and VI (see **Fig. 27**).[6] NVC at the medial side of the trigeminal root typically causes symptoms in the maxillary division, whereas NVC at the lateral side causes symptoms in the mandibular division.[26] In addition to nerve atrophy, loss of anisotropy on diffusion tensor imaging is an indicator of compression. These signs on MRI and MRA and intraoperative detection of compression are principal factors affecting the prognosis of decompressive surgery.

Schwannoma is the most common intrinsic trigeminal neoplasm and it most frequently affects the cisternal segment and Gasserian ganglion.[6] Schwannomas are typically dumbbell shaped, isointense to brain on T1WI, and hyperintense on T2WI, with more heterogeneous features in larger tumors including cystic areas with or without fluid–fluid levels and usually avid contrast enhancement. CT may depict bone remodeling or erosion at the medial aspect of the petrous bone and/or along the skull base neurovascular foramina. Malignant nerve sheath tumors should be suspected when aggressive bone destructive changes and/or rapid growth is observed.[6]

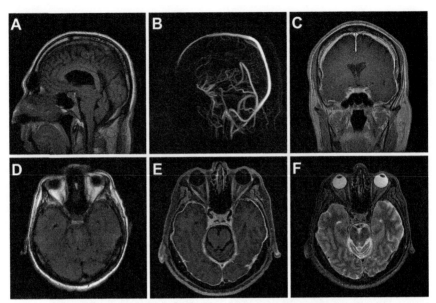

Fig. 28. Spontaneous intracranial hypotension with transtentorial herniation. Caudal dislocation of the brainstem, thick and enhancing dura, widened venous sinuses, and shortened pituitary stalk indicate intracranial hypotension on native (*A*) and contrast-enhanced T1WI (*C, E*) and ventral medial cerebral peduncle hyperintensity on T2 FLAIR (*D*) and T2WI (*F*). Sagging of the venous sinuses is shown on MR venogram (*B*). (*Courtesy of* György Várallyay, MD, Budapest, Hungary.)

Other less common intrinsic lesions include trigeminal nerve lipoma, lymphoma, and metastasis, most commonly from breast cancer, lung cancer, and melanoma.[6]

Petroclival meningiomas comprise 20% to 25% of all intracranial meningiomas.[27] They may impinge on the cisternal segment of CN V and extend into Meckel cave (**Fig. 30**). They are typically hemispheric in shape with a flat dural base and a dome-shaped medial surface that may impinge on the brainstem at the trigeminal root entry zone. Epidermoid cysts located in the prepontine cistern at the cerebellopontine angle can cause trigeminal neuralgia as a primary symptom in 40% of cases but may alternatively present with symptoms of raised ICP (see **Fig. 7**). On DWI and FLAIR sequences, epidermoid cysts are characteristically hyperintense. Therefore, the diagnosis is usually straightforward but when in doubt, CISS sequences might help with differential diagnosis by showing heterogeneous signal and hypointensity relative to CSF.[28] Also, proton MR spectroscopy demonstrates elevated lactate and lipid and an absence of amino acid peaks. In addition to epidermoid cysts, the differential diagnosis of a prepontine extra-axial lesion includes dermoid cyst (**Fig. 31**), ecchordosis physaliphora, chordoma, chondrosarcoma, neurenteric cyst, and arachnoid cyst.

The cisternal segment of CN VII extends from the lateral caudal pons into the porus acusticus and runs adjacent to fibers of CN VIII. The nerve fibers of CN VII are large enough to be seen on most standard brain MRIs and are best seen on T2WI where the nerve will seem hypointense against a background of hyperintense CSF (**Fig. 32**). The intracanalicular segment of the nerve extends from the porus acusticus to the apex of the internal auditory canal. From there, CN VII fibers run between the cochlea and the utricle of the semicircular canals, turning posteriorly and inferiorly to enter the facial canal. CN VIII fibers heading to the cochlea run anteriorly in the

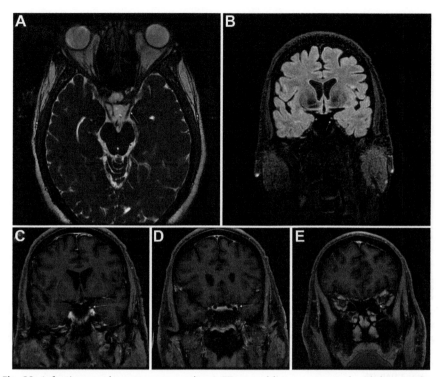

Fig. 29. Infectious oculomotor nerve palsy. A 57-year-old man presented with hearing loss, followed by unresponsiveness, and pupil-involved left CN III palsy secondary to community-acquired pneumococcal meningitis and additional CSF findings of acute neuroinvasive WNV. The course of enlarged and enhancing left CN III (marked by arrow on all images) could be followed from cisternal segment to medial rectus muscle on axial FIESTA (*A*), coronal T2 FLAIR (*B*), and CE fat-suppressed coronal T1WI (*C–E*). Patient's visual functions recovered but 5 weeks after initial presentation developed lower back pain, and MRI showed cauda equina and lumbosacral nerve root enhancement (not shown). This immunocompetent patient had both cranial and peripheral neuropathies in association with simultaneous bacterial and viral infections. WNV, West Nile virus.

internal auditory canal, whereas the fibers heading to the semicircular canals divide into superior, inferior, and posterior branches and run posteriorly. The fibers of CN VII exit the facial canal at the stylomastoid foramen after which the fibers branch and travel to their target organs.

Damage to nerve fibers of CN VII can result in a variety of clinical deficits including ipsilateral facial weakness with associated labial dysarthria, hyperacusis (from impaired innervation to the stapedius muscle), glandular dysfunction from damage to parasympathetic fibers, and loss of taste from the anterior two-thirds of the tongue. The cisternal segment of CN VII can be damaged by compression, trauma, infiltration, demyelination, infection, or idiopathic mechanisms as in Bell palsy. Damage to nerve fibers of CN VIII can result in clinical deficits including ipsilateral deafness and disequilibrium. The cisternal segment of CN VIII can be damaged by compression, trauma, infiltration (see **Fig. 32**), demyelination, or infection.

Tumors of the cerebellopontine angle, including meningiomas and schwannomas, can affect the function of CNs VII and VIII. Although both meningiomas and schwannomas are extra-axial and typically show homogenous avid contrast enhancement,

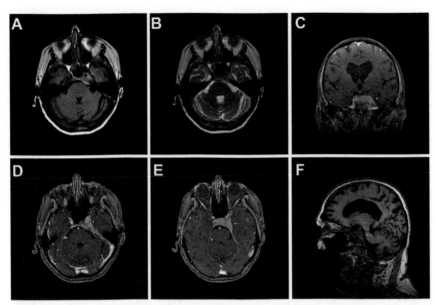

Fig. 30. Petroclival meningioma affecting the trigeminal nerve. A 75-year-old patient with history of memory loss and dizziness. Left prepontine dural-based mass lesion with extension into the cavernous sinus and Meckel cave (marked by arrow on *A, C–F*), affecting CN V, is depicted on axial FLAIR and T2WI (*A, B*). Enhancement of the meningioma could be seen on T1WI (*C–E*) after contrast administration. The meningioma is recognizable on sagittal T1WI (*F*).

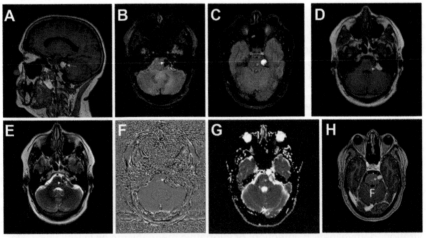

Fig. 31. Prepontine dermoid cyst causing compressive left CN V and VII neuropathy. A 64-year-old patient with history of left facial and tongue numbness. Left lateral prepontine extra-axial mass (marked by arrow on *A–H*) has the same imaging characteristics as fat, hyperintense on T1WI (*A, D*), at the level of the vestibulocochlear nerve calcification seen on SWI amplitude and phase images (hypointense region on *B* and *F*). The lesion is hyperintense on axial T2 FLAIR (*C*), heterogeneous on axial T2WI, and does not enhance with gadolinium on T1WI (*H*), and there is no significant restriction on ADC map (*G*).

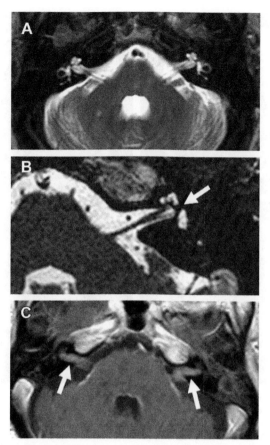

Fig. 32. The facial-vestibulocochlear nerve complex. (*A*) Axial T2WI showing the cisternal and intracanalicular segments of the left facial-vestibulocochlear nerve complex as well as the cochlea and semicircular canals within the temporal bones. (*B*) Axial SSFP image showing more detail of facial-vestibulocochlear nerve complex extending from the lateral pons into the internal auditory canal. The division of the nerve into cochlear (anterior) and vestibular (posterior) branches can be seen, and the expected location of the facial nerve fibers as they enter the facial canal is indicated by the arrow. (*C*) An axial T1WI following intravenous administration of gadolinium contrast shows abnormal enhancement of bilateral cisternal and intracanalicular segments of the facial-vestibulocochlear nerve complex in a patient with leptomeningeal carcinomatosis. Abnormal enhancement of the leptomeninges is also noted on the surface of the pons and middle cerebellar peduncles.

they can be differentiated by the fact that meningiomas tend to have a dural tail and can extend into the porus acusticus, whereas schwannomas arise from the nerve itself and typically grow out of the porus acusticus (**Fig. 33**). The presence of bilateral CN VIII schwannomas is a clue to the diagnosis of neurofibromatosis type II. Similar to CN V, discussed earlier, the cisternal segments of CNs VII and III can occasionally be compressed by an adjacent artery.

The axons of CN IX, the glossopharyngeal nerve, originate in the ipsilateral postero-lateral medulla. CN IX has a variety of functions including innervation of the stylophar-yngeus muscle, parasympathetic innervation to the parotid gland, visceral sensory input from the carotid body and sinus, sensory input from the pharynx and posterior

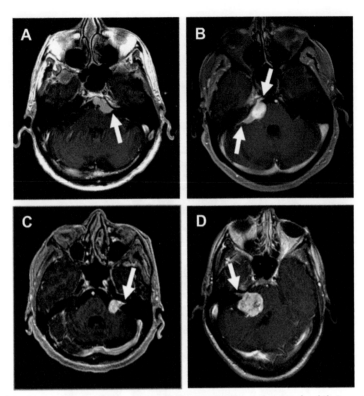

Fig. 33. Meningioma and schwannoma of the cerebellopontine angle. (*A*) An axial T1WI following intravenous administration of gadolinium contrast shows a homogenously enhancing left petroclival meningioma. The medial aspect of the mass is partially encircling the basilar artery. A dural tail adjacent to the internal auditory canal is denoted by the arrow. (*B*) An axial T1WI following intravenous administration of gadolinium contrast shows a homogenously enhancing right petroclival meningioma. Dural tails are denoted by the arrows. (*C*) An axial T1WI following intravenous administration of gadolinium contrast shows a homogenously enhancing schwannoma originating from within the left internal auditory canal (*arrow*) and extending into the cerebellopontine angle. (*D*) An axial T1WI following intravenous administration of gadolinium contrast shows a larger homogenously enhancing schwannoma originating from within the right internal auditory canal (*arrow*) and extending into the cerebellopontine angle. (*Courtesy of* Péter Barsi, MD, MD, Budapest, Hungary.)

third of the tongue, and gustatory information from the posterior third of the tongue. The axons of CN X, the vagus nerve, originate in the ipsilateral posterolateral medulla and have a variety of functions including motor parasympathetic fibers to most internal organs including the sinoatrial node of the heart, motor fibers to pharyngeal and laryngeal muscles, and gustatory information from the pharynx. The axons of CN XI, the accessory nerve, originate in the ipsilateral posterolateral medulla and innervate the sternocleidomastoid and trapezius muscles. The nerve fibers of CNs IX, X, and XI emerge into the lateral cerebellomedullary cistern and extend anterolaterally toward the jugular foramen through which they exit the skull.

Damage to the cisternal segments of CNs IX, X, and XI can produce dysphagia, guttural dysarthria, loss of taste from the posterior third of the tongue, parotid gland dysfunction, autonomic instability due to impairment of baroreceptor and chemoreceptor function, and paretic shoulder shrug and head turn. Damage can result from compression, trauma, infiltration, demyelination, or infection. Compression of the nerves can occur from tumors of the cerebellopontine angle or lesions at the jugular foramen (**Fig. 34**).

The axons of CN XII, the hypoglossal nerve, originate in the hypoglossal nucleus in the posteromedial medulla and innervate the extrinsic and intrinsic muscles of the tongue. CN XII fibers emerge from the medulla in the ipsilateral preolivary sulcus and extend anterolaterally toward the hypoglossal canal through which they exit the skull (**Fig. 35**). Damage to hypoglossal nerve fibers results in ipsilateral weakness of the tongue and associated lingual dysarthria. The cisternal segment of the hypoglossal nerve can be damaged by compression or trauma.

Intra-axial Segments

In the intra-axial segment, various lesions can occur affecting the ocular motor nuclei and fascicles including infarction, hemorrhage, demyelination, tumor, and trauma. A unilateral lesion affecting the nucleus of CN III may induce a deficit of the ipsilateral medial and inferior rectus and inferior oblique, together with a contralateral superior rectus muscle palsy. Impairment of the caudal portion of the nucleus may induce bilateral ptosis because this portion innervates both levator palpebrae muscles. Weber syndrome (CN III palsy and contralateral hemiplegia—involvement of the crus cerebri) and Claude syndrome (CN III palsy and contralateral ataxia—involvement of the red

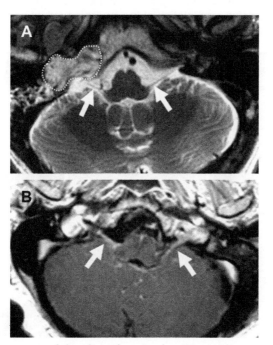

Fig. 34. Cisternal segments of the glossopharyngeal-vagus-accessory nerve complex. (*A*) An axial T2WI showing the cisternal segments of the glossopharyngeal-vagus-accessory nerve complex (*arrows*) in a patient with a paraganglioma (*dotted line*) of the right jugular fossa. (*B*) Axial T1WI following intravenous administration of gadolinium contrast shows abnormal enhancement of bilateral cisternal segments of the glossopharyngeal-vagus-accessory nerve complex (*arrows*) in a patient with leptomeningeal carcinomatosis. Abnormal enhancement of the leptomeninges is also noted on the surface of the medulla.

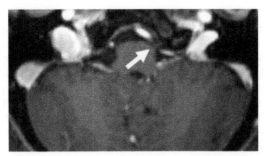

Fig. 35. Cisternal segment of the left hypoglossal nerve. An axial T1WI following intravenous administration of gadolinium contrast shows the cisternal segment of the left hypoglossal nerve (*arrow*) from its origin in the preolivary sulcus of the medulla. The contrast-enhancing left vertebral artery can be seen on either side of the nerve.

nucleus) always indicate a parenchymal lesion. Hemorrhage in the brainstem might arise from a cavernoma (**Fig. 36**). The most common causes of CN III palsy in children are intra-axial congenital, followed by traumatic and neoplastic causes. MRI of the brain and orbits with gadolinium and MRA is indicated, as associated CNS disease is often present, even among congenital cases.

CN IV is prone to traumatic damage because its nucleus and fascicles are posteriorly located and might be contused against the adjacent tentorium. CN IV palsy can be caused in hydrocephalus by dilatation of the sylvian aqueduct and downward pressure from an enlarged third ventricle.

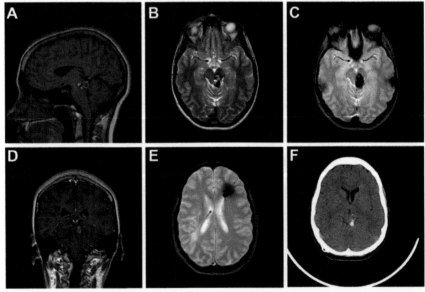

Fig. 36. Multiple congenital cavernous malformations. A 36-year-old female with diplopia secondary to hemorrhage with involvement of the upper brainstem eye movement centers, including CN III nuclei and fascicles. Cavernous malformations can be seen with mixed signal changes in left midbrain, in the left frontal periventricular white matter on sagittal native T1-weighted (*A*), axial T2-weighted (*B*), T2 gradient echo (*C, E*), and coronal T1-weighted contrast-enhanced (*D*) and axial noncontrast CT image (*F*). Arrow points to the lesion on all sequences.

Diseases affecting the parenchymal segments of CN V (the nucleus and fascicle) include ischemic lesions, inflammatory processes (**Fig. 37**), neoplasms, and cavernous angiomas. Posterior inferior cerebellar artery infarcts may affect the dorsal trigeminal nucleus and tract among others in the caudal pons and medulla; the evolving clinical picture is called Wallenberg syndrome. The signal characteristics of acute demyelinating lesions is identical to other locations in the neuraxis, low to intermediate signal intensity on T1WI, high signal intensity on T2WI and T2-FLAIR, and enhancement after intravenous administration of gadolinium; in the chronic phase contrast enhancement disappears.[12] Lesions of the intrapontine fascicular segment of the trigeminal nerve are typically linear plaques, and these can be considered distinctive MRI findings in patients with relapsing-remitting MS or clinically isolated syndrome presenting with CN V palsy[29] (**Fig. 38**).

Damage to the nuclei of CNs VII to XII can result in a variety of clinical deficits and syndromes and can result from intrapontine and intramedullary lesions including infarctions, hemorrhages, tumors, and demyelinating lesions. The coexistence of cranial neuropathies and long track signs (ie, corticospinal weakness, impairment of dorsal column-medial lemniscal or spinothalamic sensory function, or spinocerebellar dysfunction) can help localize a lesion to an intra-axial rather than extra-axial location.

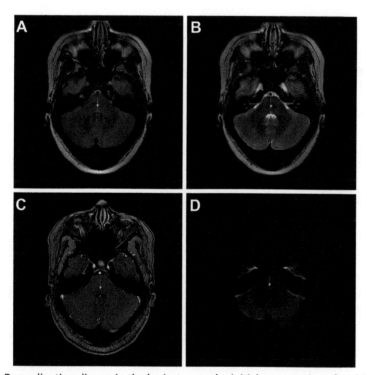

Fig. 37. Demyelinating disease in the brainstem as the initial presentation of multiple sclerosis. 26-year-old African American woman presents with acute onset of diplopia secondary to bilateral internuclear ophtalmoplegia in the setting of severe hypertension 3 weeks prior to MR examination. Axial T2 FLAIR (*A*) and T2-weighted (*B*) images show hyperintens lesions in the medial longitudinal fasciculi bilaterally and symmetrically associated with mild peripheral enhancement on 3D fat-suppressed T1WI (*C*). Mild T2-shine through was seen on DWI (*D*) but no restriction. Midline yellow arrow points to the bilateral lesions on all sequences.

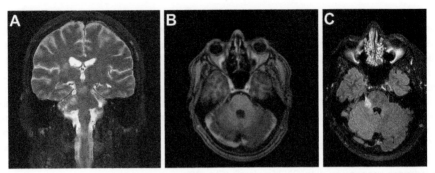

Fig. 38. Chronic demyelinating plaque affecting the trigeminal nerve fascicle, REZ, and nerve in MS in a 32-year-old man depicted on coronal T2WI (*A*), after contrast administration on axial T1WI (*B*) showing no significant enhancement and on T2 FLAIR (*C*) sequences. (*Courtesy of* György Várallyay, MD from MR Research Center at Semmelweis University, Budapest, Hungary.)

SUMMARY

Neuroimaging is the most frequently ordered ancillary test today in neurology. Neuroimaging, especially MRI, is highly sensitive for structural lesions but often nonspecific. Therefore, the most efficient way to practice patient-specific, precision medicine requires the neurologist to have neuroimaging expertise in order to translate the significance of imaging findings to the bedside.

DISCLOSURE

None.

REFERENCES

1. Blitz AM, Macedo LL, Chonka ZD, et al. High-resolution ciss mr imaging with and without contrast for evaluation of the upper cranial nerves. segmental anatomy and selected pathologic conditions of the cisternal through extraforaminal segments. Neuroimaging Clin N Am 2014;24(1):17–34.
2. Blitz AM, Choudhri AF, Chonka ZD, et al. Anatomic considerations, nomenclature, and advanced cross-sectional imaging techniques for visualization of the cranial nerve segments by MR imaging. Neuroimaging Clin N Am 2014;24(1):1–15.
3. Gillig PM, Sanders RD. Cranial nerve II: vision. Psychiatry (Edgmont) 2009;6(9):32–7.
4. Viallon M, Vargas M-I, Delavelle J, et al. Imaging of the optic nerve. Eur J Radiol 2010;74(2):299–313.
5. Ferreira T, Verbist B, van Buchem M, et al. Imaging the ocular motor nerves. Eur J Radiol 2010;74(2):314–22.
6. Borges A, Casselman J. Imaging the trigeminal nerve. Eur J Radiol 2010;74(2): 323–40.
7. Dodds NI, Atcha AW, Birchall D, et al. Use of high-resolution MRI of the optic nerve in Graves' ophthalmopathy. Br J Radiol 2009;82(979):541–4.
8. Szatmáry G. Imaging in patients with visual symptoms. Continuum (Minneap Minn) 2016;22(5, Neuroimaging):1499–528.
9. Szatmáry G. Neuro-ophthalmologic complications of neoplastic leptomeningeal disease. Curr Neurol Neurosci Rep 2013;13(12):404.

10. Whitman MC, Engle EC. Ocular congenital cranial dysinnervation disorders (CCDDs): insights into axon growth and guidance. Hum Mol Genet 2017; 26(R1):R37–44.
11. Digre KB, Lombardo NT, Frohman L. The neuro-ophthalmology virtual educational library (NOVEL). Neuroophthalmology 2007;31(5–6):175–8.
12. Brass SD, Zivadinov R, Bakshi R. Acute demyelinating optic neuritis: a review. Front Biosci 2008;13:2376–90.
13. Chen JJ, Flanagan EP, Jitprapaikulsan J, et al. Myelin oligodendrocyte glycoprotein antibody-positive optic neuritis: clinical characteristics, radiologic clues, and outcome. Am J Ophthalmol 2018;195:8–15.
14. Kidd DP, Burton BJ, Graham EM, et al. Optic neuropathy associated with systemic sarcoidosis. Neurol Neuroimmunol Neuroinflamm 2016;3(5):e270.
15. Bilgin G, Al-Obailan M, Bonelli L, et al. Aggressive low-grade optic nerve glioma in adults. Neuroophthalmology 2014;38(6):297–309.
16. Kiratli H, Tarlan B. Primary optic nerve sheath meningioma. Expert Rev Ophthalmol 2010;5(4):423–6.
17. Chandra P, Purandare N, Shah S, et al. Somatostatin receptor SPECT/CT using 99m TC labeled hynic-toc aids in diagnosis of primary optic nerve sheath meningioma. Indian J Nucl Med 2017;32(1):63.
18. Christmas NJ, Mead MD, Richardson EP, et al. Secondary optic nerve tumors. Surv Ophthalmol 1991;36(3):196–206.
19. Gonçalves ACP, Gebrim EMMS, Monteiro MLR. Imaging studies for diagnosing Graves' orbitopathy and dysthyroid optic neuropathy. Clinics (Sao Paulo) 2012; 67(11):1327–34.
20. Ferreira TA, Saraiva P, Genders SW, et al. CT and MR imaging of orbital inflammation. Neuroradiology 2018;60(12):1253–66.
21. Chen JS, Mukherjee P, Dillon WP, et al. Restricted diffusion in bilateral optic nerves and retinas as an indicator of venous ischemia caused by cavernous sinus thrombophlebitis. AJNR Am J Neuroradiol 2006;27(9):1815–6.
22. Sivak-Callcott JA, Livesley N, Nugent RA, et al. Localised invasive sino-orbital aspergillosis: characteristic features. Br J Ophthalmol 2004;88(5):681–7.
23. Vaphiades MS, Roberson GH. Imaging of oculomotor (third) cranial nerve palsy. Neurol Clin 2017;35(1):101–13.
24. Elmalem VI, Hudgins PA, Bruce BB, et al. Underdiagnosis of posterior communicating artery aneurysm in noninvasive brain vascular studies. J Neuroophthalmol 2011;31(2):103–9.
25. Nazir SA, Murphy SA, Siatkowski RM. Recurrent para-infectious third nerve palsy with cisternal nerve enhancement on MRI. J Neuroophthalmol 2004;24(1):96–7.
26. Yoshino N, Akimoto H, Yamada I, et al. Trigeminal neuralgia: evaluation of neuralgic manifestation and site of neurovascular compression with 3D CISS MR imaging and MR angiography. Radiology 2003;228(2):539–45.
27. Diluna ML, Bulsara KR. Surgery for petroclival meningiomas: a comprehensive review of outcomes in the skull base surgery era. Skull Base 2010;20(5):337–42.
28. Nagasawa D, Yew A, Safaee M, et al. Clinical characteristics and diagnostic imaging of epidermoid tumors. J Clin Neurosci 2011;18(9):1158–62.
29. Swinnen C, Lunskens S, Deryck O, et al. MRI characteristics of trigeminal nerve involvement in patients with multiple sclerosis. Mult Scler Relat Disord 2013;2(3): 200–3.

Neuroimaging of Multiple Sclerosis Mimics

Yathish Haralur, MD[a],*, Laszlo L. Mechtler, MD[b,1]

KEYWORDS

- MS mimics primary angiitis of CNS • Marchiafava-Bignami • Hashimoto encephalitis
- Neuro-Behçet • Limbic encephalitis • Susac syndrome • Neurosarcoidosis
- Bickerstaff brainstem encephalitis

KEY POINTS

- Multiple sclerosis mimics are one of the most commonly encountered clinical entities in the day to day life of a Neurologist.
- Understanding the neuro-imaging characteristics of these entities helps us to differentiate with confidence the MS variants and its mimics.
- In this chapter we discuss some of the common MS mimics and their imaging characteristics and ways to differentiate from MS and its variants.

INTRODUCTION

Multiple sclerosis (MS) is the most common immune-mediated disease of the central nervous system (CNS) and is characterized by demyelinating lesions of the brain and the spinal cord. It is extremely important that the appropriate imaging modalities are used for the proper diagnosis of this entity, which helps clinicians plan a therapeutic strategy in a timely manner to prevent further inflammation-mediated destruction of the white matter, leading to permanent disability. MRI has expanded the knowledge of lesion morphology, axonal degeneration with neuronal loss, progressive cerebral atrophy, and therapeutic responses to various immunomodulatory and immunosuppressive agents, and has allowed clinicians to scrutinize complications of therapies for MS. Neuroimaging has had the single greatest impact on the understanding and treatment of MS and its variants.

Although it is imperative that clinicians make the diagnosis of MS, it is also equally important that they recognize other CNS disorders in which the lesions are similar to MS lesions, commonly known as MS mimics. The differential diagnoses of MS include

Disclosures: None.
[a] Neuro-Hospitalist Program, Mississippi Baptist Medical Center, Jackson, MS, USA; [b] Dent Neurological Institute, Buffalo, NY, USA
[1] Present address: 3980 Sheridan Drive, Buffalo, NY 14226.
* Corresponding author. Hospitalist Program, 1225 N state St, 6th floor, Jackson, MS, 39202.
E-mail address: yathish.h.s@gmail.com

entities that lead to demyelination but are caused by other disorders, such as vascular, infectious, genetic, metabolic, granulomatous, and other immune-mediated conditions. In younger, typical populations, without other coexisting conditions, it is usually straightforward to make the diagnosis of MS. However, in older populations and in the presence of secondary disorders, diagnostic challenges prevail, which may lead to prolonged evaluation and delayed treatment. Therefore, understanding the morphologies of these lesions and typical MRI appearances in conjunction with the clinical picture helps with the proper diagnosis.

This article discusses the neuroimaging characteristics of various differential diagnoses (ie, MS mimics).

Primary Angiitis of the Central Nervous System

Primary angiitis of the CNS (PACNS), or primary CNS vasculitis, is a type of vasculitis characterized by fibrinoid necrosis of the small arteries and veins less than 200 μm in diameter in the meningeal and the parenchymal regions of the CNS. These patients commonly present with headaches, encephalopathy, seizures, signs of meningeal irritation, and focal neurologic deficits resulting from ischemic or hemorrhagic lesions[1] (**Figs. 1** and **2**).

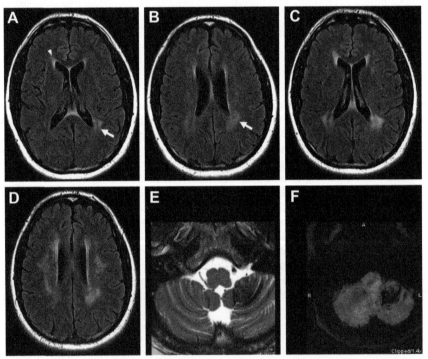

Fig. 1. Primary CNS vasculitis. A 40-year-old man who presented with disequilibrium, fatigue, and malaise initially suspected and later biopsy confirmed to be primary CNS vasculitis. Axial fluid-attenuated inversion recovery (FLAIR) images at the level of atria (*A*) and corona radiata (*B*) show bilateral periventricular confluent white matter hyperintensities (*arrows/arrow head*) in the frontal and parietal lobes. The follow-up images (*C, D*) 3 years later show symmetric progression. Parenchymal hematoma involving the left anterior inferior cerebellar region (*E, F*).

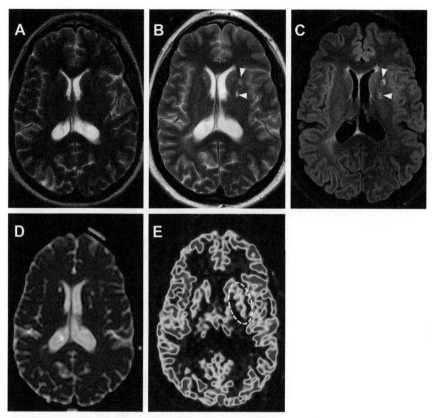

Fig. 2. Primary CNS vasculitis. A 25-year-old woman with headaches. Baseline T2-weighted axial scan (*A*) from 2013 shows no focal abnormality in the basal ganglia. The follow-up images from 2017 (*B–E*) show lacunar lesions in the basal ganglia, predominantly on the left (*arrowheads*). The lesions are hyperintense on T2 (*B*), have hyperintense margins on FLAIR (*C*), and show increased diffusion on apparent diffusion coefficient (ADC) map (*D*), consistent with chronic abnormalities. Pseudocontinuous arterial spin labeling (*E*) shows lower relative cerebral blood flow in the area of the left putamen (*circled area*).

Neuroimaging characteristics

- Neuroimaging in the initial stages can be normal but can show progressive confluent white matter lesions.
- Multiple ischemic lesions not restricted to any single vascular territory.
- Large intraparenchymal hematomas.
- Leptomeningeal enhancement.

Morphology of the lesions

- T2 and fluid-attenuated inversion recovery (FLAIR) images: multiple cortical and subcortical, confluent or discrete areas of T2 hyperintensities may be seen.
- T1-weighted (precontrast and postcontrast) imaging sequences: areas of hypointense lesions, which are either small or large, are noted with variable contrast enhancement. Leptomeningeal inflammation may show contrast enhancement.

> **Box 1**
> **Diagnostic criteria for Hashimoto encephalitis**
>
> Diagnosis can be made when all 6 of the following criteria have been met:
> 1. Encephalopathy with seizures, myoclonus, hallucinations, or strokelike episodes
> 2. Subclinical or mild overt thyroid disease (usually hypothyroidism)
> 3. Brain MRI normal or with nonspecific abnormalities
> 4. Presence of serum thyroid (thyroid peroxidase, thyroglobulin) antibodies
> 5. Absence of well-characterized neuronal antibodies in serum and cerebrospinal fluid (CSF)
> 6. Reasonable exclusion of alternative causes
>
> *Data from* Castillo P, Woodruff B, Caselli R, et al. Steroid-responsive encephalopathy associated with autoimmune thyroiditis. Archives of Neurology. 2006; 63(2):197–202.

- Diffusion weighted imaging (DWI)/apparent diffusion coefficient (ADC): areas of infarctions may show restricted diffusion.
- Susceptibility-weighted imaging: large parenchymal hemorrhages or microhemorrhages show blooming artifacts on the susceptibility-weighted images.

Hashimoto Encephalopathy

Hashimoto encephalopathy (HE)/Hashimoto encephalitis is a type of immune-mediated encephalopathy caused by antibodies associated with Hashimoto thyroiditis (anti–thyroid peroxidase antibody [TPOAb] and/or antithyroglobulin antibody

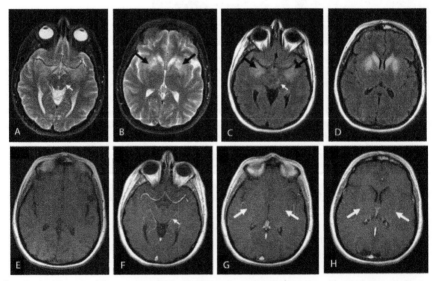

Fig. 3. A 37-year-old woman with Hashimoto encephalopathy. Brain MRI performed 6 months after the onset of symptoms. Axial T2 (*A, B*) and axial FLAIR (*C, D*) show symmetric and bilateral areas of abnormal high signal on T2-weighted and FLAIR images involving the mesial temporal lobes, caudate nuclei, and putamen (*black arrows*). The basal ganglia lesions are minimally hyperintense on T1-weighted images (*E*). These lesions have fine serpiginous enhancement on T1-weighted postcontrast images (*G, H*) (*white arrows*). In addition, a left midbrain lesion, hyperintense on T2-weighted and FLAIR images (*A, C*), shows no enhancement of gadolinium (*F*) (*small white arrow*).

[TgAb]). HE is most often characterized by a subacute onset of altered mental status, seizures, and myoclonus[2] (**Box 1, Fig. 3**).

Neuroimaging characteristics

- Typically, there are no abnormal findings on neuroimaging.[3–6]
- Nonspecific changes within the subcortical white matter are usually seen in about half of the patients, which may be incidental findings or may resemble chronic ischemic microangiopathy. Some of the lesions may show resolution.
- Demyelinating lesions may be seen within the basal ganglia and hippocampi, which may be bilateral and symmetric. Demyelinating lesions may be seen in the brain stem.
- Bilateral hippocampal lesions and meningeal enhancement may be seen.

Morphology of the lesions

- T2-weighted and FLAIR image sequences: nonspecific discrete T2 hyperintensities in subcortical white matter. Large discrete T2 hyperintensity resembling a demyelinating plaque may be seen in the deep gray structures and brain stem. Irregular T2 hyperintensities involving both the hippocampi may also be seen.
- T1-weighted precontrast and postcontrast image sequences. The nonspecific T2 changes do not show gadolinium enhancement. Meningeal enhancement may be seen in some cases.

Marchiafava-Bignami Disease

Marchiafava-Bignami disease is a rare disorder characterized by demyelination followed by necrosis of the corpus callosum secondary to toxic (alcohol) and metabolic (vitamin B deficiency) causes. Neurologic manifestations include dementia, dysarthria, aphasia, hemiparesis, ataxia, or apraxia that are not fully explained by the characteristic corpus callosum and centrum semiovale alone[7] (**Figs. 4 and 5**).

Neuroimaging characteristics

- Corpus callosum is classically involved, with the lesions extending into adjacent centrum semiovale and corona radiata. It typically starts in the body during the initial stages of the disease and later spreads anteriorly into the genu and posteriorly into the splenium.[8]
- Compared with MS, Marchiafava-Bignami has symmetric and confluent lesions within the corpus callosum; in contrast, the MS lesions are discrete, multiple ovoid lesions arranged in radial fashion (Dawson's fingers)

Morphology of the lesions

- T2-weighted and FLAIR images: in acute-phase, confluent hyperintensities within the corpus callosum are seen. The subacute phase shows hypointensity on T2 caused by hemosiderin deposition. The chronic stage shows cystic lesions hyperintense on T2 and dark on FLAIR.[8–10]
- T1-weighted images: hypointensities during the acute phase and chronic cystic lesions appear well circumscribed and hypointense.
- Diffusion-weighted imaging (DWI) and ADC sequences: true restricted diffusion, bright on DWI and dark on ADC, is seen in the acute stage.
- Magnetic resonance (MR) spectroscopy: here is a progressive decrease in N-acetyl aspartate (NAA)/creatine (Cr) ratio, which may recover partially by a year.

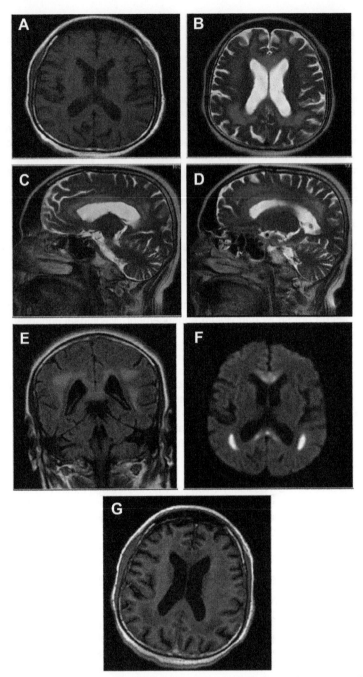

Fig. 4. Marchiafava-Bignami. A 45-year-old chronic alcoholic patient presenting with seizures, altered sensorium, and bilateral lower limb paresis. T1-weighted (*A*) image shows hypointense corpus callosum and periventricular white matter with corresponding T2-weighted (*B–D*) and FLAIR (*E*) images showing hyperintense signal with true restricted diffusion on diffusion-weighted imaging (DWI) (*F*). No postcontrast enhancement is seen (*G*). (*From* Logan, C., Asadi, H., Kok, et al. (2017), Neuroimaging of chronic alcohol misuse. J Med Imaging Radiat Oncol, 61: 435–440. https://doi.org/10.1111/1754-9485.12572; with permission.)

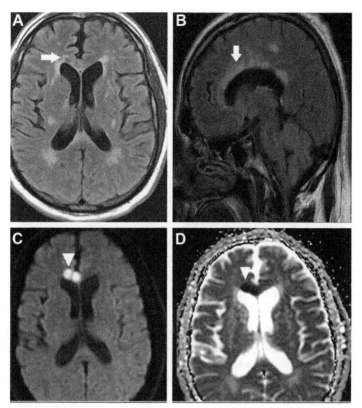

Fig. 5. Marchiafava-Bignami. A 58-year-old man with chronic alcoholism, drinking a bottle of whisky a day for more than 20 years, presenting with progressive memory decline and gait instability. Axial and sagittal FLAIR (*A*, *B*) showing areas of T2 hyperintensities involving the corpus callosum (*white arrows*). MRI showing high signal on axial DWI (*C*) and low signal on ADC (*D*) consistent with cytotoxic edema (*arrowheads*).

Neuro-Behçet Disease

Behçet disease is a rare form of vasculitis commonly affecting small vessels and less commonly medium-sized and large arteries. It is characterized by orogenital ulcers, uveitis, arthritis, and gastrointestinal manifestations. A neurologic manifestation, also called as neuro-Behçet disease (NBD), is a CNS parenchymal inflammatory syndrome commonly affecting the brain stem and basal ganglia and may involve hemispheres or the spinal cord[1,11] (**Box 2, Fig. 6**).

Neuroimaging characteristics

- Parenchymal disease: lesions resembling the demyelinating process mainly involving the brain stem and basal ganglia.[12–14] It may also involve spinal cord and cerebral white matter, resembling MS lesions, without specific predilection toward periventricular white matter. The lesions may be focal or multifocal in distribution.
- Cranial neuropathy: optic neuritis is the commonest of the cranial neuropathies. Other cranial nerves may be involved as well.

Box 2
International consensus recommendation criteria for neuro-Behçet disease diagnosis

a. Definite NBD meets all of the following 3 criteria:
   1. Satisfies the (current accepted) International Study Group criteria for Behçet disease
   2. Neurologic syndrome[a] (with objective neurologic signs) recognized to be caused by Behçet disease and supported by relevant and characteristic abnormalities seen on either or both:
      a. Neuroimaging
      b. CSF
   3. No better explanation for the neurologic findings

b. Probable NBD meets 1 of the following 2 criteria in the absence of a better explanation for the neurologic findings:
   1. Neurologic syndrome as in definite NBD, with systemic Behçet disease features but not satisfying the International Study Group criteria
   2. A noncharacteristic neurologic syndrome occurring in the context of International Study Group criteria–supported Behçet disease

[a] Parenchymal syndromes: cerebral, brainstem, myelopathic, optic nerve, multifocal (diffuse). Nonparenchymal syndromes: cerebral venous thrombosis, intracranial hypertension syndrome, acute meningeal syndrome.
From Kalra S, et al. Diagnosis and management of Neuro-Behçet's disease: international consensus recommendations. J Neurol 2014;261(9); with permission.

- Vascular manifestations: arteritis of small vessels is common, but medium and large vessel arteritis may also be seen. Dural venous sinus thrombosis is common in children, whereas adults usually manifest parenchymal disease.
- Meningoencephalitis may appear normal on MRI, occasionally showing meningeal enhancement.

Morphology of the lesions

a. Parenchymal NBD
   1. Acute/subacute stage
      - T1-weighted images: hypointense to isointense lesions with patchy contrast enhancement.
      - T2-weighted and T2 FLAIR sequences: confluent hyperintense lesions mainly in brain stem and basal ganglia, occasionally in spinal cord.
      - Diffusion-weighted images: hyperintensity may be caused by true restricted diffusion or T2 shine-through.
      - MR spectroscopy - Decreased NAA peak in the acute stage, which normalizes when lesion resolve.
   2. Chronic stage:
      - T2-weighted images show discrete, nonspecific white matter, especially in the brainstem, with resolution of contrast enhancement with or without atrophy.
b. Nonparenchymal NBD
   1. MR or computed tomography (CT) venography may show evidence of cerebral sinus or vein thrombosis.
   2. Meningeal enhancement on postcontrast T1 images represents meningitis.

Limbic Encephalitis

Limbic encephalitis (LE) refers to an autoimmune inflammatory process involving the structures of the limbic system, commonly caused by a paraneoplastic process

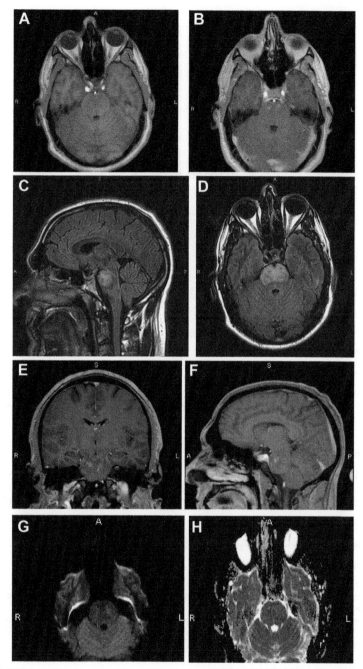

Fig. 6. A 38-year-old man presenting with recurrent diplopia and recurrent oral ulcers. Axial pre (*A*) and post (*B*) contrast T1-weighted MRI sequences show isointense areas with patchy contrast enhancement within the pons. Sagittal (*C*) and axial (*D*) FLAIR sequences show confluent hyperintense lesions within the pons. Postcontrast coronal (*E*) and sagittal (*F*) T1-weighted images show patchy enhancement within the pons. Axial diffusion-weighted image (*G*) shows hyperintensity within the left pons, which is isointense on the ADC (*H*) axial image. Complete resolution of the pontine lesions after immunosuppressive therapy as seen on axial T1-weighted precontrast (*I*) and postcontrast (*J*) images and axial FLAIR (*K*) sequences.

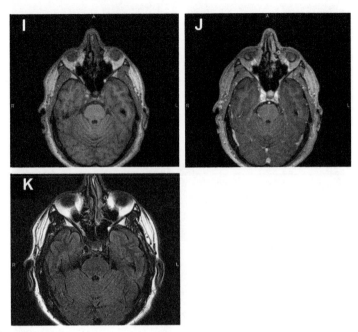

Fig. 6. (*continued*).

but can occur as an autoimmune syndrome without a cancer association. LE most commonly presents with rapidly progressive short-term memory loss, psychiatric symptoms, and seizures[15] (**Box 3**, **Fig. 7**).

Neuroimaging characteristics

- Imaging findings may be normal during the early course of the disease.[9,16–22]
- The perivascular inflammation and demyelination are similar to MS, but usually associated with fever and monophasic. In contrast, MS lesions are separated

---

Box 3
Diagnostic criteria

1. Pathologic demonstration of LE, or

2. All 4 of the following:
   a. Symptoms of short-term memory loss, seizures, or psychiatric symptoms suggesting the involvement of limbic system
   b. Less than 4 years between the onset of neurologic symptoms and the cancer diagnosis
   c. Exclusion of metastasis, infection, metabolic and nutritional deficits, stroke, and side effects of therapy that may cause limbic encephalopathy
   d. At least 1 of the following:
      i. CSF with inflammatory findings
      ii. MRI FLAIR or T2 unilateral or bilateral temporal lobe hyperintensities
      iii. Electroencephalogram (EEG) with epileptic or slow activity focally involving the temporal lobes

From Gultekin SH, Rosenfeld MR, Voltz R, et al. Paraneoplastic limbic encephalitis: Neurological symptoms, immunological findings and tumor association in 50 patients. Brain. 2000;123:1481–94; with permission.

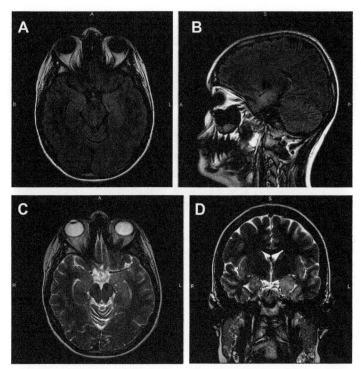

Fig. 7. A 28-year-old with short-term memory loss with biopsy-positive and glutamic acid decarboxylase (GAD) 65–positive autoimmune encephalitis in the setting of papillary carcinoma of thyroid. Axial (*A*) and sagittal (*B*) FLAIR image sequences show hyperintensities in the bilateral hippocampus and the mesial temporal lobe areas. Axial (*C*) and coronal (*D*) T2-weighted image sequences show hyperintensities in the bilateral hippocampal and the mesial temporal lobe areas.

in time and space, are much more diffusely distributed, and typically are not associated with fever.

- Cortical thickening of the mesial temporal lobes, commonly bilateral, is noted in 60% of cases.
- Bilateral basal ganglia are frequently involved.

Morphology of the lesions

- T2-weighted and FLAIR images: irregular areas of hyperintensities are noted within the mesial temporal and basal ganglia.
- T1-weighted precontrast and postcontrast images: the precontrast lesions are isointense with patchy contrast enhancement.
- DWI and ADC: hyperintense on diffusion-weighted images with no ADC correlate (T2 shine-through)

Susac syndrome

Susac syndrome is a microangiopathic process with a triad of encephalopathy, sensorineural hearing loss, and visual disturbances[1] (**Figs. 8–10**).

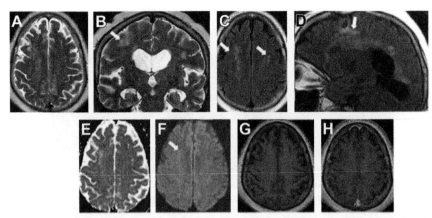

Fig. 8. Susac syndrome. A 71-year-old man with biopsy-positive Susac syndrome showing discrete hyperintensities (*arrows*) in the region of the periventricular deep white matter and centrum semiovale on axial (*A*) and sagittal (*B*) T2-weighted images and on axial (*C*) and sagittal (*D*) FLAIR image sequences. Axial DWI (*F*) shows hyperintensity with axial ADC hyperintensity (*E*) T2 shine-through. Axial precontrast (*G*) and postcontrast (*H*) T1-weighted images show hypointense lesions with no enhancement.

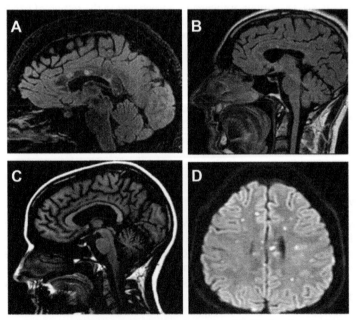

Fig. 9. Susac syndrome. Sagittal FLAIR image sequence (*A, B*) showing typical corpus callosum hyperintense snowball lesions, icicles, and spokes in the genu, body, and the splenium. Sagittal T1-weighted (*C*) images showing black holes. Axial DWI (*D*) showing several areas of restricted diffusion in the corpus callosum and centrum semiovale.

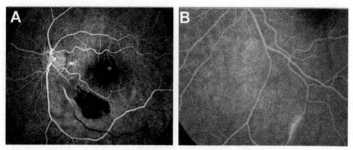

Fig. 10. Susac syndrome. Fluorescein angiography. (*A*) Branch retinal artery occlusions and vessel wall hyperfluorescence. (*B*) Segmental vessel wall hyperfluorescence and leakage.

Neuroimaging characteristics

- The characteristic lesions on MRI, known as snowballs, represent microinfarctions/microischemias of the central corpus callosum fibers.[2] Other characteristic lesions include linear infarcts (spokes) and upper fiber infarcts (icicles).
- Internal capsule infarctions can be seen, in a string-of-beads pattern. Fluorescein angiography and tonal audiometry can provide important clues, in patients who currently do not have visual or auditory symptoms, toward making a diagnosis of Susac syndrome.
- Branch retinal artery occlusions and segmental vessel wall hyperfluorescence are pathognomonic findings.

Morphology of the lesions

- T2-weighted and FLAIR images: discrete hyperintensities involving the corpus callosum resembling the snowball appearance.
- T1-weighted images: the corpus callosal lesions appear hypointense on the T1-weighted images without contrast enhancement.
- DWI/ADC: hyperintense DWI with no ADC hypointensity (T2 shine-through). True restricted diffusion (with low ADC) may be seen in acute microinfarcts.

Cerebral Autosomal Dominant Arteriopathy with Subcortical Infarcts and Leukoencephalopathy

Cerebral autosomal dominant arteriopathy with subcortical infarcts and leukoencephalopathy (CADASIL) is an autosomal dominant microangiopathy caused by the mutations in the NOTCH3 gene with age-dependent clinical manifestations. The earliest of the manifestations is migraine with auras, usually presenting within the third decade of life, with subcortical lacunar infarcts occurring by the fifth decade and the neuropsychiatric manifestations later as the microangiopathy progresses[23] (**Fig. 11**).

Neuroimaging characteristics

- Confluent white matter changes involving the centrum semiovale and corona radiata.[24–30]
- External capsule and subcortical region of the anterior temporal lesions are classic.
- Lacunar infarcts are seen involving the subcortical regions, especially the gray-white junction.

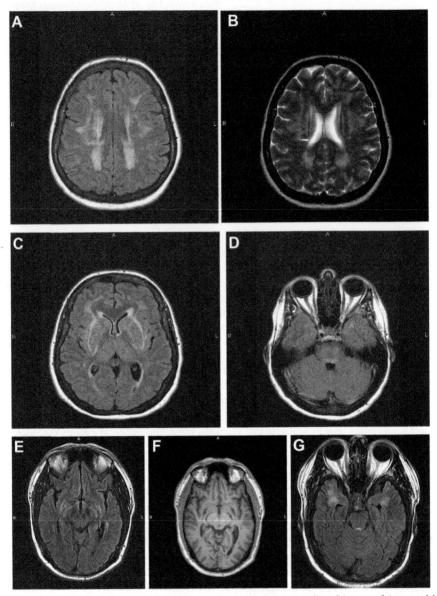

Fig. 11. CADASIL. A 45-year-old white woman with long-standing history of intractable migraines, cognitive impairment, and depression diagnosed with CADASIL positive for NOTCH3 gene sequence. Axial FLAIR (*A*) and T2-weighted (*B*) image sequences showing confluent hyperintensities involving the centrum semiovale and corona radiata appearing as mirror images of each other. Axial FLAIR image sequences showing hyperintensities in the external capsules (*C*) and anterior temporal lobes (*D*) are classic MRI findings. A 48-year-old man with presenting with migraines diagnosed with CADASIL. Axial FLAIR (*E*) sequence showing lacunar infarcts, seen as ovoid, circumscribed, hyperintense lesions arranged in a linear fashion, and axial T1-weighted sequences (*F*) showing the lacunar infarcts seen as well-circumscribed areas of hypointensities (*black holes*). Axial FLAIR image (*G*) showing anterior temporal lesions. A 27-year-old with family history of CADASIL involving multiple family members on paternal side who presented with migraines and was later diagnosed with CADASIL. FLAIR axial (*H*) and sagittal (*I*) image sequences show hyperintensities within the anterior part of the temporal regions. Axial FLAIR (*J*) and T2-weighted (*K*) image sequences showing external capsular lesion appearing earlier in the disease course.

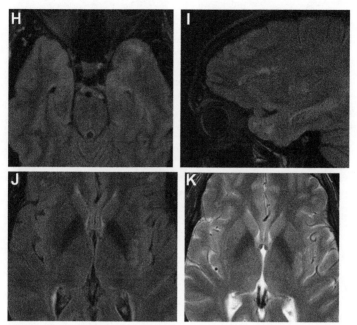

Fig. 11. (*continued*).

- Cerebral microhemorrhages are an important feature with no characteristic distribution.
- Cerebral atrophy is usually seen in advanced disease with neurocognitive decline.
- Optic nerve and spinal cord lesions are characteristic of MS, whereas CADASIL is more likely to involve anterior temporal lobes.

Characteristic MRI findings

- T2-weighted and FLAIR sequences:
  - Confluent hyperintensities involving the centrum semiovale and corona radiata appear as mirror images of each other.
  - The external capsular lesions appear as linear hyperintensities.
  - Lacunar infarcts are seen as rounded, circumscribed, hyperintense lesions arranged in a linear fashion.
- T1-weighted sequences: lacunar infarcts are seen as well-circumscribed areas of hypointensity (black holes).
- Gradient echo/susceptibility-weighted sequences: microhemorrhages are seen as well-circumscribed, ovoid areas of hypointensities (susceptibility artifacts) measuring 2 to 5 mm.
- Diffusion weighted: acute lacunar infarcts may show restricted diffusion.

Neurosarcoidosis

CNS complication (neurosarcoidosis) is seen in about 5% of the patients with sarcoidosis, involving both central and peripheral nervous systems with various clinical

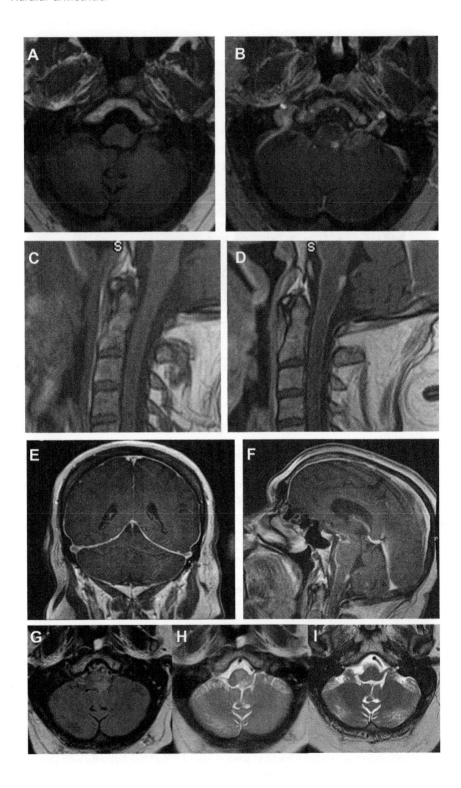

manifestations based on the location. There is cranial neuropathy, especially involving the optic nerve and facial nerve; neuroendocrine manifestations when the hypothalamus and the pituitary are involved; myelopathic symptoms (sensory, motor, and autonomic); signs of meningitis/encephalitis from pachymeningeal/leptomeningeal involvement; and inflammatory peripheral neuropathy resembling Guillain-Barré syndrome[31] (Fig. 12).

Neuroimaging characteristics

- Parenchymal involvement: parenchymal lesions may appear as small, discrete lesions indistinguishable from MS.
- Meningeal involvement:
  - Pachymeningeal disease may involve both supratentorial and infratentorial regions that show thickening with contrast enhancement.
  - Leptomeningeal disease may appear normal, thickening with contrast enhancement.
- Pituitary involvement: may show thickening with enhancement of the pituitary stalk.
- Cranial nerve involvement may show enlargement/enhancement in the acute stage and atrophy in the chronic stage. Optic neuritis in sarcoidosis may be indistinguishable from that in MS.
- Ventriculomegaly caused by communicating hydrocephalus.
- Spinal lesions:
  - Cord lesions usually involving the subpial regions
  - Thickening with enhancement of the spinal nerve roots, especially the cauda equine.

Morphology of the lesions

- T2 weighted and : parenchymal lesions are hyperintense, nodular, and discrete. They may extend from the leptomeninges, periventricular regions (indistinguishable from MS), or the subpial regions when involving the spinal cord.
- T1-weighted postcontrast images: the discrete parenchymal lesions may show contrast enhancement in the acute stage. Leptomeningeal or pachymeningeal enhancement may be diffuse or focal. Pituitary involvement shows thickening with enhancement of the infundibulum. Optic and facial neuropathy may show contrast enhancement in the acute phase. Cauda equine involvement shows enhancement, thickening, and clumping of the nerve roots.

◀━━━

Fig. 12. Neurosarcoidosis. Axial T1-weighted precontrast (A) and postcontrast (B) images show a homogeneously contrast-enhancing mass in posterior part of the left medulla. There is thickening and enhancement of the left glossopharyngeal nerve. Sagittal precontrast (C) and postcontrast (D) T1-weighted images show leptomeningeal enhancement of the brain stem and the upper part of the cervical spine. Coronal (E) and sagittal (F) T1 postcontrast image sequence shows pachymeningeal enhancement involving the cerebral convexity and tentorium cerebella. Also seen is leptomeningeal enhancement anterior to the brain stem (B) and (D). Axial FLAIR (G) and T2-weighted (H) image sequence showing the lesion in the posterior part of the left medulla. Thickening of the left glossopharyngeal nerve is noted on the axial T2 image sequence (I).

Lyme Disease

Lyme disease of the nervous system, also known as neuroborreliosis, is a tick-borne illness that is caused, at least in the United States, by a spirochetal organism, *Borrelia burgdorferi*. Neurologic manifestations may include lymphocytic meningitis, cranial neuropathies, peripheral neuropathies mimicking Guillain-Barré syndrome, multiple mononeuropathies, encephalomyelitis, and cerebellar ataxia.

Neuroimaging characteristics

- Occult lesions may be seen in brain and spinal cord.[32–39]
- The severity of the white matter lesions is mild, resembling nonspecific lesions as seen in chronic ischemic microangiopathy. In contrast, in MS the demyelination is moderate to severe, causing damage of the parenchyma.
- MRI may show rare tumefactive white matter lesions.
- Antibiotic treatment may cause resolution of the MRI lesions.

Lesion morphology

- T2-weighted and FLAIR image sequences: irregular discrete areas of hyperintensities in the subcortical and juxtacortical regions are noted in lyme disease. The MS lesions are periventricular in distribution, and tend to be well-defined ovoid lesions.
- T1-weighted image sequences: may be normal but can show discrete areas of hypointensities

CHRONIC LYMPHOCYTIC INFLAMMATION WITH PONTINE PERIVASCULAR ENHANCEMENT RESPONSIVE TO STEROIDS

Chronic lymphocytic inflammation with pontine perivascular enhancement responsive to steroids (CLIPPERS) is a distinct radiological, clinical, neuropathologic, biopsy-proven entity.[40] It presents with gait ataxia, dysarthria, pseudobulbar affect, facial paresthesia/hypoesthesia, spasticity, diplopia (occasionally episodic), and other signs of brainstem and cerebellar involvement.[40–42] CLIPPERS is a young entity and debate still exists whether it is underdiagnosed. Differential diagnosis

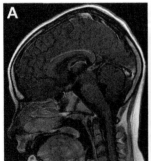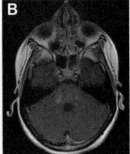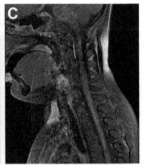

Fig. 13. CLIPPERS: MRI features of a patient at her initial presentation at 10 years of age. Sagittal T1 (*A*) brain MRI with gadolinium showing nodular enhancements peppering the pons and upper cervical spinal cord; axial T1 brain (*B*) MRI showing contrast enhancement in midbrain and cerebellar peduncles; sagittal T1 spine (*C*) MRI showing diffuse nodular enhancement in cervical and thoracic spine.

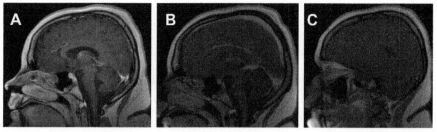

Fig. 14. CLIPPERS. Sagittal T1 brain (*A*) MRI with gadolinium at the age of 14 years showing resolution of the previously seen enhancements and atrophy of pons, midbrain, and cerebellum; sagittal T1 brain (*B, C*) MRI at the age of 15 years showing radiological relapse involving brain stem and periventricular white matter.

includes other MS mimics discussed earlier in this article. Pathologically, CLIPPERS is characterized by perivascular and diffuse parenchymal T-cell infiltrate with intact myelin[40] (**Figs. 13–15**).

Neuroimaging of Chronic Lymphocytic Inflammation with Pontine Perivascular Enhancement Responsive to Steroids

- Classic MRI appearance is peppering in the pons, referring to a pattern of curvilinear, punctate enhancement in the pons and extending variably into adjacent craniocaudal structures.[40]
- It can involve spinal cord in a linear distribution of the punctate enhancement extending down into the cervical and thoracic spinal cord.

Lesion Morphology

- T2-weighted and FLAIR image sequences: irregular and punctate patchy T2 hyperintensities.[40–49]
- T1 precontrast and postcontrast: multiple, punctate, patchy, linear regions of contrast enhancement relatively confined to pons.
- Susceptibility-weighted images: prominent veins in the brainstem and cerebellum.

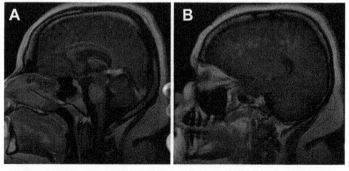

Fig. 15. CLIPPERS. Sagittal T1 post contrast (A and B) brain MRI at the age of 15 years when she had a clinicalrelapse showing multiple nodular enhancements involving cerebral hemispheres, brainstem, and upper cervical spinal cord.

- Perfusion-weighted imaging (dynamic susceptibility-weighted imaging): shows lower values of relative cerebral blood flow and relative cerebral blood volume compared with age-matched controls.
- Magnetic resonance spectroscopy: shows reduced NAA/Cr ratio in the pons and bilateral thalami.
- PET-CT: shows minimal hypermetabolism, hence differentiating it from lymphoma.

Bickerstaff Brainstem Encephalitis

Bickerstaff brainstem encephalitis (BBE) was initially described in 1951 as inflammatory disorder of the CNS and peripheral nervous system.[46] This condition has clinical features as seen in both Guillain-Barré syndrome and Miller Fischer syndrome. BBE is radiologically very similar to CLIPPERS but lesions of BBE are usually isolated to the brainstem, with no rostrocaudal extension. The classic peppering noted in the latter has not been reported in BBE.[46] However, it is important to look for and rule out other secondary causes, including infectious, paraneoplastic, granulomatous, other autoimmune disorders, such as lupus.

Routine MRI sequences in conjunction with advance neuroimaging modalities, including PET-CT scans, MR spectroscopy, and MR/CT perfusion scans and arterial spin labeling scans, provide more information about in vivo morphology without having to obtain biopsy of these lesions. These imaging findings, along with the clinical assessment and other laboratory analyses, are invaluable in establishing the correct diagnosis and differentiating MS from other conditions, which aids physicians in formulating treatment plans.

REFERENCES

1. Dimberg EL. Rheumatology and neurology. Continuum (Minneap Minn) 2017; 23(3):691–721. Available at: http://journals.lww.com/continuum/Fulltext/2017/06000/Rheumatology_and_Neurology.9.aspx.
2. Lublin FD, Reingold SC, Cohen JA, et al. Defining the clinical course of multiple sclerosis: The 2013 revisions. Neurology 2014. https://doi.org/10.1212/WNL.0000000000000560.
3. Chong JY, Rowland LP, Utiger RD. Hashimoto encephalopathy: Syndrome or myth? Arch Neurol 2003;60(2):164–71.
4. Castillo P, Woodruff B, Caselli R, et al. Steroid-responsive encephalopathy associated with autoimmune thyroiditis. Arch Neurol 2006;63(2):197–202.
5. Forchetti CM, Katsamakis G, Garron DC. Autoimmune thyroiditis and a rapidly progressive dementia: global hypoperfusion on SPECT scanning suggests a possible mechanism. Neurology 1997;49(2):623.
6. Ramalho J, Castillo M. Hashimoto's encephalopathy. Radiol Case Rep 2011; 6(1):445.
7. Brust JCM. Persistent cognitive impairment in substance abuse. Continuum (Minneap Minn) 2004;10(5):144–50.
8. Gambini A, Falini A, Moiola, et al. Marchiafava-Bignami disease: longitudinal MR imaging and MR spectroscopy study. AJNR Am J Neuroradiol 2003;24(2): 249–53.
9. Bano S, Mehra S, Yadav SN, et al. Marchiafava-Bignami disease: Role of neuroimaging in the diagnosis and management of acute disease. Neurol India 2009; 57(5):649–52.

10. Tozakidou M, Stippich C, Fischmann A. Teaching neuroimages: radiologic findings in Marchiafava-Bignami disease. Neurology 2011;77:e67.
11. Koc Y, Gullu I, Akpek G, et al. Vascular involvement in Behcet's disease. J Rheumatol 1992;19(3):402–10.
12. Lee SH, Yoon PH, Park SJ, et al. MRI findings in neuro-behçet's disease. Clin Radiol 2001;56(6):485.
13. Akman-Demir G, Serdaroglu P, Tasçi B. Clinical patterns of neurological involvement in Behçet's disease: evaluation of 200 patients. The Neuro-Behçet Study Group. Brain 1999;122(Pt 11):2171.
14. Uluduz D, Kürtüncü M, Yapıcı Z, et al. Clinical characteristics of pediatric-onset neuro-Behçet disease. Neurology 2011;77(21):1900–5.
15. Tüzün E, Dalmau J. Limbic encephalitis and variants: classification, diagnosis and treatment. Neurologist 2007;13:261–71.
16. Oyanguren B, Sánchez V, González FJ, et al. Limbic encephalitis: a clinical-radiological comparison between herpetic and autoimmune etiologies. Eur J Neurol 2013;20(12):1566–70.
17. Kelley BP, Patel SC, Marin HL, et al. Autoimmune encephalitis: pathophysiology and imaging review of an overlooked diagnosis. AJNR Am J Neuroradiol 2017; 38(6):1070–8.
18. Susac JO. Susac's syndrome The triad of microangiopathy of the brain and retina with hearing loss in young women. Neurology 1994;44(4):591.
19. Vodopivec I, Venna N, Rizzo JF 3rd, et al. Clinical features, diagnostic findings, and treatment of Susac syndrome: a case series. J Neurol Sci 2015;357(1):50–7.
20. Marrodan M, Correale J, Alessandro L, et al. Susac syndrome: a differential diagnosis of white matter lesions. Mult Scler Relat Disord 2017;15:42–6.
21. Demir MK. Case 142: Susac syndrome. Radiology 2009;250(2):598–602.
22. Grygiel-Górniak B, Puszczewicz M, Czaplicka E. Susac syndrome - Clinical insight and strategies of therapy. Eur Rev Med Pharmacol Sci 2015;19(9): 1729–35.
23. Majersik JJ. Inherited and uncommon causes of stroke. Continuum (Minneap Minn) 2017;23(1):211–37.
24. Auer DP, Pütz B, Gössl C, et al. Differential lesion patterns in CADASIL and sporadic subcortical arteriosclerotic encephalopathy: MR imaging study with statistical parametric group comparison. Radiology 2001;218(2):443–51.
25. O'Sullivan M, Jarosz JM, Martin RJ, et al. MRI hyperintensities of the temporal lobe and external capsule in patients with CADASIL. Neurology 2001;56(5): 628–34.
26. Van den Boom R, LesnikOberstein SA, Ferrari MD, et al. Cerebral autosomal dominant arteriopathy with subcortical infarcts and leukoencephalopathy: MR imaging findings at different ages–3rd-6th decades. Radiology 2003;229(3): 683–90.
27. Van den Boom R, LesnikOberstein SAJ, van Duinen SG, et al. Subcortical lacunar lesions: an MR imaging finding in patients with cerebral autosomal dominant arteriopathy with subcortical infarcts and leukoencephalopathy. Radiology 2002; 224(3):791–6.
28. LesnikOberstein SA, van den Boom R, van Buchem, et al. Cerebral microbleeds in CADASIL. Neurology 2001;57(6):1066–70.
29. Dichgans M, Holtmannspötter M, Herzog J, et al. Cerebral microbleeds in CADASIL: a gradient-echo magnetic resonance imaging and autopsy study. Stroke 2002;33(1):67–71.

30. Peters N, Holtmannspötter M, Opherk C, et al. Brain volume changes in CADASIL: A serial MRI study in pure subcortical ischemic vascular disease. Neurology 2006;66(10):1517–22.
31. Aksamit A. Neurosarcoidosis. Continuum (Minneap Minn) 2008;14:181–96.
32. Logigian EL, Kaplan RF, Steere AC. Chronic neurologic manifestations of lyme disease. N Engl J Med 1990;323(21):1438–44.
33. Steinbach JP, Melms A, Skalej M, et al. Delayed resolution of white matter changes following therapy of B burgdorferi encephalitis. Neurology 2005;64(4): 758–9.
34. Halperin JJ. Nervous system manifestations of Lyme disease. Rheum Dis Clin North Am 1989;15(4):635–47.
35. Fernandez RE, Rothberg M, Ferencz G, et al. Lyme disease of the CNS: MR imaging findings in 14 cases. AJNR Am J Neuroradiol 1990;11(3):479–81. Available at: http://www.ajnr.org/content/11/3/479.abstract.
36. Morgen K, Martin R, Stone RD, et al. FLAIR and magnetization transfer imaging of patients with post-treatment Lyme disease syndrome. Neurology 2001;57(11):1980–5.
37. Lycklama G, Thompson A, Filippi M, et al. Spinal-cord MRI in multiple sclerosis. Lancet Neurol 2003;2:555–62.
38. Filippi M. In-vivo tissue characterization of multiple sclerosis and other white matter diseases using magnetic resonance based techniques. J Neurol 2001;248: 1019–29.
39. Agosta F, Rocca MA, Benedetti B, et al. MR imaging assessment of brain and cervical cord damage in patients with neuroborreliosis. AJNR Am J Neuroradiol 2006;27(4):892–4. Available at: http://www.ajnr.org/content/27/4/892.abstract.
40. Pittock SJ, Jan D, Krecke KN, et al. Chronic lymphocytic inflammation with pontine perivascular enhancement responsive to steroids (CLIPPERS). Brain 2010;133(9):2626–34.
41. Simon NG, Parratt JD, Barnett MH, et al. Expanding the clinical, radiological and neuropathological phenotype of chronic lymphocytic inflammation with pontine perivascular enhancement responsive to steroids (CLIPPERS). J Neurol Neurosurg Psychiatry 2012;83(1):15–22.
42. Dudesek A, Rimmele F, Tesar, et al. CLIPPERS: Chronic lymphocytic inflammation with pontine perivascular enhancement responsive to steroids. Review of an increasingly recognized entity within the spectrum of inflammatory central nervous system disorders. Clin Exp Immunol 2014;175(3):385–96.
43. Kastrup O, Van De Nes J, Gasser T, et al. Three cases of CLIPPERS:A serial clinical, laboratory and MRI follow-up study. J Neurol 2011;258(12):2140–6.
44. Pesaresi I, Sabato M, Desideri I, et al. 3.0T MR investigation of CLIPPERS: Role of susceptibility weighted and perfusion weighted imaging. Magn Reson Imaging 2013;31(9):1640–2.
45. Sempere AP, Mola S, Martin-Medina P, et al. Response to immunotherapy in CLIPPERS: clinical, MRI, and MRS follow-up. J Neuroimaging 2011;23(2):254–5.
46. Hou X, Wang X, Xie B, et al. Horizontal eyeball akinesia as an initial manifestation of CLIPPERS: Case report and review of literature. Medicine 2016;95(34):e4640.
47. Taieb G, Duflos C, Renard D, et al. Long-term outcomes of CLIPPERS (chronic lymphocytic inflammation with pontine perivascular enhancement responsive to steroids) in a consecutive series of 12 patients. Arch Neurol 2012;69:847–55.
48. Ferreira RM, Machado G, Souza AS, et al. CLIPPERS-like MRI findings in a patient with multiple sclerosis. J Neurol Sci 2013;327:61–2.
49. Bickerstaff ER, Cloake PCP. Mesencephalitis and Rhombencephalitis. Br Med J 1951;2(4723):77–81.

Neuroimaging of Normal Pressure Hydrocephalus and Hydrocephalus

Patrick M. Capone, MD, PhD[a,b,c],*, John A. Bertelson, MD[d,e],
Bela Ajtai, MD, PhD[f]

KEYWORDS

- Idiopathic normal pressure hydrocephalus • Magnetic resonance imaging
- Computerized tomography • Ventricular shunting • Dementia

KEY POINTS

- Idiopathic normal pressure hydrocephalus (iNPH) is a potentially reversible cause of dementia.
- Estimated to be present in approximately 6% of individuals older than 80 years.
- Clinical guidelines exist based on clinical trials for the evaluation and treatment of these patients.
- Evaluation is based on clinical features of the patient and morphologic evaluation with computed tomography and/or MRI.
- Imaging features of iNPH emphasize hydrocephalus and disproportionately enlarged subarachnoid spaces excessive of any underlying cerebral atrophy and increased intraventricular cerebrospinal fluid flow rates and volumes.

There are few neurologic syndromes that have proved more vexing for the neurologist than idiopathic normal pressure hydrocephalus (iNPH).Since the initial description of the clinical triad of gait apraxia, urinary incontinence, and dementia in the setting of occult hydrocephalus in 1965, the potential of a treatable cause for dementia has generated extensive scientific interest and debate with a wide range of strong proponents and equally strong skeptics.[1–3] Secondary hydrocephalus subsequent to central nervous system (CNS) infections, neoplastic processes, hemorrhage, or trauma is a

Disclosures: None.
[a] Virginia Commonwealth University, Richmond, VA, USA; [b] Department of Neurology and Medical Imaging, Winchester Medical Center, 1840 Amherst Street, Winchester, VA 22601, USA; [c] Winchester Neurological Consultants, Inc., 125-A Medical Circle, Winchester, VA 22601, USA; [d] Texas Tech Health Sciences Center, Lubbock, TX, USA; [e] UT Austin Dell Medical School, 1600 West 38th Street, Suite 308, Austin, TX 78731, USA; [f] Dent Neurologic Institute, 3980A Sheridan Drive, Amherst, NY 14226, USA
* Corresponding author. Winchester Neurological Consultants, Inc., 125-A Medical Circle, Winchester, VA 22601, USA.
E-mail address: patrickcapone1952@gmail.com

well-recognized phenomenon that has shown more consistent benefit from cerebrospinal fluid (CSF) shunting. iNPH is much more problematic, and there remains considerable debate as to the cause, anatomic features, and the risks and benefits of shunting.[2,3] The importance of a potentially treatable cause for dementia generated extensive scientific interest. There were 1429 publications on this topic identified between 1965 and 2012.[4] The clinical features of iNPH have significant overlap with multiple neurodegenerative disorders, including parkinsonian syndromes, dementia of the Alzheimer type, and leukoaraiosis. Even with modern imaging techniques, differentiating iNPH from hydrocephalus ex vacuo is challenging due to considerable anatomic overlap.[5] This is not a minor clinical issue: The prevalence of probable NPH has been estimated with a range of figures at 0.2% in individuals between the ages of 70 and 79 years and at 5.9% for individuals aged 80 and 27 years or older in Sweden and 21.9/100,000 and an incidence of 5.5/10,000 in Norway and is equally common in both sexes.[6,7] Shunting complications are not insignificant. A systematic review of 44 studies demonstrated a complication rate of 38%. Shunt complications included subdural hemorrhages or effusions, infections, seizures, focal neurologic deficits, shunt malfunction, and death. Twenty-two percent of patients required additional surgery with 6% resulting in permanent neurologic deficits or death.[8]

The American Academy of Neurology has published practice guidelines regarding iNPH, and there are US, International, and Japanese guidelines established for the evaluation and treatment of iNPH.[4,9,10] US and international guidelines have provided a classification of possible, probable, and definite categories. Definite iNPH are those patients who show significant improvement with shunting.

The initial guidelines were published in 2005 for probable iNPH[10] (**Box1**).

More recent Japanese/International guidelines were published in 2012[5] (**Box2**)

Brain morphology assessments with computed tomography (CT) or MRI as per the clinical guidelines includes Evans' index, which is the ratio of the maximum width of the frontal horns to the maximum width of the inner table of the cranium. Measurements greater than 0.3 are considered hydrocephalus (**Fig. 1**).

Tight high convexities and midline subarachnoid structures such as the obscuration of sulci on coronal T1-weighted sequences along with adjacent medial surfaces are the morphologic features that suggest iNPH (**Fig. 2**).

Box 1
Criteria for probable idiopathic normal pressure hydrocephalus

1. Insidious onset

2. Age greater than 40 years

3. Duration of at least 3 to 6 months

4. No prior event known to cause secondary hydrocephalus, and no other neurologic, psychiatric, or medical cause to explain the clinical symptoms

5. Brain imaging to include computed tomography or MRI demonstrating ventricular enlargement not attributable to atrophy or congenital enlargement

6. Included a requirement of Evans' index of greater than 0.3, enlargement of the temporal horns not attributable to atrophy, with no obstructive lesions, and a callosal angle of 40° or more

7. Evidence of periventricular signal changes not attributable to microvascular ischemic changes or demyelination

8. Evidence of an aqueductal or fourth ventricular flow void on MRI.

Box 2
Japanese/International guidelines for probable idiopathic normal pressure hydrocephalus

1. More than one of the clinical triad of gait disturbance, cognitive impairment, and urinary incontinence

2. Age of 60 years or greater

3. Ventricular dilatation by Evans' index of greater than 0.3

4. The exclusion of an alternative cause for the hydrocephalus or an alternative explanation for the patient's clinical findings

5. Normal CSF with an opening pressure of 200 mm of water or less

6. Either disproportional enlargement of the subarachnoid space hydrocephalus (DESH) on neuroimaging or improvement of symptoms after CSF tap or a drainage test

7. Neuroimaging features described as DESH would include features such as narrowing of the sulci and arachnoid spaces over the high convexities or midline surfaces, widening of the sylvian fissures and basilar cisterns, focal dilatation of sulci not attributable to atrophy, and included criteria on how measurements of the callosal angle and Evans' index to be consistently determined

---

The callosal angle is another morphologic feature that is frequently measured, using coronal views that are perpendicular to the anterior and posterior commissure with the coronal CT or MRI centered through the posterior commissure (**Fig. 3**). Patients with iNPH have smaller angles (less than 90°) than those with ventriculomegaly from atrophy or normal controls (100°–120°).[4]

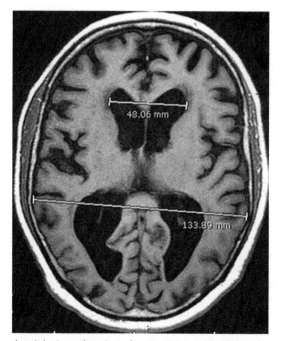

Fig. 1. T1-weighted axial view showing the maximum diameter of the horns and the maximum inner skull diameter in the slice above the foramen of Monro. The ratio is termed Evans' index.

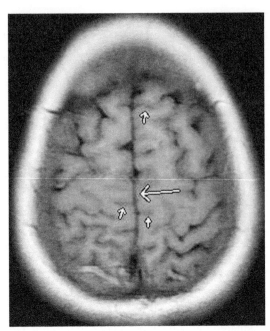

Fig. 2. T1-weighted axial view of the high convexity sulci is relatively obscured with the small arrows pointing to the narrowed sulci and a tight interhemispheric fissure with the large arrow.

Other features of disproportionate enlarged subarachnoid space hydrocephalus (DESH) include assessing the cingulate sulcus on a midsagittal T2-weighted MRI view. In a normal patient, the anterior half is narrower or equal to the posterior half. Patients with probable iNPH have narrowing of the posterior half of the cingulate sulcus as compared with the anterior (**Fig. 4**).

Sylvian fissures widening disproportionate to the other sulci and fissures is a frequent feature on iNPH (**Fig. 5**).

Focally widened sulci in the absence of generalized atrophy are also called transport sulci (**Fig. 6**).

The third ventricular walls in the normal individuals generally bow inward (waistlike) but become parallel or bow outward in iNPH[11] (**Fig. 7**).

The presence of signal flow voids in the aqueduct and fourth ventricle (**Fig. 8**) has been suggested as a possible indicator of increased flow due to iNPH and has been referenced in several studies in the past although it has not been found to be a reliable marker, particularly in its greater presence with newer higher-field MRIs that may produce similar flow voids on normal studies. More recent studies are utilizing cine phase MRI for assessment of flow velocities and stroke volume.[11]

The following is an example of patient management of iNPH with additional cine phase MRI (**Fig. 9**): a 76-year-old patient presents with a 3-year history of progressive gait decline. Her ambulation has been getting progressively slow and unsteady, with decreasing stride length. Because of her difficulties, she started using a cane and later had to switch to a walker. Eventually for longer distances and transportation she required a wheelchair. During the course of the past 1 year, she also developed urinary incontinence. Her family also reported a 5-year history of cognitive slowing. Initial MRI

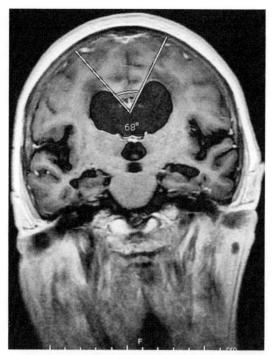

Fig. 3. T1-weighted coronal view through the posterior commisure perpendicular to the anterior and posterior commissure planes.

of her brain revealed enlarged third and lateral ventricles, out of proportion to the size of the superficial CSF spaces.

A subsequent MRI scan of the head was obtained, using a quantitative CSF flow sequence in the axialplane, oriented perpendicular to the cerebral aqueduct, for calculation of the flow velocities and total CSF flux through the cerebral aqueduct (absolute aqueductal stroke volume).

The technique uses phase contrast imaging for the evaluation of the aqueductal CSF flow. The measurements are carried out with cardiac gating, using either chest leads or finger plethysmography.

During one cardiac cycle, the CSF moves caudally in the aqueduct during systole and cephalad during diastole. The caudal and cephalad flow volumes are similar, within about 5% of each other, but with anet caudal motion (big step forward, smaller step back), resulting in net CSF motion from the third to the fourth ventricle. Most currently used MRI equipments include software that calculates theforward and reverse volumes, the sum of which represents the absolute aqueductal stroke volume.

Traditionally, larger stroke volumes are thought to indicate higher likelihood of shunt responsiveness. In the patient presented here, the absolute aqueductal stroke volumes, on 2 separate measurements, were 518 and 434 µL, respectively, indicating high probability of success with shunting.

For further evaluation, the patient underwent a diagnostic spinal tap trial and later a 72-hour lumbardrain trial, after which she showed improvement of her symptoms.

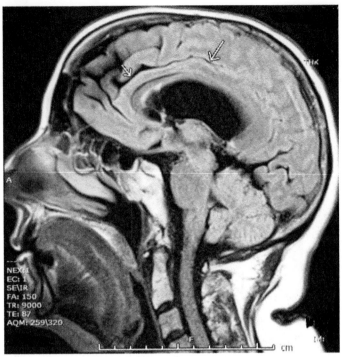

Fig. 4. T1-weighted sagittal view through the midline with short arrow pointing to the anterior cingulate sulcus and the longer arrow to the more posterior sulcus.

The technique uses phase contrast imaging for the evaluation of the aqueductal CSF flow. The measurements are carried out with cardiac gating, using either chest leads or finger plethysmography.

During one cardiac cycle, the CSF moves caudally in the aqueduct during systole and cephalad during diastole. The caudal and cephalad flow volumes are similar, within about 5% of each other, but with a net caudal motion (big step forward, smaller step back), resulting in net CSF motion from the third to the fourth ventricle, the sum of which represents the absolute aqueductal stroke volume.

Larger stroke volumes are thought to indicate higher likelihood of shunt responsiveness. In the patient presented here, the absolute aqueductal stroke volumes, on 2 separate measurements, were 518 and 434 μL, respectively, indicating high probability of success with shunting.

CSF taps have been generally reported in studies using high-volume lumbar taps of 30–50 mL or by external lumbar drainage tests over several days (300–500 mL) followed by objective testing of clinical functions including gait and cognition.[4]

Guidelines in 2005 indicated that a positive tap of 40 to 50 mL had a higher degree of certainty of a favorable response to shunting than clinical examination but not an exclusionary test due to a low sensitivity of (26%–61%) and that prolonged external drainage in excess of 300 mL was associated with a high sensitivity of (50%–10%) and a positive predictive value of (80%–100%). Those guidelines recommended external drainage testing for patients with possible iNPH not improving with high-volume taps.[12]

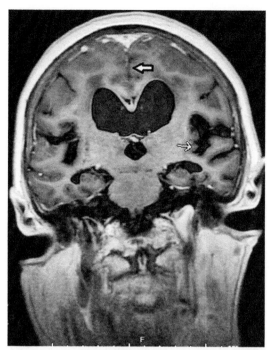

Fig. 5. T1-weighted coronal view with a small arrow directed at a widely enlarged sylvan fissure and a larger arrow pointing to a very disproportionally narrowed interhemispheric fissure.

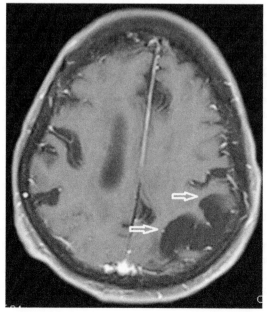

Fig. 6. T1-weighted axial view with small arrows directed at disproportionally focally widened sulci.

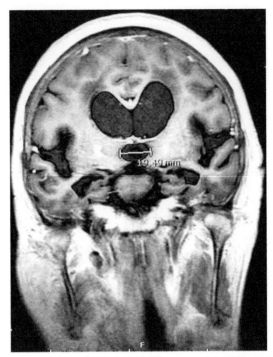

Fig. 7. T1-weighted coronal view through the widest segment of the third ventricle, which shows a midline measurement in the image and is markedly bowed.

A recent study challenged the need for high-volume taps and found no evidence that high-volume CSF removal affected gait testing.[13]

A systematic review of these studies demonstrated a 59% (range 24%–100%) of improvement in patients after shunting and 29% (range 10%–100%) experiencing prolonged or significant improvement.[8]

Gait apraxia is generally reported as the most responsive to shunting, with dementia and urinary incontinence less so.[8,14] The absence of gait disturbance or its onset after the onset of dementia predicts a poor response to shunting.[14,15]

There have been several clinical trials using ever increasing numbers of morphologic imaging markers in an attempt to improve the accuracy for selection of patients with probable NPH for shunting.[6,16–19] Most of these studies use different aspects of DESH along with Evans' index and the callosal angle. These morphometric signs seem to enhance the diagnostic selection process.

In a study using 13 morphometric markers for a pool of 168 patients with probable NPH, 68% showed improvement with shunting although none of the 13 MRI markers were statistically significant predictors of improvement of the shunting process.[19] The study also indicates that although morphometric markers may be indications of iNPH, the absence of any of these markers in a given patient did not exclude the possibility that they would, in fact, benefit from shunting.[19]

The morphometric markers correlated with symptom severity in only a limited degree but were not prognostic of their response to shunting. Numerous other techniques have been reported to attempt to improve diagnostic accuracy and the predictability of a shunting response such as supplementing morphometric measures with volumetric MRI,[20] assessment of diffusion tensor imaging profiles to evaluate for

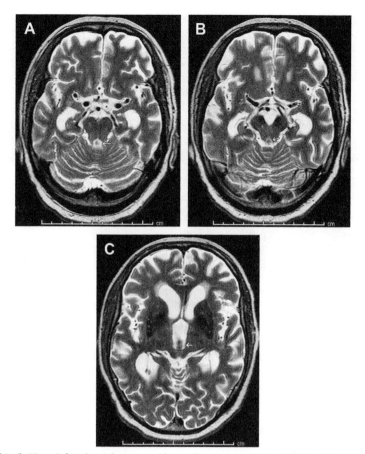

Fig. 8. (A–C) T2-weighted axial views with small arrows pointing to the "flow void sign" that is present in the fourth ventricle in (A), the aqueduct in (B), and the third ventricle in (C).

NPH by neural track distortion,[21] and MR elastography to assess increased brain stiffness.[22] There are multiple techniques to assess cerebral blood flow, which is thought to have decreased in iNPH, including arterial spin labeling, MR perfusion,[23] CT perfusion techniques,[24] and nuclear medicine techniques such as single-photon emission computed tomography to assess cerebral perfusion.[25]

MR spectroscopy in a pilot study reportedly demonstrated that NAA/Cr correlated with cognitive impairment in this patient population and significantly increased after shunting[26] CSF flow studies and stroke volume.[11,27–29] Glymphatic with intrathecal gadolinium–enhanced MRI has been recently reported as a potential new diagnostic technique.[30] Nuclear studies such as ^{18}F-flutemetamol PET imaging have been utilities for assessment of amyloid to better distinguish Alzheimer with possible NPH.[31] CSF biomarker such as beta-amyloid peptide 1-42, tau, and sulfatide levels have also been suggested in small studies to help distinguish iNPH from other neurovegetative disorders but have not shown wider utilization.[32–34]

CSF flow studies, either with assessment of flow rates by phase contrast MRI or with the presence of flow voids, had not, however, clearly established diagnostic utility. Cisternography was determined to be of no diagnostic value for iNPH. Cerebral blood

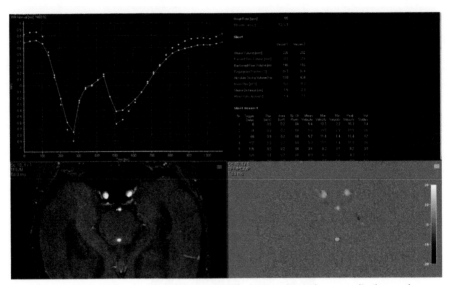

Fig. 9. A quantitative CSF flow study in the axial plane, oriented perpendicular to the cerebral aqueduct, for calculation of the flow velocities and total CSF flux through the cerebral aqueduct (absolute aqueductal stroke volume).

flow studies were shown to be of use for distinguishing iNPH from other causes of dementia.[4]

There are numerous theories to explain the iNPH syndrome. Guidelines indicated that leukoaraiosis was, in fact, more often seen in iNPH than in healthy individuals, although was not a prerequisite for the diagnosis. Population-based studies demonstrated vascular risk factors and white matter lesions with a statistical relationship to the clinical and imaging features of iNPH.[35] It has been proposed that reduced venous compliance with iNPH, as has been demonstrated with MR flow quantitation studies of the superior sagittal sinus, results in preferential reabsorption via the subependymal into the deep system and impaired CSF reabsorption through arachnoid granulations.[36]

Patients with shunt-responsive iNPH are reported to have both hyperdynamic CSF flow and deep white matter ischemia.[11] Patients with NPH have statistically larger intracranial volumes and have had dilated ventricles for years before they become symptomatic, and it has been suggested that they may have had benign external hydrocephalus as infants.[37] It has been speculated that these individuals may be more dependent on the parallel glymphatic pathway of CSF reabsorption to supplement the usual fourth ventricle outflow into the arachnoid granulation reabsorption.[11]

Microscopic flows of CSF through the brain parenchyma termed the glymphatic system have recently been a topic of research related to NPH. The glymphatic system is a convective fluid transport through the interstitial spaces mediated by Aquaporin-4 channels at astrocytic perivascular end feet. Impaired transport with accumulations of cellular waste such as amyloid and tau aggregation has been proposed as having a role in Alzheimer and other conditions.[38] Glymphatic CSF transport depends on arterial pulsation. Syndromes such as iNPH with reduced intracranial compliance have restricted arterial pulsations. Impaired glymphatic function could be behind the comorbidity seen with Alzheimer and iNPH.[39]

Impaired glymphatic clearance has been demonstrated in both animal models of NPH and human models with iNPH.[11,30]

SUMMARY

iNPH remains a challenging but important neurologic syndrome. The syndrome's complexity has resulted in a multitude of scientific evaluations that have provided new insights into the range of anatomy and dynamic changes that take place in the CNS, the risk factors, and the implications. The focus of this article is to demonstrate the neuroimaging features that have been shown to better select patients with the clinical triad of iNPH who may benefit from shunting. These morphologic features also provide insights into the pathophysiology of this syndrome.

REFERENCES

1. Adams RD, Fisher CM, Hakim S, et al. Symptomatic occult hydrocephalus with "normal" cerebrospinal-fluid pressure: a treatable syndrome. N Engl J Med 1965;273:117–26.
2. Espay AJ, Da Prat GA, Dwivedi AK, et al. Deconstructing normal pressure hydrocephalus: ventriculomegaly as early sign of neurodegeneration. Ann Neurol 2017;82:503–13.
3. Saper CB. Is there even such a thing as "idiopathic normal pressure hydrocephalus"? Ann Neurol 2017;82:514–5.
4. Mori E, Ishikawa M, Kato T, et al, Japanese Society of Normal Pressure Hydrocephalus. Guidelines for management of idiopathic normal pressure hydrocephalus: second edition. Neurol Med Chir (Tokyo) 2012;52:775–809.
5. Neill R. Graff-Radford Is normal pressure hydrocephalus becoming less idiopathic? Neurology 2016;86:588–9.
6. Jaraj D, Rabiei K, Marlow T, et al. Prevalence of idiopathic normal pressure hydrocephalus. Neurology 2014;82(16):1449–54.
7. Brean A, Eide P. Prevalence of probable idiopathic normal pressure hydrocephalus in a Norwegian population. ActaNeurolScand 2008;118:48–53.
8. Hebb A, Cusimano M. Idiopathic normal pressure hydrocephalus: a systematic review of diagnosis and outcome. Neurosurgery 2001;49:1166–86.
9. Halperin J, Kurlan R, Schwab J, et al. Practice guideline: idiopathic normal pressure hydrocephalus: response to shunting and predictors of response. Neurology 2015;85:2063–71.
10. Relkin N, Marmarou A, Klinge P, et al. Diagnosing idiopathic nor- mal-pressure hydrocephalus. Neurosurgery 2005;57(3 Suppl):S4–16 [discussion: ii-v].
11. Bradley WG Jr. CSF flow in the brain in the context of normal pressure hydrocephalus. AJNR 2015;36(5):831–8.
12. Marmarou A, Bergsneider M, Klinge P, et al. The value of supplemental prognostic tests for the preoperative assessment of idiopathic normal-pressure hydrocephalus. Neurosurgery 2005;57:S17–28.
13. Thakur S, Serulle Y, Miskin N, et al. Lumbar puncture test in normal pressure hydrocephalus: does the volume of CSF removed affect the response to tap? AJNR 2017;38:1456.
14. Klassen BT, Ahlskog JE. Normal pressure hydrocephalus: how often does the diagnosis hold water? Neurology 2011;77(12):1119–25.
15. Black P. Idiopathic normal-pressure hydrocephalus: results of shunting in 62 patients. J Neurosurg 1980;52:371–7.
16. Hashimoto M, Masatsune I, Mori E, et al. Diagnosis of idiopathic normal pressure hydrocephalus is supported by MRI-based scheme: a prospective cohort study. Cerebrospinal Fluid Res 2010;7:18.

17. Virhammar J, Laurell K, Cesarini KG, et al. Preoperative prognostic value of MRI findings in 108 patients with idiopathic normal pressure hydrocephalus. AJNR Am J Neuroradiol 2014;35:2311–8.
18. Kojoukhova1 M, Koivisto M, Korhonen R, et al. Feasibility of radiological markers in idiopathic normal pressure hydrocephalus. ActaNeurochir 2015;157:1709–19.
19. Agerskov S, Wallin M, Hellstrom P, et al. Absence of disproportionately enlarged subarachnoid space hydrocephalus, a sharp callosal angle, or other morphologic MRI markers should not be used to exclude patients with idiopathic normal pressure hydrocephalus from shunt surgery. AJNR Am J Neuroradiol 2019; 40:74–9.
20. Miskin N, Patel H, Franceschi A, et al. Diagnosis of normal-pressure hydrocephalus: use of traditional measures in the era of volumetric MRimaging. Radiology 2017;285(1):197–205.
21. Keong N, Pena A, Price S, et al. Diffusion tensor imaging profiles reveal specific neural tract distortion in normal pressure hydrocephalus. PLoSOne 2017;12: e0181624.
22. Fattahi N, Arani A, Perry A, et al. Elastographydemonstrates increased brain stiffness in normal pressure hydrocephalus. AJNR Am J Neuroradiol 2016;37:462–7.
23. Virhammar J, Laurell K, Ahlgren A, et al. Arterial spin-labeling perfusion mr imaging demonstrates regional CBFdecrease in idiopathic normal pressure hydrocephalus. AJNR Am J Neuroradiol 2017;38:2081–8.
24. Ziegelitz D, Arvidsson J, Hellström P. Pre-and postoperative cerebral blood flow changes in patients with idiopathic normal pressure hydrocephalus measured by computed tomography (CT)-perfusion. J CerebBlood Flow Metab 2016;36(10): 1755–66.
25. Sasaki H, Ishii K, Kono A, et al. Cerebral perfusion pattern of idiopathic normal pressure hydrocephalus studied by SPECT and statistical brain mapping. Ann Nucl Med 2007;21(1):39–45.
26. del MarMatarín M, Pueyo R, Poca M, et al. Post-surgical changes in brain metabolism detected by magnetic resonance spectroscopy in normal pressure hydrocephalus: results of a pilot study. J NeurolNeurosurgPsychiatry 2007;78:760–3.
27. Miskin N, Serulle Y, Wu W, et al. Post-shunt gait improvement correlates with increased cerebrospinal fluid peak velocity in normal pressure hydrocephalus: A retrospective observational phase contrast magnetic resonance imaging study. Int J Sci Stud 2015;3:48–54.
28. Bradley W, Scalzo D, Queralt J, et al. Normal-pressure hydrocephalus: evaluation with cerebrospinal fluid flow measurements at MR imaging. Radiology 1996;198: 523–9.
29. Scollato A, Tenenbaum R, Bahl G, et al. Changes in aqueductalCSF stroke volume and progression of symptoms in patients with unshunted idiopathic normal pressure hydrocephalus. AJNR Am J Neuroradiol 2008;29:192–7.
30. Ringstad G, Vatnehol S, Eide P. Glymphatic MRI in idiopathic normal pressure hydrocephalus. Brain 2017;140(10):2691–705.
31. Rinne J, Wong D, Wolk D, et al. [18F]Flutemetamol PET imaging and cortical biopsy histopathology for fibrillar amyloid b detection in living subjects with normal pressure hydrocephalus:
pooled analysis of four studies. Acta Neuropathol 2012;124(6):833–45.
32. Lins H, Wichart I, Bancher C, et al. Immunoreactivities of amyloid b peptide (1–42) and total t protein in lumbar cerebrospinal fluid of patients with normal pressure hydrocephalus. J NeuralTransm 2004;111:273–80.

33. Kudo T, Mima T, Hashimoto R. Tau protein is a potential biological marker for normal pressure hydrocephalus. Psychiatry Clin Neurosciences 2000;54: 199–202.
34. Tullberg M, Månsson J, Fredman P. CSF sulfatide distinguishes between normal pressure hydrocephalus and subcortical arteriosclerotic encephalopathy. J NeurolNeurosurgPsychiatry 2000;69:74–81.
35. Jaraj D, Agerskov S, Rabiei K, et al. Vascular factors in suspected normal pressure hydrocephalus: A population-based study. Neurology 2016;86:592–9.
36. Bateman G. The pathophysiology of idiopathic normal pressure hydrocephalus: cerebral ischemia or altered venous hemodynamics? AJNR Am J Neuroradiol 2008;29(1):198–203.
37. Bradley W, Safar F, Hurtado CJ. Increased intracranial volume: a clue to the etiology of idiopathic normal-pressure hydrocephalus? AJNR Am J Neuroradiol 2004;25:1479–84.
38. Iliff J, Wang M, LiaoY BA, et al. A paravascular pathway facilitates CSF flow through the brain parenchyma and the clearance of interstitial solutes, including amyloid β. SciTransl Med 2012;4(147):147ra111.
39. Cabral D, Beach T, Vedders L. Frequency of Alzheimer's disease pathology at autopsy in patients with clinical normal pressure hydrocephalus. Alzheimer's Dement 2011;7(5):509–13.

Neuroimaging of Acute Stroke

Ashutosh P. Jadhav, MD, PhD[a],*, Shashvat M. Desai, MD[a], David S. Liebeskind, MD[b], Lawrence R. Wechsler, MD[a]

KEYWORDS

- Stroke • Ischemic stroke • Neuroimaging • Infarction • Hemorrhage
- Thrombectomy

KEY POINTS

- Computed tomography (CT) of the head is the first line of neuroimaging for patients suspected of having a stroke.
- CT head can identify hemorrhage and its severity and location; it can also be used to rule out hemorrhage and administer thrombolytic therapy and approximate ischemic stroke burden using ASPECTS score.
- CT angiography detects occlusion and/or dissection in extracranial and intracranial arteries and perfusion imaging can detect blood flow and cerebral perfusion characteristics. CTA and CTP are essential to select patients for late window thrombectomy and to rule out stroke mimics.
- MRI is an advanced tool of neuroimaging that can reliably detect hemorrhagic and ischemic stroke with specific uses.

INTRODUCTION

Acute stroke is a major cause of mortality and the leading cause of adult disability in the United States.[1] In adults, 87% of acute stroke is caused by compromised blood flow with resultant ischemia, whereas the remainder of acute stroke is secondary to intracranial hemorrhage.[1] Tissue injury is typically rapid and often irreversible and thus expedited triage, diagnosis, and treatment are critical components to optimizing outcome.[2,3] Imaging contributes to rapid triage and facilitates prompt potentially tissue-saving therapy.

COMPUTED TOMOGRAPHY

Computed tomography (CT) head is typically the favored initial diagnostic approach for acute stroke because the test is performed quickly with low cost.[4] In addition,

[a] Neurology, University of Pittsburgh, 200 Lothrop Street, Pittsburgh, PA 15222, USA;
[b] Neurology, University of California Los Angeles, 635 Charles E Young Drive South, Suite 225, Los Angeles, CA 90095, USA
* Corresponding author.
E-mail address: Jadhav.library@gmail.com

Neurol Clin 38 (2020) 185–199
https://doi.org/10.1016/j.ncl.2019.09.004
0733-8619/20/© 2019 Elsevier Inc. All rights reserved.

neurologic.theclinics.com

CT imaging is tolerated by most patients and there are few contraindications. As such, CT scanners have become widely available. CT imaging uses radiation to measure tissue density. Higher density structures are manifest as brighter with higher Hounsfield units (HU). Typical HU measurement ranges relevant to intracranial tissue include: fat (−100 to −50), water (0), blood (30–45), gray matter (37–45), white matter (20–30), and bone (700–3000).

In the setting of acute stroke, CT may appear normal but skilled observers often identify subtle abnormalities indicative of early ischemia signifying either impending or irreversible brain injury. Early ischemic changes (EIC) include sulcal effacement, edema, and hypoattenuation and subtle changes may be difficult to appreciate. Adjustment of window settings can improve lesion conspicuity; for example, by centering at the mean attenuation of gray and white matter, it has been shown that diagnostic accuracy is improved. Specifically, adjusting windows from the standard settings of 35 HU center and 100 HU width level to a center level of 35 HU and a width of 30 HU (stroke window) improved detection of EIC from 18% versus 70% in one study.[5]

Alberta Stroke Program Early Computed Tomography Score

The extent of EIC in the distribution of the left middle cerebral artery (MCA) is broadly dichotomized as less or more than one-third of the MCA territory; however, this approach is limited by marked lack of agreement between experienced clinicians. This limitation prompted the development of a more systematic approach where the MCA territory was divided into 10 topographic regions (insular ribbon, head of caudate, posterior limb of the internal capsule, putamen, and six cortical regions). The Alberta Stroke Program Early CT Score (ASPECTS) is a quantitative score in which points are subtracted for areas with hypoattenuation. A normal scan is assigned an ASPECTS score of 10 and a completed infarct leads to an ASPECTS score of 0.[6] The score has been applied as a continuous measurement and a dichotomized score. ASPECTS score of 0 to 7 versus 8 to 10 has been shown to have prognostic value among patients treated with intravenous alteplase (intravenous tissue plasminogen activator [IV-tPA]) for acute ischemic stroke within 3 hours of symptoms onset, and higher rates of recanalization.[7] Furthermore, ASPECTS score of 7 or less is associated with a higher likelihood of thrombolytic-related parenchymal hemorrhage.[8] **Fig. 1** demonstrates a patient with an ASPECTS score of 2 and another patient with an ASPECTS score of 10.

Hyperdense sign

Organized clot, typically rich in red blood cell (RBC),[9] can manifest on CT head as a hyperattenuation or "hyperdensity" in the involved artery, commonly the MCA (**Fig. 2**) or basilar artery. The impression of a hyperdense vessel sign is confounded

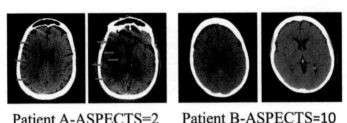

Patient A-ASPECTS=2   Patient B-ASPECTS=10

Low ASPECTS=High Stroke burden   High ASPECTS=Low Stroke burden

Fig. 1. Two patients with acute right middle cerebral artery occlusion (M1). Arrows refer to topographic regions with hypodense signal on CT head.

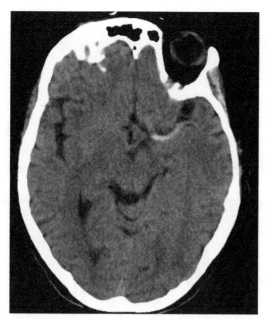

Fig. 2. Hyperdense vessel sign on noncontrast CT head involving the left middle cerebral artery.

by false positives. By measuring the absolute attenuation in affected and normal vessels, accuracy is highest when the affected MCA has an HU of 43 or higher or when there is a ratio of greater than 1.2 with the contralateral MCA (or >1.4 when compared with the basilar artery).[10] Similarly, hyperattenuation in the basilar artery can indicate the presence of occlusion with a range of 40 to 42 HU corresponding to a sensitivity of up to 78%, a specificity of up to 83%, and accuracy up to 80%.[11] The presence of a hyperdense vessel sign has been associated with more severe neurologic deficit and poor functional outcome and cerebral damage, edema and mass effect, and hemorrhagic conversion.[12] Resolution of the hyperdense vessel sign after reperfusion therapy is associated with vessel recanalization and favorable outcome.[13]

Posterior Circulation Alberta Stroke Program Early Computed Tomography Score
The extent of EIC in the posterior circulation caused by a basilar artery occlusion is assessed with the posterior circulation ASPECTS (pc-ASPECTS) score. Two points each are subtracted for EIC in midbrain or pons and one point each for EIC in left or right thalamus, cerebellum, or posterior cerebral artery (PCA)-territory, respectively.[14] pc-ASPECTS scoring system has been depicted in **Fig. 3**A.[14] pc-ASPECTS score of less than 8 has been associated with reduced likelihood of a good outcome in patients with basilar artery occlusion despite recanalization.[15] **Fig. 3**B demonstrates noncontrast CT head of a patient with an acute distal basilar occlusion and pc-ASPECTS score of 7 (cerebellum [1 point] and midbrain [2 points] involvement).

Computed Tomography Angiography

CT angiography (CTA) is a specialized CT head involving the introduction of an intravenous contrast during imaging. This technique specifically enhances visualization of

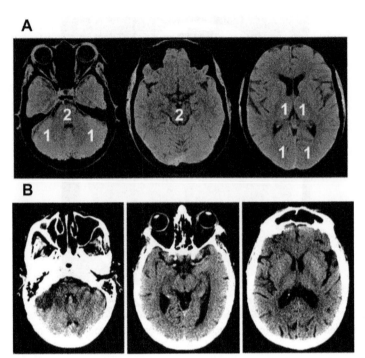

Fig. 3. (A) pc-ASPECTS scoring system. (B) pc-ASPECTS score of 7 for a patient with distal basilar occlusion. ([A] *From* Puetz V, Sylaja PN, Coutts SB, et al. Extent of hypoattenuation on CT angiography source images predicts functional outcome in patients with basilar artery occlusion. *Stroke* 2008; 39: 2485–90; with permission.)

the cerebral vasculature, extracranial and intracranial arteries and veins. CTA is a powerful tool in the triage and diagnosis of acute stroke, ischemic and hemorrhagic.

Although CT head is the only investigation required before IV-tPA administration, many centers routinely perform CTA to diagnose carotid stenosis, intracranial atherosclerosis, and/or large vessel occlusion. Acute CTA findings have triage and acute and secondary prevention implications for acute ischemic stroke. Diagnosis of carotid stenosis or large vessel occlusion at a primary stroke center in patients within the appropriate time window warrants consideration of immediate transfer to an interventional neurology center for advanced care including carotid stenting and/or mechanical thrombectomy.

Clinical trials that proved the superiority of mechanical thrombectomy over medical management for large-vessel occlusion stroke used CTA for patient selection because of its high sensitivity and specificity in diagnosing large-vessel occlusion.[16–22] Beyond confirmation of large-vessel occlusion (**Figs. 4** and **5**), CTA also can provide information regarding collateral blood flow (**Fig. 6**)[23] and clot burden and characteristics. Additionally, extracranial carotid artery stenosis (**Figs. 7** and **8**) and aortic arch anatomy may be delineated on CTA.

Computed Tomography Perfusion

CT perfusion is a specialized application of conventional CT imaging using advanced software processing. Using contrast material, CT perfusion enables real-time

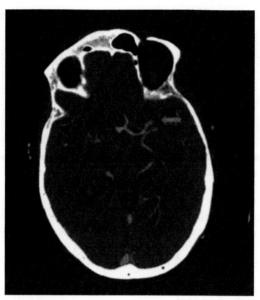

Fig. 4. Left middle cerebral artery occlusion on CTA. The arrow indicates the site of occlusion in the left middle cerebral artery.

visualization of cerebrovascular physiology parameters, including cerebral blood flow, cerebral blood volume, and mean transit time through brain parenchyma. CT perfusion imaging can assess the volume of irreversibly ischemic brain tissue (core) and brain tissue suffering from hypoperfusion (penumbra). Volume of parenchyma with relative cerebral blood flow of less than 30% (compared with contralateral hemisphere) is superior to other parameters for measuring infarcted brain tissue.[19] Volume of time to peak to more than 6 seconds (T max >6) corresponds more accurately to hypoperfused brain parenchyma (penumbra) destined to go on to infarction if not reperfused.[24] These thresholds may vary with post-software processing algorithms and degree of smoothing but were used in major clinical trials for patient selection. In **Fig. 9**, a right MCA M1 occlusion patient with an ischemic core volume of 47 mL (relative cerebral blood flow <30%) and penumbral volume of 259 mL (T max >6 seconds) is shown.

Late window thrombectomy trials, including a subset of the DAWN and the DEFUSE-3 trials, used CT perfusion or MR perfusion to measure ischemic core volume (DAWN and DEFUSE-3) and penumbra (DEFUSE-3) to select patients for

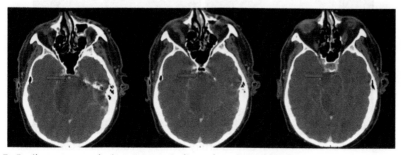

Fig. 5. Basilar artery occlusion. Arrows indicate location of basilar artery occlusion.

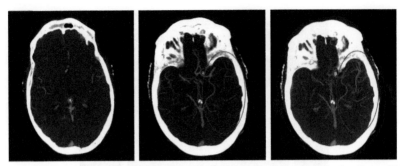

Fig. 6. Collateral status on multiphase CTA. Circled region denotes area of collateral blood supply.

thrombectomy. Both trials were successful and established that salvageable tissue is key to achieving good outcomes in large vessel occlusion (LVO) strokes beyond 6 hours of last known well.[20,21] Recently published late window trials for administration of IV-tPA beyond 4.5 hours of last known well also used CT perfusion.[25]

Future of Computed Tomography Head, Computed Tomography Angiography, and Computed Tomography Perfusion

Mobile stroke unit

Mobile stroke units (MSU) are specialized emergency ambulances equipped with a CT scanner. They have the ability to bring neuroimaging to the patient, rather than bringing the patient to a neuroimaging center, allowing treatment with IV-tPA in the field and reducing time from stroke onset to treatment. Initial experience with MSUs around the world has confirmed that they can reduce time from emergency medical service activation to therapy initiation decision.[26] However, studies are underway to detect clinical benefit of MSUs and optimum deployment in diverse resource environments.[27,28] **Fig. 10** demonstrates CT head (with left hyperdense sign and no intracranial hemorrhage) acquired in an MSU.

Flat-panel computed tomography

Conventional multislice scanners yield high-quality images that can readily exclude the presence of hemorrhage and identify EIC. However, there is increasing interest

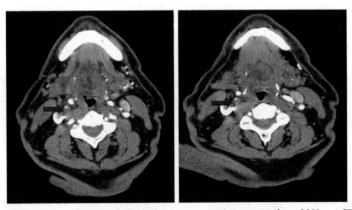

Fig. 7. Right extracranial internal carotid artery stenosis greater than 90% on CTA. Arrow indicates internal carotid artery stenosis.

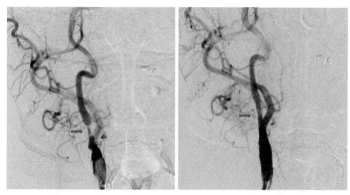

Fig. 8. Right extracranial internal carotid artery stenosis greater than 90% on digital subtraction angiography. Arrow indicates region of stenosis.

in flat-panel CT because this technique is performed directly on the angiosuite table. As such this allows parenchymal imaging to be directly performed immediately before, during, and immediately after angiography. In particular, this allows patient diversion away from the time-consuming congestion of emergency room triage.[29]

Automated computed tomography analysis

Like other fields of medicine, neuroimaging and automation have come together. Various platforms are exploring the utility and efficacy of deep machine learning and image processing algorithms to process and interpret neuroimaging to assist radiologists and neurologists. Automated CT analysis aims to exclude hemorrhage, identify ischemia and its extent (ASPECTS and/or approximate ischemic volume), and detect presence of large-vessel occlusion. The primary objective of such technology is to screen quickly and continuously triage a large number of neuroimages, and notify the on-call neurologist.[30,31]

Computed tomography perfusion for intracranial occlusion detection

Angiographic reconstruction from whole-brain CT perfusion has been used for detection of intracranial vessel occlusion. In one study, CT perfusion–based angiographic

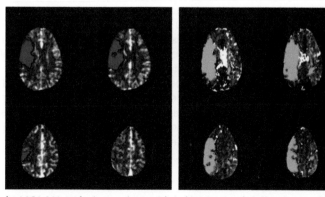

Fig. 9. Right MCA M1 occlusion patient with ischemic core (*pink*) volume of 47 mL (relative cerebral blood flow <30%) and penumbral volume (*green*) of 259 mL (T max >6 seconds).

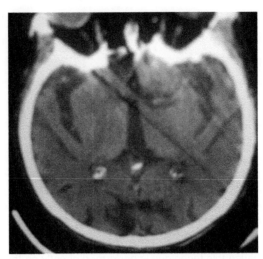

Fig. 10. Left MCA hyperdense vessel sign on CT head acquired from a mobile stroke unit.

reconstruction reached 94% sensitivity and 100% positive predictive value for detecting intracranial arterial occlusion.[32] CT perfusion can also assist in confirming suspected distal vessel occlusion (anterior circulation occlusion distal to M2 segment) on CTA.[33]

MRI

MRI is an advanced tool for neuroimaging in acute stroke. Conventional MRI sequences (T1 and T2) along with diffusion (DWI) and perfusion (PWI) weighted imaging have the advantage of detecting early ischemia over conventional CT. MRI sequences, including gradient recalled echo (GRE), are noninferior to CT for acute hemorrhage and are superior to CT for detecting chronic hemorrhage with almost 100% sensitivity.[34]

Diffusion-Weighted Imaging

DWI is built on the principle of MRI to be able to detect water molecule movement between two closely spaced radiofrequency pulses. Failure of the sodium-potassium pump following ischemia results in increased accumulation of intracellular water, which is detected by DWI within less than 30 minutes of ischemia onset. DWI is superior to CT for acute ischemic stroke diagnosis in the acute window following stroke onset.[35] DWI sensitivity for ischemia detection is nearly 90%, but this number may decrease for minor strokes. Acute DWI lesion volumetric analysis corresponds well with the size of ischemic core during large vessel occlusion (LVO) stroke. **Fig. 11** shows DWI MRI ischemic core volume of two patients after 2 hours of acute MCA-M1 occlusion.

High signal on DWI images may occur due to high T2 signal, referred to as T2 "shine through", that is not attributable to restricted diffusion. This should be distinguished from true restricted diffusion. A lesion having high signal on DWI and low signal on ADC (Apparent Diffusion Coefficient), is likely caused by abnormal tissue including vasogenic edema or cyst. Hence, ADC can differentiate between T2 shine through and ischemia.

Perfusion-Weighted Imaging

Although DWI can accurately delineate irreversibly damaged brain parenchyma, PWI can provide information regarding extent of reversible ischemia. Two broad

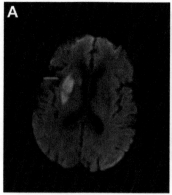
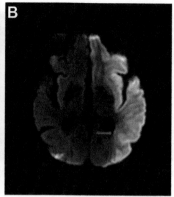

Patient
Right MCA-M1 Occlusion
Stroke Onset- 2 h
Ischemic Core Volume- 7 mL

Patient
Left MCA-M1 Occlusion
Stroke Onset- 2 h
Ischemic Core Volume- 163 mL

Fig. 11. DWI ischemic core volume after middle cerebral artery M1 occlusion. (A) Slow Progressor (B) Fast Progressor. Arrows indicate region of DWI restriction.

methods of obtaining MR perfusion are available: with contrast enhancement using gadolinium (similar to CT perfusion); and without contrast enhancement, using continuous arterial spin labeling, a technique especially useful in pediatric and renal failure subgroups. PWI is done alongside standard MRI and MR angiography (MRA). Relative

---

Box 1
Current American Heart Association/American Stroke Association guidelines related to neuroimaging for acute stroke

- All patients admitted to hospital with suspected acute stroke should receive brain imaging evaluation on arrival to hospital.

- In most cases, noncontrast CT provides the necessary information to make decisions about acute management (Class 1B).

- Systems should be established so that brain imaging studies can be performed within 20 minutes of arrival in the emergency department (Class 1B).

- Recommended door-to-needle time is less than 45 to 60 minutes (Class 1B). It may be useful for primary stroke centers to develop the capability of performing emergency noninvasive intracranial vascular imaging to most appropriately select patients for transfer for endovascular intervention and to reduce the time to endovascular thrombectomy (EVT) (Class IIB).

- For patients who otherwise meet criteria for EVT, a noninvasive intracranial vascular study is recommended during the initial imaging evaluation of the acute stroke patient (Class IA).

- CT perfusion and/or DWI MRI is required to selection patients for mechanical thrombectomy in the 6 to 24 hours window after stroke onset (Class IA).

- Evaluation of extracranial carotid and vertebral arteries (Class IIA), along with collateral visualization (Class IIB) using CTA/MRA, is reasonable.

From Powers WJ, Rabinstein AA, Ackerson T, *et al.* 2018 Guidelines for the Early Management of Patients With Acute Ischemic Stroke: A Guideline for Healthcare Professionals From the American Heart Association/American Stroke Association. *Stroke* 2018; published online March. https://www.ahajournals.org/doi/abs/10.1161/STR.0000000000000158 (accessed Oct 1, 2018); with permission.

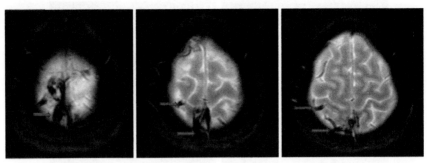

Fig. 12. Thrombosis of the posterior portion of the superior sagittal sinus. Arrow indicates regions of thrombosis.

cerebral blood flow and mean transit time maps could be generated to identify ischemic core and penumbra, respectively.

MRI Angiography

Similar to CTA, MRA has the ability to visualize extracranial and intracranial arteries and veins. In acute stroke, its primary purpose is to identity stenosis or occlusion. There are broadly two techniques for MRA: without contrast, using time of flight (TOF) and phase contrast (two or three dimensional); and contrast enhanced using gadolinium.

TOF MRA is a GRE sequence. The magnetic field induces a continuous spin in the proton of a specific region of the brain leading to signal loss. However, blood flow introduces new protons without a spin and the arising signal helps to identify the vasculature. Venous signals are selectively minimized by placing a saturation band. An alternative noncontrast technique is phase contrast MRA, where alternating phasing and rephasing of tissue with opposite magnetic field helps identify moving blood. Phase contrast MRA is better than TOF MRA at detecting sluggish flow and dissection and is obtained even after gadolinium administration. However, TOF MRA is superior for neck visualization and is done in a shorter time span. Three-dimensional TOF can provide better spatial resolution and less dispersion than two-dimensional TOF but is more susceptible to saturation effects.

A   **B**

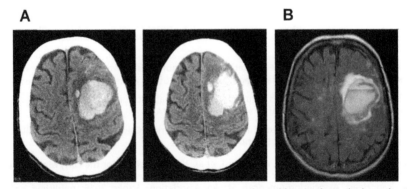

Fig. 13. (A) CT head on arrival with left parietal parenchymal hemorrhage (volume by ABC/2 = 32 mL). (B) MRI at 6 hours. CT head at 24 hours showing extension of hemorrhage (volume by ABC/2 = 39 mL).

Table 1
CT and MRI evaluations

	0–6 h	6–24 h	Beyond 24 h
Noncontrast CT head	Rule out hemorrhage before thrombolytic therapy Identify early ischemic changes Identify hyperdense vessel sign Previous infarction areas Cerebral edema: grey-white differentiation, midline shift, herniation Hemorrhage characteristics Hyperacute — Hyperdense, confluent Acute (12–48 h) — Hyperdense, with fluid level	Early subacute (72 h) Hypodense, local mass effect	Late subacute (3–20 d) Less hypodense, ring-like appearance Chronic (>8 wk) Isodense or mildly hypodense
CT angiography	Confirm intracranial large vessel occlusion Confirm extracranial carotid stenosis/occlusion Quantify collateral status in the presence of large vessel occlusion Aneurysm detection Site of hemorrhage detection		In addition to utility before acute reperfusion therapy Confirm recanalization postreperfusion therapy Secondary work-up to detect extracranial or intracranial stenosis Follow-up postaneurysm treatment
CT perfusion	Per guidelines not essential in 0–6 h for patient selection for thrombectomy Can aid diagnosis of distal vessel occlusion Can be used to confirm mismatch profile (clinical core or perfusion mismatch) May be used for patient selection for thrombolytic therapy beyond 4.5 h May be useful for patient selection for extracranial carotid occlusion	Per guidelines CT perfusion or MRI should be used for late window thrombectomy patient selection Adequately delineates ischemic core and penumbra Automated software analysis required Can aid diagnosis of distal vessel occlusion May be used for patient selection for thrombolytic therapy beyond 4.5 h	Tissue characteristics are more important than time Patients may be selected using CT perfusion for beyond 24-h thrombectomy

(continued on next page)

Table 1 (continued)			
	0–6 h	6–24 h	Beyond 24 h
MRI diffusion-weighted imaging			
Apparent diffusion coefficient	Identifies areas of restricted diffusion and cytotoxic edema in the setting of acute ischemic stroke	Identifies areas of restricted diffusion and cytotoxic edema in the setting of acute ischemic stroke	Restoration to normal apparent diffusion coefficient begins weeks and up to months after the initial infarct
GRE	Hypointensity indicative of acute hemorrhage or chronic blood products. Age cannot be determined on this sequence. Hemorrhage characteristics		
	Hyperacute	Acute (1–3 days)	Early subacute (3–7 days)	Late subacute (7–14 days)	Chronic (>2 weeks)
T1 weighted	Hypointense or isointense	Hypointense with hyperintense rim	Hyperintensity	Hyperintensity	Hypointensity
T2 weighted	Hyperintense	Hypointense with hyperintense rim	Hypointensity	Hyperintensity	Hypointensity
GRE	Severe hypointensity	Severe hypointensity	Hypointensity	Hypointensity	Hyperintense or isointense center surrounded by hypointense rim

Contrast-enhanced MRA uses gadolinium as contrast. T1 sequence is made shorter (<10 ms) and opacified vessels become hyperintense. It must be performed in a short time interval requiring adequate coordination with the bolus of contrast. This technique is similar to CTA. Contrast-enhanced MRA images the contrast and detailed vascular anatomy is seen, compared with TOF or phase contrast MRA, which rely on physiologic perfusion of the tissue.

Based on data from randomized controlled trials and registry-level data, guidelines have been published for the optimal use of neuroimaging for stroke management, including recognition, triage, and patient selection (**Box 1**).

VENOUS IMAGING

Cerebral venous thrombosis (CVT) is an uncommon cause of stroke (0.5%–1%), but is an important cause in the young and is frequently misdiagnosed or diagnosed after significant delays. Venous infarcts typically do not follow an arterial distribution, often extend to the cortical surface, and are more likely to be hemorrhagic.

Neuroimaging plays a central role in identifying CVT. Noncontrast CT head is the first line of neuroimaging. It helps to rule out other more common causes of arterial occlusion or hemorrhage. Hyperdensity of cortical vein or dural sinus on CT head is the primary sign of CVT. Another diagnostic sign is the filled delta sign, appearing as a dense triangle caused by thrombosis of the posterior aspect of the superior sagittal sinus. CT head in CVT is abnormal only in about a third of patients. Additionally, ischemic areas may be observed on CT and they do not conform to usual arterial distribution. Contrast-enhanced CT may show an "empty delta" sign, characterized by a filling defect within the dural sinus.

MRI for CVT is more sensitive. A "hyperintense vein sign" may be seen on MRI. Signal from the thrombus depends on the time from onset of thrombus formation. In the first week, T1 signal is isointense and T2 signal is hypointense because of deoxyhemoglobin. In the second week, hyperintense T1 and T2 signal are caused by presence of methemoglobin. Secondary MRI signs include edema and/or infarction. Hemorrhagic conversion may also be observed. CT or MR venography may be useful to delineate the venous system and identify a flow void. In the acute phase, it may not always be possible to distinguish a flow void from a flow-related signal. T2-weighted GRE is useful and highly sensitive for CVT diagnosis compared with other MRI sequences (**Fig. 12**). Additional techniques include catheter-based cerebral venography.

HEMORRHAGE

About 15% to 20% of acute strokes are caused by intracerebral hemorrhage. Noncontrast CT head as a part of first-line acute stroke neuroimaging is commonly used and has high sensitivity for detecting intracerebral hemorrhage. Quantitative hemorrhage assessment using CT is done using the ABC/2 method (**Fig. 13**). Age of the hematoma is determined by evaluating the density using HU on CT or the intensity on MRI sequences (**Table 1**).[36]

SUMMARY

Vascular neurology and stroke is rapidly evolving. Acute reperfusion therapy including tPA and endovascular thrombectomy are increasingly being offered, even in late time window strokes. Neuroimaging plays a central role in stroke management from recognition of stroke and its type, triage, and patient selection for treatment.

DISCLOSURES

The authors have nothing to disclose.

REFERENCES

1. Stroke Facts | cdc.gov. Available at: https://www.cdc.gov/stroke/facts.htm. Accessed October 24, 2018.
2. Desai SM, Rocha M, Jovin TG, et al. High variability in rate of neuronal loss- time is brain, re-quantified. Stroke Press 2019;50:34–7.
3. Saver Jeffrey L. Time is brain—quantified. Stroke 2006;37:263–6.
4. Wardlaw JM, Seymour J, Cairns J, et al. Immediate computed tomography scanning of acute stroke is cost-effective and improves quality of life. Stroke 2004;35: 2477–83.
5. Mainali S, Wahba M, Elijovich L. Detection of early ischemic changes in noncontrast CT head improved with "stroke windows". ISRN Neurosci 2014;2014. https://doi.org/10.1155/2014/654980.
6. Pexman JH, Barber PA, Hill MD, et al. Use of the Alberta Stroke Program Early CT Score (ASPECTS) for assessing CT scans in patients with acute stroke. AJNR Am J Neuroradiol 2001;22:1534–42.
7. Demchuk Andrew M, Hill MD, Barber PA, et al. Importance of early ischemic computed tomography changes using ASPECTS in NINDS rtPA stroke study. Stroke 2005;36:2110–5.
8. Vora NA, Gupta R, Thomas AJ, et al. Factors predicting hemorrhagic complications after multimodal reperfusion therapy for acute ischemic stroke. AJNR Am J Neuroradiol 2007;28:1391–4.
9. Brinjikji W, Duffy S, Burrows A, et al. Correlation of imaging and histopathology of thrombi in acute ischemic stroke with etiology and outcome: a systematic review. J Neurointerv Surg 2017;9:529–34.
10. Chrzan R, Gleń A, Urbanik A. How to avoid false positive hyperdense middle cerebral artery sign detection in ischemic stroke. Neurol Neurochir Pol 2017;51: 395–402.
11. Connell L, Koerte IK, Laubender RP, et al. Hyperdense basilar artery sign-a reliable sign of basilar artery occlusion. Neuroradiology 2012;54:321–7.
12. Li Q, Davis S, Mitchell P, et al. Proximal hyperdense middle cerebral artery sign predicts poor response to thrombolysis. PLoS One 2014;9. https://doi.org/10.1371/journal.pone.0096123.
13. Mair G, von Kummer R, Morris Z, et al. Effect of alteplase on the CT hyperdense artery sign and outcome after ischemic stroke. Neurology 2016;86:118–25.
14. Puetz V, Sylaja PN, Coutts SB, et al. Extent of hypoattenuation on CT angiography source images predicts functional outcome in patients with basilar artery occlusion. Stroke 2008;39:2485–90.
15. Werner MF, López-Rueda A, Zarco FX, et al. Value of posterior circulation ASPECTS and Pons-Midbrain Index on non-contrast CT and CT angiography source images in patients with basilar artery occlusion recanalized after mechanical thrombectomy. Radiologia 2019;61:143–52.
16. Berkhemer OA, Fransen PSS, Beumer D, et al. A randomized trial of intraarterial treatment for acute ischemic stroke. N Engl J Med 2015;372:11–20.
17. Jovin TG, Chamorro A, Cobo E, et al. Thrombectomy within 8 hours after symptom onset in ischemic stroke. N Engl J Med 2015;372:2296–306.
18. Goyal M, Demchuk AM, Menon BK, et al. Randomized assessment of rapid endovascular treatment of ischemic stroke. N Engl J Med 2015;372:1019–30.

19. Campbell BCV, Mitchell PJ, Kleinig TJ, et al. Endovascular therapy for ischemic stroke with perfusion-imaging selection. N Engl J Med 2015;372:1009–18.
20. Nogueira RG, Jadhav AP, Haussen DC, et al. Thrombectomy 6 to 24 hours after stroke with a mismatch between deficit and infarct. N Engl J Med 2018;378: 11–21.
21. Albers GW, Marks MP, Kemp S, et al. Thrombectomy for stroke at 6 to 16 hours with selection by perfusion imaging. N Engl J Med 2018;378:708–18.
22. Saver JL, Goyal M, Bonafe A, et al. Stent-retriever thrombectomy after intravenous t-PA vs. t-PA alone in stroke. N Engl J Med 2015;372:2285–95.
23. Yang C-Y, Chen Y-F, Lee C-W, et al. Multiphase CT angiography versus single-phase CT angiography: comparison of image quality and radiation dose. AJNR Am J Neuroradiol 2008. https://doi.org/10.3174/ajnr.A1073.
24. Olivot J-M, Mlynash M, Thijs VN, et al. Optimal Tmax threshold for predicting penumbral tissue in acute stroke. Stroke 2009;40:469–75.
25. Thomalla G, Simonsen CZ, Boutitie F, et al. MRI-guided thrombolysis for stroke with unknown time of onset. N Engl J Med 2018;379:611–22.
26. Bowry R, Parker S, Rajan SS, et al. Benefits of stroke treatment using a mobile stroke unit compared with standard management: the BEST-MSU study run-in phase. Stroke 2015;46:3370–4.
27. BEnefits of stroke treatment delivered using a mobile stroke unit - Full Text View - ClinicalTrials.gov. Available at: https://clinicaltrials.gov/ct2/show/NCT02190500. Accessed November 24, 2018.
28. 'Mobile Stroke-Unit' for reduction of the response time in ischemic stroke - Full Text View - ClinicalTrials.gov. Available at: https://clinicaltrials.gov/ct2/show/NCT00792220. Accessed June 4, 2019.
29. Doerfler A, Gölitz P, Engelhorn T, et al. Flat-panel computed tomography (DYNA-CT) in neuroradiology. From high-resolution imaging of implants to one-stop-shopping for acute stroke. Clin Neuroradiol 2015;25(Suppl 2):291–7.
30. Gillebert CR, Humphreys GW, Mantini D. Automated delineation of stroke lesions using brain CT images. Neuroimage Clin 2014;4:540–8.
31. Guberina N, Dietrich U, Radbruch A, et al. Detection of early infarction signs with machine learning-based diagnosis by means of the Alberta Stroke Program Early CT score (ASPECTS) in the clinical routine. Neuroradiology 2018;60:889–901.
32. Frölich AMJ, Psychogios MN, Klotz E, et al. Angiographic reconstructions from whole-brain perfusion CT for the detection of large vessel occlusion in acute stroke. Stroke 2012;43:97–102.
33. Becks MJ, Manniesing R, Vister J, et al. Brain CT perfusion improves intracranial vessel occlusion detection on CT angiography. J Neuroradiol 2019;46:124–9.
34. Kidwell CS, Chalela JA, Saver JL, et al. Comparison of MRI and CT for detection of acute intracerebral hemorrhage. JAMA 2004;292:1823–30.
35. Mitomi M, Kimura K, Aoki J, et al. Comparison of CT and DWI findings in ischemic stroke patients within 3 hours of onset. J Stroke Cerebrovasc Dis 2014;23:37–42.
36. Macellari F, Paciaroni M, Agnelli G, et al. Neuroimaging in intracerebral hemorrhage. Stroke 2014;45:903–8.

Neuroimaging of Deep Brain Stimulation

Lorand Eross, MD, PhD, FIPP[a],*, Jonathan Riley, MD[b], Elad I. Levy, MD, MBA[c], Kunal Vakharia, MD[c]

KEYWORDS

- Deep brain stimulation • Diffusion tensor imaging • Functional imaging
- Neuromodulation

KEY POINTS

- Advances in functional neurosurgery were supported in the last decade by modern imaging and innovations in neurotechnology.
- DBS targeting changed from indirect targeting by the technical advancement of MRI technology to direct targeting.
- DTI of white matter fibers helps to understand the effect of DBS, improves surgical outcome, and became an imaging tool in human translational neuroscience.
- Parcellation of cortical and subcortical structures let functional neurosurgeons get detailed functional anatomic differences of the targeted structures and led to more precise targeting in DBS therapy.

INTRODUCTION

Deep brain stimulation (DBS) is an invasive neuromodulation technique that reintroduced quality of life for thousands of patients with movement disorders in the last 25 years. Especially in Parkinson disease (PD), more than 80% improvement is achievable in motor scores and kinetic performance in the implanted patients. This tremendous increase is based on recent inventions of the neurotechnological industry and caused by the introduction of modern MRI. Indirect targeting based on ventriculography has been changed to direct targeting on MRI sequences. This article summarizes many of the new techniques and technologies developed in MRI for stereotactic and functional neurosurgery and DBS. We also emphasize the advantages of the new imaging techniques for clinical practice and translational research.

[a] Department of Functional Neurosurgery, Center of Neuromodulation, National Institute of Clinical Neurosciences, Amerikai út 57, Budapest 1145, Hungary; [b] Department of Neurosurgery, Jacobs School of Medicine and Biomedical Sciences, University Buffalo Medical, 955 Main Street, Buffalo, NY 14203, USA; [c] Department of Neurosurgery, Jacobs School of Medicine and Biomedical Sciences, University Buffalo, 955 Main Street, Buffalo, NY 14203, USA
* Corresponding author.
E-mail address: l.g.eross@gmail.com

Neurol Clin 38 (2020) 201–214
https://doi.org/10.1016/j.ncl.2019.09.005
0733-8619/20/© 2019 Elsevier Inc. All rights reserved.

INTRODUCTION OF TAILORED MRI TECHNIQUES IN SURGICAL PLANNING

To increase optimal placement of DBS electrodes several MRI sequences have been introduced to achieve more precise targeting, and advancements in magnetic field strength have also resulted in higher resolution images. The introduction of proton density imaging provides high contrast rate between the intramedullary lamina and the intranuclear gray, making it possible to distinguish between the internal part of the globus pallidus (GPi) and external part of the globus pallidus, making the stereotactic target for dystonia (DT) and in some cases of PD more identifiable.[1] T2,[2] susceptibility weighted imaging, and quantitative susceptibility mapping[3] can identify the iron content within the subthalamic nucleus (STN), red nucleus, the GP, and the substantia nigra making them more distinguishable from the surrounding regions, thus providing optimal target identification in PD. Although the latter technique (quantitative susceptibility mapping) (**Fig. 1**) requires several steps of post-processing to occur for optimal outcome, it can also differentiate calcification from iron content relying on their diamagnetic and paramagnetic qualities. Double inversion recovery sequences using different inversion times can create two image sets in the same coregistered space, one with nulled white matter signal and another with nulled cerebrospinal fluid intensity. On the resulting images the intramedullary lamina within the GP or other important anatomic markers, such as mammillothalamic tract, are clearly differentiated (eg, making the anterior nucleus of the thalamus [ANT] more outlined for epilepsy DBS) (**Fig. 2**).[4–6]

Emerging targets, such as the pedunculopontine nucleus in postural instability and gait disorder, has also been observed on tailored ultrahigh-field 7-T MP2RAGE images as intermediate-intensity structure between the hypointense periaqueductal gray and hyperintense fiber tracts of the medial lemniscus.[7,8]

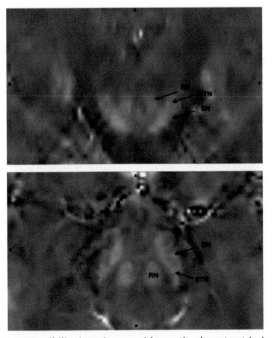

Fig. 1. Quantitative susceptibility imaging provides optimal contrast in iron-rich structures, delineating the STN for targeting in PD. RN, red nucleus; SN, substantia nigra.

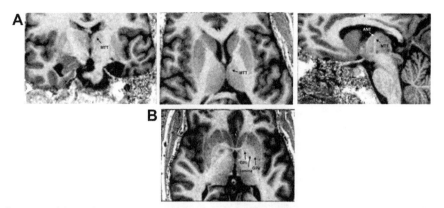

Fig. 2. Dual inversion recovery sequences outline white matter tracts and intramedullary laminae. (*A*) Mammillothalamic tract. (*B*) Intramedullary lamina bordering the GPi and external part of the globus pallidus. GPe, external part of the globus pallidus; MTT, mammillothalamic tract.

Diffusion tensor imaging (DTI) and tractography provide a noninvasive method to visualize important white matter connections within the brain. Several options and mathematical models exist to reconstruct diffusion gradients within the examined voxels,[9–11] thus simple and more refined interpretations exist to calculate white matter fiber orientations.[12–17] Although modeling of crossing fibers and connectivity probabilities are also available, higher resolution images require immense calculations, making their daily use more time consuming, thus mainly restricting probabilistic tractography for research purposes only. Recent advancements in the underlying architecture of graphic processing units provide an option for task parallelization,[18] thus reducing the required time for calculations. Until graphic processing units–based modeling is widely available, deterministic tractography and modeling of principal diffusion orientations are suitable options for a simpler interpretation of individual anatomic relations.

ADVANCEMENTS IN MOVEMENT DISORDERS

Since the first implantation carried out by Benabid and coworkers[19] several advancements have occurred to take DBS surgery in movement disorders several steps further from its infancy. Ventriculography and the use of standard coordinates have been replaced by modern MRI and individually tailored therapeutic plans. Not only has the targeting been refined, but robot-assisted procedures have also been introduced to achieve the best clinical outcome (**Fig. 3**).[20,21]

CLINICAL RATIONALE OF THE STEREOTACTIC TARGETS IN MOVEMENT DISORDERS

The three main therapeutic targets (the internal part of the GPi, the ventral intermediate nucleus [VIM], and the STN) where in the center of constant debates between clinicians and researchers because each provides certain benefits for patients after electrode implantation in PD, DT, or essential tremor. For example, although VIM stimulation can achieve significant benefit in tremor-dominant PD or essential tremor, it only has moderately sufficient long-term impact on rigidity and none on bradykinesia in PD[22]; thus, these patients still require elevated doses of levodopa substitution,

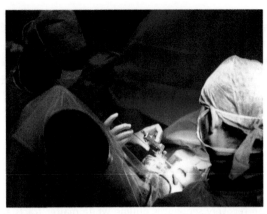

Fig. 3. Robot-assisted DBS results in more accurate electrode placement.

resulting in unwanted dyskinesia. Because GPi is the main "output" to the thalamus from the basal ganglia, and because of the decrease of dopamine release in substantia nigra and the resulting hyperactive inhibitory state of the GPi providing thalamic inactivation, its high-frequency stimulation could result in favorable outcomes in akinetic-rigid type of PD.[23] GPi is also the favorable target in DT. Stimulation of the STN, however, might result in optimal tremor control, while also resulting in sustained decrease of rigidity and bradykinesia, but ventromedial misplacement of the electrodes could induce hyperactivity, mania, depression, and suicidal intent.[24]

THE ROLE OF CONNECTIVITY PATTERNS AND DIFFUSION TENSOR IMAGING IN MOVEMENT DISORDERS

Although proper visualization of the STN, the GPi or the VIM is crucial to achieve the best clinical results, several centers still favor intraoperative electrophysiology during implantation to maintain an optimal target point within the microstructure of the nuclei.[25,26] Recent studies have emphasized that the STN, the GPi, and the VIM all connect to distinct cortical areas, which can explain unwanted side effects observed in, for example, ventromedial STN stimulation. Most optimal results in STN stimulation were achieved in dorsolateral electrode placements, within the nucleus or near the caudal zona incerta.[27,28] Recent studies established DTI and tractography to be an essential tool to identify these sweet spots in each disease.[29] Tracer studies conducted in primates are in agreement with recent DTI studies showing a clear orientation of limbic, associative, and sensorimotor connections aligned on the ventromedial-dorsolateral axis in the STN.[30] Noninvasive mapping of the target structures provides an early insight to their internal configuration, thus resulting in individually tailored preoperative plans. Observed beta activity and recorded local field potentials also correlate with disease severity in PD providing a biologic marker for electrode placement.[31–34] Several of the aforementioned noninvasive or electrophysiologic measurements conclude that the most optimal point within the STN resides within the sensorimotor portion of the nucleus. Reconstruction of the activated tissue volume and the activated fiber tracts suggest that reduction of clinical symptoms was achievable in those cases when fibers projecting to the supplementary motor cortex or primary motor cortex were stimulated.[35]

Clear definition of the optimal target within the GPi is yet to be found using noninvasive methods, although some suggest that identification of the posteroventrolateral portion of the GPi projecting to the thalamus and the sensorimotor system is the key for the most beneficial effect.[36,37] Cervical, segmental, or generalized DT all benefit from the stimulation within this location.

Recent studies on 7-T MRI provided high-resolution images from the thalamic nuclei, but availability of these systems in general patient care is still far off. DTI and probabilistic tractography-based parcellation of the thalamus showed an invaluable tool to distinguish nuclei and their projections.[1,38] Several studies have also emphasized that identifying and targeting the dentate-rubro-thalamic tract, arising from the cerebellum and projecting to the primary motor cortex after entering the thalamus, results in favorable tremor control in essential tremor or PD, but progressive gait ataxia has also been connected to maladaptive response to stimulation within this region (**Fig. 4**).[39–41]

DEEP BRAIN STIMULATION FOR EPILEPSY

One-third of the population of the 66 million epilepsy patients worldwide suffer from drug-resistant epilepsy. Those who have focal seizures or focal lesions are good candidates for resective surgery. Those who are neither successfully treated by drugs and ketogenic diet nor optimal candidates for resective surgery are potential candidates for neuromodulation. Neuromodulation of epilepsy could be noninvasive or invasive. The invasive neuromodulative techniques could stimulate peripheral nerves, such as vagal nerve stimulation, or they can target the central nervous system. Although many cortical and subcortical targets were used over the last decades, evidence collected from extensive clinical research supports only the ANT as a suggested target. The centromedian nucleus of the thalamus and the hippocampus are under investigation in pivotal studies.[42] ANT-DBS showed the most benefit in bitemporal epilepsy in the SANTE study.[43,44] Centromedian nucleus DBS was popularized by the Velasco group for generalized epilepsy.[45,46]

Future applications of imaging shift the focus from DBS in epilepsy based on indirect targeting and atlas-based stereotactic coordinates. The Wahren-Schaltenbrand atlas, one of the most widely used worldwide, was based on cadaver samples from three individuals.[47–49] The anatomic variation of the anterior nucleus has been previously described in anatomic studies by Van Buren and Borke in 1972,[50] and modern imaging proved the accuracy of these findings. Delineation of the anterior thalamus

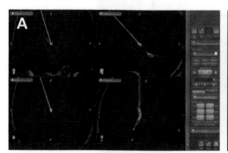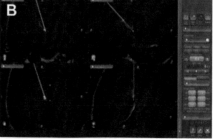

Fig. 4. Visualization of dentate-rubro-thalamic tract carried out using probabilistic tractography might provide the optimal target for DBS in essential tremor. Its place can highly differ from standard stereotactic coordinates. (*A*) Location of dentate-rubro-thalamic target, which provided optimal tremor control during surgery. (*B*) Standard target according to anterior copmissure - posterior comissure (AC-PC) coordinates differed by 4.8 mm (*red dot*).

was a challenge until the introduction of short tau inversion recovery sequences on 3-T MRI machines. Inversion recovery sequences with a short inversion time, at the point where difference in longitudinal magnetization is at its maximum at the border of white matter and gray matter, generates superior contrast between the observed structures. Möttönen and colleagues[51] measured the degree of anatomic variation and overlap in the location of ANT in an anterior comissure (AC) - posterior comissure (PC)-based coordinate system between individuals and found extensive individual variability. ANT location was based on the contrast between the gray matter of ANT and the white matter of mammillothalamic tract. Their study demonstrated the weaknesses of the ventriculography-based indirect AC-PC targeting. They found that the AC-PC-based targeting used in epilepsy DBS, because of the variability of the location of human anterior thalamic nucleus, can result in inconsistencies and it can influence outcome analysis of the therapies. Therefore, they suggest that direct visualization is superior to indirect targeting. The introduction of dual inversion recovery provides sufficient benefit over short tau inversion recovery because movement-related artifacts can hinder the acquisition of the latter, thus requiring the scan to be done under general anesthesia. Dual inversion recovery does not have this drawback and the acquisition is carried out on awake patients as well within 7 to 8 minutes.

The exact knowledge of the postoperative location of the active contact is essential for comparative analysis of surgical outcomes (**Fig. 5**).[52] We should also emphasize that the ANT not only measures a mere $10 \times 5 \times 4$ mm, it also contains three separate nuclei with different cortical connections. In the future, high-field MRI parcellation of these subregions within the ANT might provide higher accuracy in selective targeting and could probably improve patient selection and DBS outcome. Superresolution track density images (TDI) developed by Calamante group substantially improved the visualization of white matter tracts. The sensitivity of TDI further improved with 7-T field MRI.[53] They conclude that the use of 7-T superresolution TDI can reveal structures beyond the resolution of the acquired imaging voxel. This technique was able to visualize even thalamocortical connections, such as septum pellucidum tract.[54] Direct visualization of the Papez circuit with 7-T superresolution MRI tractography provides hope for the possibility of superselective targeting in DBS epilepsy.[55]

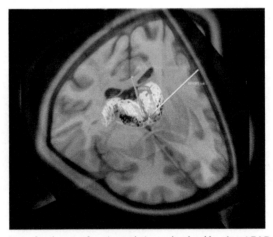

Fig. 5. Reconstruction of volume of activated tissue (*red orb*) using LEAD DBS toolbox provides a useful tool for electrode localization, DBS electrodes implanted in the anterior nucleus of the thalamus (ANT, *light blue*).

In cases of patients diagnosed with different types of epileptic seizures and syndromes, it was already recognized that they would benefit from DBS using different targets and various types of electrodes.[42]

DEEP BRAIN STIMULATION FOR PSYCHIATRIC INDICATIONS

The Austrian physician Gottlieb Burckhardt was the first to pioneer neurosurgical intervention, in the form of trephination and topectomy, for psychiatric indications in the late 1880s.[56] Although the subsequent presentation of his findings was not well received, this initial work was foundational to the subsequent efforts of Moniz and Lima, beginning in 1935, to introduce the prefrontal leukotomy (commonly known as the frontal lobotomy).[57] Rapid popularization of this procedure would come to serve as a cautionary tale for the introduction of new surgical therapies. Adoption of the prefrontal leucotomy was spurred by a lack of effective contemporary psychiatric therapies, the minimally invasive nature of the procedure, and marketing and showmanship by such practitioners as Freeman and Watts. The application of this procedure was largely carried with broad and poorly studied indications and without attempts at careful clinical follow-up. By the time a Congressional report on psychosurgery was released in 1977 that cautioned the careful application of surgery for psychiatric indications, such procedures had largely fallen out of favor in lieu of the advent of effective antipsychotic and antidepressant medication.[58] Ironically, the significant decline in the use of neurosurgical intervention for psychiatric disorders coincided with rapid advancements in the principles and techniques of stereotactic neurosurgical interventions and lesioning procedures. A demonstrated ability to precisely target a lesion or modulate specific tissues would ultimately provide the foundation for a new paradigm of neurosurgical intervention.

AN IMAGE-BASED RATIONALE FOR INTERVENTION

The most common psychiatric indication currently explored for surgical intervention is depression. Several intracranial targets have recently been attempted. These include the nucleus accumbens,[59] lateral habenula,[60] inferior thalamic peduncle,[61] ventral capsule/ventral striatum (VC/VS),[62] and subgenual cingulate.[63] The latter two targets have been explored in randomized controlled trials and are instructive because of a differing basis for exploration. The VC/VS target received a Humanitarian Device Exemption from the Food and Drug Administration in 2009 for the treatment of refractory obsessive-compulsive disorder (OCD).[64] This target, chosen as a variation of prior lesioning target for OCD, was observed to have the parallel benefit of improvement in mood when stimulated for treatment of OCD.

The subgenual cingulate (Brodmann area 25) was chosen for clinical investigation based on concordant findings implicating this area in PET studies demonstrating alterations observed in depressed mood.[65,66] Further evaluations demonstrated normalization with medical management, cognitive therapy, and transcranial magnetic stimulation.

CONTEMPORARY RANDOMIZED CLINICAL TRIAL RESULTS FOR DEPRESSION

Based on the previously mentioned open label studies, two separate randomized clinical trials have been recently completed for depression: the RECLAIM (VC/VS)[67] and the BROADEN (subgenual cingulate)[68] trials. Both trials were terminated before planned enrollment completion. The blind was broken for an interim analysis on the RECLAIM trial following enrollment of 30 out of 208 planned patients. Twenty-nine of 30 patients had completed the blinded phase; there was a 14.3% response rate in the sham group and 20% response rate. The blinded stimulation period began 4 weeks following implant and randomization. Given a less than expected response at the end of the blinded phase in this interim analysis, enrollment was terminated. The BROADEN trial was designed to enroll 201 patients and to detect effect with a 40% response in the active group and a 15% response in the sham group. A futility analysis conducted after the blinded phase in the first 90 patients (6 months of stimulation) demonstrated a response in only 17% in the sham group and 20% in the active group. The assessment demonstrated a 17% chance of demonstrating a response difference between groups if carried to completion. The sponsor elected to terminate the trial. In the open-label follow-up phase, response was detected in 53% at 18 months and 49% at 24 months.

Multiple reasons have been posited for poorer than expected outcomes in these trials. These include lack of efficacy of DBS at these targets, a prolonged placebo effect and shorter than appropriate blinded phase, trial interaction effects (greater than usual caregiver attention provided to participants), suboptimal outcome measurement tools, inadequate lead targeting strategies, and patient selection concerns (given heterogeneity of depression). Functional neuroimaging techniques have shown promise to address these latter concerns.

A CONNECTOME-BASED TARGETING APPROACH

Throughout the BROADEN study, investigators worked to further tailor the intracranial lead placement targeting strategy that was used. A DTI-based analysis of responders and nonresponders demonstrated a characteristic pattern of connectivity in the vicinity of the active treatment electrode contact. Specifically, responders were observed to have electrode placement at a location representing the confluence of the (1) forceps minor, (2) medial aspect of the uncinate fasciculus, (3) the cingulum bundle, and (4) frontostriatal fibers connecting to deep subcortical nuclei (eg, nucleus accumbens, VS).[69] The same connectivity pattern was not observed in nonresponders. Since the initial retrospective investigation, this methodology has been developed into a tool capable of clinical intraoperative targeting application.[70] Furthermore, this approach was prospectively applied to 11 patients in the BROADEN trial. Eight of 11 were responders at conclusion of the blinded phase (6 months) and 82% at 1 year. Therefore, the subset of patients targeted with the DTI-based connectivity "fingerprint," had substantially improved response.

The recent past has seen significantly increased activity in exploration of DBS for psychiatric disorders, namely depression and OCD. Despite negative outcomes, the two recent randomized controlled trials for depression have been instructive for future investigative efforts. Significant advances in connectome-based targeting show promise toward selection of surgical candidates and optimization of patient response to stimulation therapy. Such strategies may be used in concert with additional functional imaging techniques that predict a response to intervention[71] and ongoing efforts to better biologically subtype psychiatric disorders,[72] thereby improving patient selection. The climate of recent industry partnership for DBS for psychiatric disorders, regulatory body interest in better characterizing the biologic substrate and subtypes of psychiatric disorders (eg, NIMH RDoC program), improving imaging-based diagnostic and targeting tools, and the significant knowledge obtained from the recent trials all provide encouragement for a future role for DBS for selected treatment-refractory psychiatric disorders.

DEEP BRAIN STIMULATION FOR TREATMENT OF CHRONIC PAIN

Intracranial stimulation for the treatment of chronic pain disorders has been explored in the context of motor cortex stimulation[73-75] and DBS at multiple subcortical targets.

DBS targets have included the VS/anterior limb of the interal capsule,[76] ventral posterolateral thalamic nucleus,[77–79] periaqueductal/periventricular brainstem nucleus,[78] and dorsal anterior cingulate cortex.[80,81] DBS was most effective for phantom limb pain, stump pain, failed back surgery syndrome (FBSS), cranial and facial pain, including anesthesia dolorosa and plexopathies. Poststroke pain is successful if the pain presented as a burning hyperesthesia. The possible misinterpretation and methodologic limitations of published studies and the difficulty to compare it with alternatives, clouds the potential of DBS in the treatment of chronic pain.[82] Although multiple prospective studies demonstrate the utility of this intervention in selected patients, significant questions remain. One such question includes trying to understand whether preintervention imaging may help to determine likely responders to intracranial stimulation. 11C–diprenorphine PET-based studies have helped to demonstrate that the subsequent response to motor cortex stimulation may be predicted by the preoperative number of opioid receptors.[83] Similar PET-based studies of DBS following periaqueductal stimulation have been used to document an increased release of endogenous opioids.[84] Functional MRI-based evidence of likely responders in patients with postlaminectomy syndrome receiving trial stimulation is identified with characteristic activation-deactivation patterns.[85] Additional roles explored for functional neuroimaging for intracranial stimulation include targeting optimization for lead placement and clinical outcome prediction. Tractography-based efforts have explored both. DTI has been explored as a means of facilitating selective preoperative targeting of fiber tracts when anatomic imaging alone cannot sufficiently identify a subcortical nuclei and a means to postoperatively confirm lead placement in the ventral posterolateral thalamic nucleus,[86] dorsal anterior cingulate cortex,[87] periaqueductal,[88] and spinothalamic tract at the level of the posterior limb of the internal capsule.[89]

There are multiple case series supporting a role for intracranial stimulation for chronic pain syndromes. Currently five clinical trials are registered in the United States; four in France; and one in Denmark, which is suspended. Challenges that exist toward understanding the efficacy of DBS for treatment-refractory chronic pain include diagnostic heterogeneity, prolonged placebo effect in neurostimulation randomized controlled trials, prominent trial-related treatment interactions (eg, significant increased attention by care providers and research personnel), and difficulty in recruiting a sufficient number of similar patients. The previously mentioned studies demonstrate that advanced neuroimaging techniques hold promise to help preemptively stratify stimulation responders, preoperatively revise implant strategies for targets that are not directly visible on anatomic imaging, and allow for confirmation of adequate postoperative lead positioning.

SUMMARY

Modern imaging opens new advancements for stereotactic and functional neurosurgery. The weaknesses of indirect targeting because of the great individual variability of the patient's brain became evident. Direct targeting improves accuracy and in DBS surgery can improve outcome. Direct targeting with new MRI sequences and with the MRI-compatible neurotechnological devices allowed comparative analysis for surgical outcome in cases of multicentric studies, which is essential to improve DBS therapy.

ACKNOWLEDGMENTS

The authors acknowledge the support of the Hungarian Brain Research Program and the work of Dr László Halász, PhD fellow and neurosurgical resident at Department of

Functional Neurosurgery and Center of Neuromodulation, National Institute of Clinical Neurosciences in Budapest.

DISCLOSURE

The authors receives funding from Hungarian Brain Research Program 2017-1.2.1-NKP-2017-00002.

REFERENCES

1. Behrens TEJ, Johansen-Berg H, Woolrich MW, et al. Non-invasive mapping of connections between human thalamus and cortex using diffusion imaging. Nat Neurosci 2003;6(7):8.
2. Dormont D, Ricciardi KG, Tande D, et al. Is the subthalamic nucleus hypointense on T2- weighted images? A correlation study using MR imaging and stereotactic atlas data. AJNR Am J Neuroradiol 2004;25(9):1516–23.
3. Schäfer A, Forstmann BU, Neumann J, et al. Direct visualization of the subthalamic nucleus and its iron distribution using high-resolution susceptibility mapping. Hum Brain Mapp 2012;33(12):2831–42.
4. Ryan ME. Utility of double inversion recovery sequences in MRI. Pediatr Neurol Briefs 2016;30(4):26.
5. Wattjes MP, Lutterbey GG, Gieseke J, et al. Double inversion recovery brain imaging at 3T: diagnostic value in the detection of multiple sclerosis lesions. AJNR Am J Neuroradiol 2007;28(1):54–9.
6. Sudhyadhom A, Haq IU, Foote KD, et al. A high resolution and high contrast MRI for differentiation of subcortical structures for DBS targeting: the fast gray matter acquisition T1 inversion recovery (FGATIR). Neuroimage 2009;47(Suppl 2): T44–52.
7. Wang J-W, Cong F, Zhuo Y, et al. 7.0T ultrahigh-field MRI directly visualized the pedunculopontine nucleus in Parkinson's disease patients. Clinics (Sao Paulo) 2019;74:e573.
8. Wang J-W, Zhang Y-Q, Zhang X-H, et al. Deep brain stimulation of pedunculopontine nucleus for postural instability and gait disorder after Parkinson disease: a meta-analysis of individual patient data. World Neurosurg 2017;102:72–8.
9. Woolrich MW, Jbabdi S, Patenaude B, et al. Bayesian analysis of neuroimaging data in FSL. Neuroimage 2009;45(1):S173–86.
10. Tournier J-D, Calamante F, Connelly A. Robust determination of the fibre orientation distribution in diffusion MRI: non-negativity constrained super-resolved spherical deconvolution. Neuroimage 2007;35(4):1459–72.
11. Jbabdi S, Sotiropoulos SN, Savio AM, et al. Model-based analysis of multishell diffusion MR data for tractography: how to get over fitting problems. Magn Reson Med 2012;68(6):1846–55.
12. Hosey TP, Harding SG, Carpenter TA, et al. Application of a probabilistic double-fibre structure model to diffusion-weighted MR images of the human brain. Magn Reson Imaging 2008;26(2):236–45.
13. Jeurissen B, Leemans A, Jones DK, et al. Probabilistic fiber tracking using the residual bootstrap with constrained spherical deconvolution. Hum Brain Mapp 2011;32(3):461–79.
14. Jenkinson M, Beckmann CF, Behrens TEJ, et al. FSL. Neuroimage 2012;62(2): 782–90.
15. Tournier J-D, Calamante F, Connelly A. MRtrix: diffusion tractography in crossing fiber regions. Int J Imaging Syst Technol 2012;22(1):53–66.

16. Leemans A, Sijbers J, Verhoye M, et al. Mathematical framework for simulating diffusion tensor MR neural fiber bundles. Magn Reson Med 2005;53(4):944–53.
17. Behrens TEJ, Berg HJ, Jbabdi S, et al. Probabilistic diffusion tractography with multiple fibre orientations: what can we gain? Neuroimage 2007;34(1):144–55.
18. Hernández M, Guerrero GD, Cecilia JM, et al. Accelerating fibre orientation estimation from diffusion weighted magnetic resonance imaging using GPUs. PLoS One 2013;8(4):e61892.
19. Benabid AL, Pollak P, Gao D, et al. Chronic electrical stimulation of the ventralis intermedius nucleus of the thalamus as a treatment of movement disorders. J Neurosurg 1996;84(2):203–14.
20. Goia A, Gilard V, Lefaucheur R, et al. Accuracy of the robot-assisted procedure in deep brain stimulation. Int J Med Robot 2019;e2032. https://doi.org/10.1002/rcs.2032.
21. Ho AL, Pendharkar AV, Brewster R, et al. Frameless robot-assisted deep brain stimulation surgery: an initial experience. Oper Neurosurg (Hagerstown) 2019. https://doi.org/10.1093/ons/opy395.
22. Benabid AL, Pollak P, Seigneuret E, et al. Chronic VIM thalamic stimulation in Parkinson's disease, essential tremor and extra-pyramidal dyskinesias. Acta Neurochir Suppl (Wien) 1993;58:39–44.
23. Liu Y, Li W, Tan C, et al. Meta-analysis comparing deep brain stimulation of the globus pallidus and subthalamic nucleus to treat advanced Parkinson disease. J Neurosurg 2014;121(3):709–18.
24. Patel AS. Deep brain stimulation target selection in an advanced Parkinson's disease patient with significant tremor and comorbid depression. Tremor Hyperkinetic Mov 2017;7. https://doi.org/10.7916/D8KD23NZ.
25. Neumann W-J, Turner RS, Blankertz B, et al. Toward electrophysiology-based intelligent adaptive deep brain stimulation for movement disorders. Neurother J Am Soc Exp Neurother 2019;16(1):105–18.
26. Winter M, Costabile JD, Abosch A, et al. Method for localizing intraoperative recordings from deep brain stimulation surgery using post-operative structural MRI. Neuroimage Clin 2018;20:1123–8.
27. Blomstedt P, Stenmark Persson R, Hariz G-M, et al. Deep brain stimulation in the caudal zona incerta versus best medical treatment in patients with Parkinson's disease: a randomised blinded evaluation. J Neurol Neurosurg Psychiatry 2018;89(7):710–6.
28. Plaha P, Ben-Shlomo Y, Patel NK, et al. Stimulation of the caudal zona incerta is superior to stimulation of the subthalamic nucleus in improving contralateral parkinsonism. Brain 2006;129(Pt 7):1732–47.
29. Lambert C, Zrinzo L, Nagy Z, et al. Confirmation of functional zones within the human subthalamic nucleus: patterns of connectivity and sub-parcellation using diffusion weighted imaging. Neuroimage 2012;60(1):83–94.
30. Haynes WIA, Haber SN. The organization of prefrontal-subthalamic inputs in primates provides an anatomical substrate for both functional specificity and integration: implications for basal ganglia models and deep brain stimulation. J Neurosci 2013;33(11):4804–14.
31. Little S, Brown P. The functional role of beta oscillations in Parkinson's disease. Parkinsonism Relat Disord 2014;20:S44–8.
32. Neumann W-J, Staub-Bartelt F, Horn A, et al. Long term correlation of subthalamic beta band activity with motor impairment in patients with Parkinson's disease. Clin Neurophysiol 2017;128(11):2286–91.

33. Steiner LA, Neumann W-J, Staub-Bartelt F, et al. Subthalamic beta dynamics mirror Parkinsonian bradykinesia months after neurostimulator implantation. Mov Disord 2017;32(8):1183–90.
34. Trager MH, Koop MM, Velisar A, et al. Subthalamic beta oscillations are attenuated after withdrawal of chronic high frequency neurostimulation in Parkinson's disease. Neurobiol Dis 2016;96:22–30.
35. Akram H, Sotiropoulos SN, Jbabdi S, et al. Subthalamic deep brain stimulation sweet spots and hyperdirect cortical connectivity in Parkinson's disease. Neuroimage 2017;158:332–45.
36. Rozanski VE, da Silva NM, Ahmadi S-A, et al. The role of the pallidothalamic fibre tracts in deep brain stimulation for dystonia: a diffusion MRI tractography study. Hum Brain Mapp 2017;38(3):1224–32.
37. da Silva NM, Ahmadi S-A, Tafula SN, et al. A diffusion-based connectivity map of the GPi for optimised stereotactic targeting in DBS. Neuroimage 2017;144:83–91.
38. Johansen-Berg H, Behrens TEJ, Sillery E, et al. Functional-anatomical validation and individual variation of diffusion tractography-based segmentation of the human thalamus. Cereb Cortex 2005;15(1):31–9.
39. Coenen VA, Allert N, Mädler B. A role of diffusion tensor imaging fiber tracking in deep brain stimulation surgery: DBS of the dentato-rubro-thalamic tract (DRT) for the treatment of therapy-refractory tremor. Acta Neurochir (Wien) 2011;153(8):1579–85.
40. Coenen VA, Varkuti B, Parpaley Y, et al. Postoperative neuroimaging analysis of DRT deep brain stimulation revision surgery for complicated essential tremor. Acta Neurochir (Wien) 2017;159(5):779–87.
41. Reich MM, Brumberg J, Pozzi NG, et al. Progressive gait ataxia following deep brain stimulation for essential tremor: adverse effect or lack of efficacy? Brain 2016;139(11):2948–56.
42. Cukiert A, Lehtimäki K. Deep brain stimulation targeting in refractory epilepsy. Epilepsia 2017;58(Suppl 1):80–4.
43. Fisher R, Salanova V, Witt T, et al. Electrical stimulation of the anterior nucleus of thalamus for treatment of refractory epilepsy. Epilepsia 2010;51(5):899–908.
44. Salanova V, Witt T, Worth R, et al. Long-term efficacy and safety of thalamic stimulation for drug-resistant partial epilepsy. Neurology 2015;84(10):1017–25.
45. Velasco F, Velasco AL, Velasco M, et al. Deep brain stimulation for treatment of the epilepsies: the centromedian thalamic target. Acta Neurochir Suppl 2007;97(Pt 2):337–42.
46. Velasco F, Velasco M, Jimenez F, et al. Stimulation of the central median thalamic nucleus for epilepsy. Stereotact Funct Neurosurg 2001;77(1–4):228–32.
47. Bajcsy R, Lieberson R, Reivich M. A computerized system for the elastic matching of deformed radiographic images to idealized atlas images. J Comput Assist Tomogr 1983;7(4):618–25.
48. Davatzikos C. Spatial normalization of 3D brain images using deformable models. J Comput Assist Tomogr 1996;20(4):656–65.
49. Vayssiere N, Hemm S, Cif L, et al. Comparison of atlas- and magnetic resonance imaging-based stereotactic targeting of the globus pallidus internus in the performance of deep brain stimulation for treatment of dystonia. J Neurosurg 2002;96(4):673–9.
50. Van Buren JM, Borke RC. The mesial temporal substratum of memory. Anatomical studies in three individuals. Brain 1972;95(3):599–632.
51. Möttönen T, Katisko J, Haapasalo J, et al. Defining the anterior nucleus of the thalamus (ANT) as a deep brain stimulation target in refractory epilepsy: delineation

using 3 T MRI and intraoperative microelectrode recording. Neuroimage Clin 2015;7:823–9.

52. Horn A, Li N, Dembek TA, et al. Lead-DBS v2: towards a comprehensive pipeline for deep brain stimulation imaging. Neuroimage 2019;184:293–316.

53. Calamante F, Oh S-H, Tournier J-D, et al. Super-resolution track-density imaging of thalamic substructures: comparison with high-resolution anatomical magnetic resonance imaging at 7.0T. Hum Brain Mapp 2013;34(10):2538–48.

54. Cho Z-H, Chi J-G, Choi S-H, et al. A newly identified frontal path from fornix in septum pellucidum with 7.0T MRI track density imaging (TDI): the septum pellucidum tract (SPT). Front Neuroanat 2015;9. https://doi.org/10.3389/fnana.2015.00151.

55. Choi S-H, Kim Y-B, Paek S-H, et al. Papez circuit observed by in vivo human brain with 7.0T MRI super-resolution track density imaging and track tracing. Front Neuroanat 2019;13. https://doi.org/10.3389/fnana.2019.00017.

56. Manjila S, Rengachary S, Xavier AR, et al. Modern psychosurgery before Egas Moniz: a tribute to Gottlieb Burckhardt. Neurosurg Focus 2008;25(1):E9. https://doi.org/10.3171/FOC/2008/25/7/E9.

57. Wind JJ, Anderson DE. From prefrontal leukotomy to deep brain stimulation: the historical transformation of psychosurgery and the emergence of neuroethics. Neurosurg Focus 2008;(25):E10.

58. Psychosurgery CR. Available at: https://videocast.nih.gov/pdf/ohrp_psychosurgery.pdf. Accessed August 23, 2019.

59. Bewernick BH, Hurlemann R, Matusch A, et al. Nucleus accumbens deep brain stimulation decreases ratings of depression and anxiety in treatment-resistant depression. Biol Psychiatry 2010;67(2):110–6.

60. Sartorius A, FA H. Deep brain stimulation of the lateral habenula in treatment resistant major depression. Med Hypotheses 2007;69(6):1305–8.

61. Jimenez F, Velasco F, Salin-Pascual R. A patient with a resistant major depression disorder treated with deep brain stimulation in the inferior thalamic peduncle. Neurosurgery 2005;3(585–593):585–93.

62. Malone DA, Dougherty DD, Rezai AR, et al. Deep brain stimulation of the ventral capsule/ventral striatum for treatment-resistant depression. Biol Psychiatry 2009;65(4):267–75.

63. Mayberg HS, Lozano AM, Voon V, et al. Deep brain stimulation for treatment-resistant depression. Neuron 2005;45(5):651–60.

64. HDE for OCD DBS. Available at: https://www.accessdata.fda.gov/scripts/cdrh/cfdocs/cfhde/hde.cfm?id=H050003. Accessed August 23, 2019.

65. Mayberg HS, Liotti M, Brannan SK, et al. Reciprocal limbic-cortical function and negative mood: converging PET findings in depression and normal sadness. Am J Psychiatry 1999;156(5):675–82.

66. Seminowicz DA, Mayberg HS, McIntosh AR, et al. Limbic-frontal circuitry in major depression: a path modeling metanalysis. Neuroimage 2004;22(1):409–18.

67. Dougherty DD, Rezai AR, Carpenter LL, et al. A randomized sham-controlled trial of deep brain stimulation of the ventral capsule/ventral striatum for chronic treatment-resistant depression. Biol Psychiatry 2015;78(4):240–8.

68. Holtzheimer PE, Husain MM, Lisanby SH, et al. Subcallosal cingulate deep brain stimulation for treatment-resistant depression: a multisite, randomised, sham-controlled trial. Lancet 2017;4(11):839–49.

69. Riva-Posse P, Choi KS, Holtzheimer PE, et al. Defining critical white matter pathways mediating successful subcallosal cingulate deep brain stimulation for treatment-resistant depression. Biol Psychiatry 2014;76(12):963–9.

70. Noecker AM, Choi KS, Riva-Posse P, et al. StimVision software: examples and applications in subcallosal cingulate deep brain stimulation for depression. Neuromodulation 2018;21(2):191–6.

71. McGrath CL, Kelley ME, Dunlop BW, et al. Pretreatment brain states identify likely nonresponse to standard treatments for depression. Biol Psychiatry 2014;76(7): 527–35.

72. Drysdale AT, Grosenick L, Downar J, et al. Resting-state connectivity biomarkers define neurophysiological subtypes of depression. Nat Med 2017;23(1):28–38.

73. Parravano DC, Ciampi DA, Fonoff ET. Quality of life after motor cortex stimulation: clinical results and systematic review of the literature. Neurosurgery 2019;84(2):451–6.

74. Henssen DJHA, Kurt E, van Cappellen van Walsum A-M, et al. Long-term effect of motor cortex stimulation in patients suffering from chronic neuropathic pain: an observational study. PLoS One 2018;13(1):e0191774.

75. Tsubokawa T, Katayama Y, Yamamoto T, et al. Chronic motor cortex stimulation in patients with thalamic pain. J Neurosurg 1993;78(3):393–401.

76. Lempka SF, Malone DA, Hu B, et al. Randomized clinical trial of deep brain stimulation for poststroke pain. Ann Neurol 2017;81(5):653–63.

77. Abreu V, Vaz R, Rebelo V. Thalamic deep brain stimulation for neuropathic pain: efficacy at three years' follow-up. Neuromodulation 2017;20(5):504–13.

78. Boccard SGJ, Pereira EAC, Aziz TZ. Deep brain stimulation for chronic pain. J Clin Neurosci 2015;22(10):1537–43.

79. Pereira EA, Boccard SG, Linhares P, et al. Thalamic deep brain stimulation for neuropathic pain after amputation or brachial plexus avulsion. Neurosurg Focus 2013;35:3.

80. Boccard SGJ, Prangnell SJ, Pycroft L, et al. Long-term results of deep brain stimulation of the anterior cingulate cortex for neuropathic pain. World Neurosurg 2017;106:625–37.

81. Russo JF, Sheth SA. Deep brain stimulation of the dorsal anterior cingulate cortex for the treatment of chronic neuropathic pain. Neurosurg Focus 2015;38(6):E11.

82. Farrell SM, Green A, Aziz T. The current state of deep brain stimulation for chronic pain and its context in other forms of neuromodulation. Brain Sci 2018;8(8). https://doi.org/10.3390/brainsci8080158.

83. Maarrawi J, Peyron R, Mertens P. Brain opioid receptor density predicts motor cortex stimulation efficacy for chronic pain. Pain 2013;154(11):2563–8.

84. Sims-Williams H, Matthews JC, Talbot PS, et al. Deep brain stimulation of the periaqueductal gray releases endogenous opioids in humans. Neuroimage 2017; 146:833–42.

85. Moens M, Sunaert S, Marien P, et al. Spinal cord stimulation modulates cerebral function: an fMRI study. Neuroradiology 2012;54(12):1399–407.

86. Kovanlikaya I, Heier L, Kaplitt M. Treatment of chronic pain: diffusion tensor imaging identification of the ventroposterolateral nucleus confirmed with successful deep brain stimulation. Stereotact Funct Neurosurg 2014;92(6):365–71.

87. Boccard SGJ, Fernandes HM, Jbabdi S, et al. Tractography study of deep brain stimulation of the anterior cingulate cortex in chronic pain: key to improve the targeting. World Neurosurg 2016;86:361–70.e1-3.

88. Owen SL, Heath J, Kringelbach M, et al. Pre-operative DTI and probabilisitic tractography in four patients with deep brain stimulation for chronic pain. J Clin Neurosci 2008;15(7):801–5.

89. Hunsche S, Sauner D, Runge MJ, et al. Tractography-guided stimulation of somatosensory fibers for thalamic pain relief. Stereotact Funct Neurosurg 2013; 91(5):328–34.

Neuro-ultrasonography

Ryan Hakimi, DO, MS, FNCS, NVS[a],*, Andrei V. Alexandrov, MD, RVT[b], Zsolt Garami, MD[c,d]

KEYWORDS

- TCD • Transcranial Doppler ultrasonography • Vasospasm • Neurosonology
- Subarachnoid hemorrhage • Neurocritical care • Optic nerve sheath diameter
- Emboli detection

KEY POINTS

- Transcranial Doppler ultrasonography (TCD) is a noninvasive, bedside, portable tool for assessment of cerebral hemodynamics and detection of focal stenosis, arterial occlusion, monitoring the treatment effect of intravenous tissue plasminogen activator and assessment of vasomotor reactivity.
- Modern TCD head frames allow continuous hands-free emboli detection, allowing risk stratification and assessment of treatment efficacy in several cardiovascular disease processes.
- TCD is an excellent screening tool for vasospasm in aneurysmal subarachnoid hemorrhage because of its high sensitivity and negative predictive value.
- The use of intraoperative TCD during carotid endarterectomy and stenting allows optimal intraoperative hemodynamic management while minimizing the risk for brain ischemia.

TRANSCRANIAL POWER MOTION DOPPLER AND SPECTRAL DISPLAY

Transcranial Doppler ultrasonography (TCD) is a noninvasive, portable, bedside tool for assessment of cerebral hemodynamics (**Box 1**). The instrument displays spectral waveforms that represent the depth, direction, and intensity of the blood flow through the intracranial vasculature. Although the instrument does not measure blood flow directly, the parameters that it does calculate do correlate with cerebral blood flow (CBF).

In the past, TCD machines were only able to display a spectral waveform. The operator was left to deduce which vessel was being insonated by attempting to obtain the

[a] Director, Neuro ICU, Inpatient Neurology, and TCD Services, Greenville Memorial Hospital, Prisma Health-Upstate, University of South Carolina School of Medicine-Greenville, 200 Patewood Drive, Suite B350, Greenville, SC 29615, USA; [b] Department of Neurology, The University of Tennessee Health Science Center, 855 Monroe Avenue, Suite 415, Memphis, TN 38163, USA; [c] Institute for Academic Medicine, Research Institute, Houston, TX, USA; [d] Vascular Ultrasound Laboratory, Houston Methodist Hospital, Weill Cornell Medical College, 6550 Fannin Street, Suite 1401, Houston, TX 77030, USA
* Corresponding author.
E-mail address: Ryan.hakimi@prismahealth.org

Neurol Clin 38 (2020) 215–229
https://doi.org/10.1016/j.ncl.2019.09.006
0733-8619/20/© 2019 Elsevier Inc. All rights reserved.

same waveform or an inverted version of the same waveform using a variety of different approaches, termed windows, at different depths. With the addition of power motion–mode Doppler (PMD), sonographers are able to obtain the spectral waveform as well as knowing the depth of the insonated vessel, the direction of flow relative to the probe, and the intensity of the signal (**Box 2, Figs. 1** and **2**).

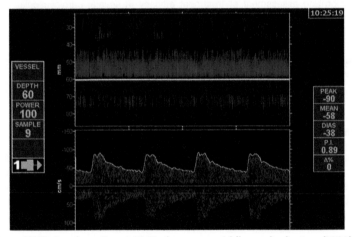

Fig. 1. Normal TCD signals on Power M Mode screen: middle cerebral artery (MCA) (red: 40–60 mm), anterior cerebral artery (ACA) (blue: 60–70 mm), contralateral ACA (red: 70–80 mm), and Contralateral MCA (blue: 80–90 mm). (*From* Garami Z, Alexandrov AV. Neurosonology. Neurol Clin. 2009;27(1):89–108; with permission).

The temporal bone is the thinnest portion of the human skull and is located immediately superior to the tragus. A 2-MHz TCD probe is placed at this location and the intracranial arteries are insonated to produce the aforementioned spectral waveforms and physiologic parameters. The skin surface where the probe contacts the head serves as the zero depth and distances are measured from that point onward. For most adults the midline lies at approximately 70 to 80 mm. At deeper depths the contralateral vasculature is insonated, whose spectral waveforms would be expected to have the opposite direction of that obtained when imaged from the ipsilateral side.

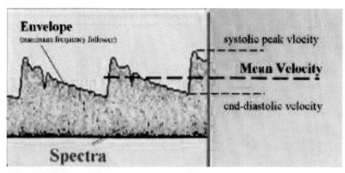

Fig. 2. Doppler velocity.

Box 2
Criteria for identification of a focal stenosis

Waveform after the area of stenosis shows delayed systolic upstroke relative to the waveform proximal to the stenosis, and:

Poststenotic MFV is greater than 100 cm/s and is 2 times the prestenotic MFV, or

Poststenotic MFV is greater than 100 cm/s and is 2 times the MFV of the contralateral homologous segment

---

EMBOLI DETECTION AND MONITORING

TCD can be used for microemboli detection. Modern TCD manufacturers have created adjustable head frames allowing the operator to affix up to 2 TCD probes to insonate vessels bilaterally, most commonly the middle cerebral arteries (MCAs), in a hands-free fashion. However, operators can increase the gait to allow each probe to insonate multiple vessels at the same time. Such technology has a vast number of applications, including risk stratification of carotid artery dissection, risk stratification of asymptomatic carotid stenosis,[1] monitoring the effect of tissue plasminogen activator (tPA) on an acutely occluded vessel, assessing the efficacy of anticoagulation in nonvalvular atrial fibrillation,[2] and risk stratifying moderate carotid artery stenosis.

INTRACRANIAL STENOSIS AND DETECTION OF FOCAL ARTERIAL OCCLUSION

TCD can detect and grade the severity of intracranial stenosis from acute thrombosis, intracranial dissection, or focal intracranial atherosclerosis. Although a variety of mean flow velocity (MFV) criteria have been used to make this assessment, the authors suggest a multistep approach, beginning by looking at the waveform morphology and MFV of the Doppler signal before and after the area of stenosis and then comparing the MFV with the contralateral homologous segment (see **Box 2; Fig. 3**).

Thrombolysis in brain ischemia classification has been created to describe residual flow or to monitor clot dissolution.[3] Such a classification allows better communication between providers about the extent of revascularization and can be used to determine the optimal systemic blood pressure in post-tPA and mechanical thrombectomy patients, and detection of reocclusion, particularly in patients under general anesthesia **(Fig. 4)**.

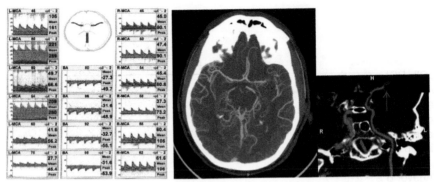

Fig. 3. Waveform morphology and MFV of the Doppler signal before (LMCA at 78 mm) and after (LMCA at 50 mm) the area of stenosis (red arrow), then comparing the MFV with the contralateral homologous segment (RMCA at 54 mm).

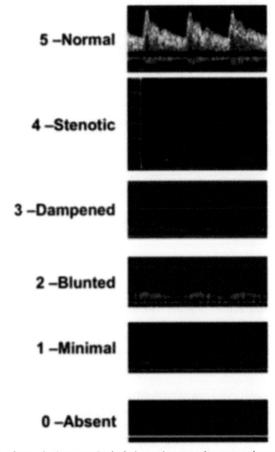

5 –Normal

4 –Stenotic

3 –Dampened

2 –Blunted

1 –Minimal

0 –Absent

Fig. 4. Detection of reocclusion, particularly in patients under general anesthesia. (*From* Garami Z, Alexandrov AV. Neurosonology. Neurol Clin. 2009; 27(1):89-108; with permission.)

CEREBRAL ARTERY VASOSPASM

Cerebral artery vasospasm, a reduction in the caliber of a cerebral artery, is a common consequence of aneurysmal subarachnoid hemorrhage (aSAH). Even now, aSAH portends a 50% mortality, chiefly caused by delayed cerebral ischemia (DCI). DCI can be prevented by identifying and appropriately treating vasospasm, which occurs in 50% to 70% of aSAH cases.[4–6] TCD can predict symptomatic vasospasm and has high sensitivity, specificity, positive and negative predictive values.[7–11] Three major neurologic bodies endorse the use of TCD in the care of patients with aSAH, namely the American Heart Association/American Stroke Association (AHA/ASA), the American Academy of Neurology (AAN), and the Neurocritical Care Society (NCS). The AHA/ASA designates the use of TCD in aSAH as class IIA/level B evidence, whereas the other 2 entities designate it as moderate-quality evidence/strong recommendation. The largest meta-analysis to date, by Kumar and colleagues,[12] reviews the use of TCD for aSAH in 17 pooled studies (2870 patients). They reported TCD evidence of vasospasm to be highly predictive of DCI, with a sensitivity of 90%, specificity of 71%, positive predictive value of 57%, and negative predictive value of 92%. The excellent sensitivity and high negative predictive value makes TCD an ideal screening tool for detecting vasospasm in aSAH.

In general, TCD is less reliable at identifying posterior circulation than anterior circulation vasospasm (because of greater anatomic variance). There are multiple published criteria for anterior circulation vasospasm. One often used set of criteria is shown in **Table 1**.

Given that each individual's baseline anatomic and physiologic parameters are different, identification of vasospasm is improved by performing daily TCD and trending the MFV, because the trends and waveform morphology are often more valuable than simply the numerical values. For example, an increase in the MFV of 50 cm/s or greater in a vessel between one day and the next is suggestive of vasospasm even if the MFV is less than 120 cm/s. Therefore, it is optimal to obtain a daily TCD, including on the day of presentation, to establish a baseline and to monitor for trends suggesting vasospasm, thereby allowing prompt treatment and prevention of DCI (**Figs. 5** and **6**).

Ideally, every TCD laboratory should be accredited by the Intersocietal Accreditation Commission (IAC), or an equivalent body, and every sonographer should be certified by the American Society of Neuroimaging (ASN), American Registry for Diagnostic Medical Sonography (ARDMS), or an equivalent body to ensure diagnostic accuracy and optimal patient care.

Table 1 Criteria for vasospasm	
Mild vasospasm 120–160 cm/s	Lindegaard ratio (MCA velocity/extracranial ICA) 3–4
Moderate vasospasm 160–200 cm/s	Lindegaard ratio (MCA velocity/extracranial ICA) 4–6
Severe vasospasm >200 cm/s	Lindegaard ratio (MCA velocity/extracranial ICA) >6

Abbreviation: ICA, internal carotid artery.

SUBCLAVIAN STEAL

Side-to-side blood pressure variance of 20 mm Hg or more is often the first sign of subclinical subclavian steal.[13] Such patients often have global atherosclerosis,

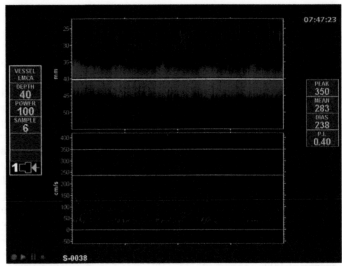

Fig. 5. Daily TCD. (*From* Garami Z, Alexandrov AV. Neurosonology. Neurol Clin. 2009; 27(1):89-108; with permission.)

Velocity Trend Report

Velocity Trend

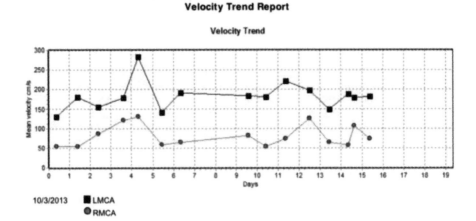

10/3/2013 ■ LMCA
● RMCA

Ratio

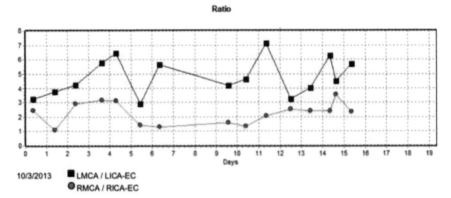

10/3/2013 ■ LMCA / LICA-EC
● RMCA / RICA-EC

Fig. 6. Velocity trend report. LICA-EC, extracranial left ICA; RICA-EC, extracranial right ICA; LMCA, left MCA; RMCA, right MCA.

including the proximal subclavian artery. This condition results in varying degrees of retrograde flow within the ipsilateral vertebral artery, limiting perfusion of the ipsilateral arm. Symptomatic subclavian steal manifests as paroxysmal vertigo, syncope, and ipsilateral arm claudication.

TCD serves as an excellent screening tool for such patients.[14] Although reported, complete reversal of vertebral artery blood flow at rest is uncommon. Therefore, in order to make the diagnosis, an ischemic cuff test is performed wherein the cuff is inflated to 20 mm Hg greater than the patient's own systolic blood pressure and maintained for a few minutes. This pressure renders the arm ischemic. During this process the ipsilateral vertebral artery is insonated. The cuff is then rapidly deflated, resulting in rapid reperfusion of the arm and varying degrees of reversal of flow in the ipsilateral vertebral artery confirming the diagnosis of subclavian steal syndrome. Most commonly these patients are treated with medical therapy. In some more advanced cases, subclavian artery stenting is required[13] (Figs. 7–9).

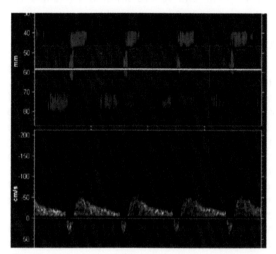

Fig. 7. Alternating flow signal in the vertebral artery (VA). PMD display: on the yellow line, red color signal, steal direction/toward the probe in systole; blue, away (normal direction) in diastole. Spectral display: negative and positive waveforms corresponding with direction changes.

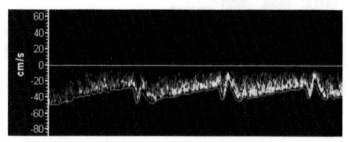

Fig. 8. Abnormal waveform in the VA indicates subclavian steal phenomenon. V-shaped cutout is the first form of the alternating flow signal. (*From* Garami Z, Alexandrov AV. Neurosonology. Neurol Clin. 2009; 27(1):89-108; with permission.)

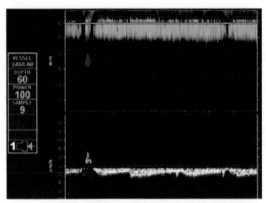

Fig. 9. Hyperemia test: overinflated blood pressure cuff released, flow reversal (*red signal*) in the vertebral-basilar system, and various waveforms returned to baseline (spectral display).

CEREBRAL CIRCULATORY ARREST

Brain death, also termed death by neurologic criteria, is the irreversible cessation of whole-brain function with sustained systemic perfusion caused by support of mechanical ventilation, medications, and various medical measures. This support was not possible until the development of mechanical ventilation and the advancement of critical care techniques, allowing patients to be systemically stable after developing cessation of brain function. Brain death remains a clinical diagnosis requiring a variety of clinical, laboratory, and respiratory criteria to be met.[15] However, in some instances, the patient is clinically unstable and cannot meet all of the necessary criteria, and thus an ancillary test is needed. The AAN only endorses 3 ancillary tests with level B or higher designation. TCD is one such test with level A evidence for use as an ancillary test for determination of brain death.

Bilateral insonation of the anterior and posterior circulation is performed through the temporal and suboccipital windows, showing reverberating flow or small systolic spikes. Absence of flow can only be used as a marker for cerebral circulatory arrest if an acoustic signal that had previously been obtained in the same patient is now absent. This finding distinguishes cerebral circulatory arrest from technical issues, such as absence of windows seen with hyperostosis of the skull (**Fig. 10**).

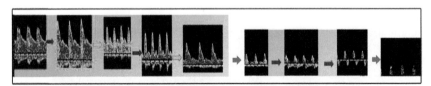

Fig. 10. TCD waveform progression from normal MCA to cerebral circulatory arrest. (*Courtesy of* A. Razumovsky, PhD.)

VASOMOTOR REACTIVITY

Vasomotor reactivity can be assessed using a variety of means, including CO_2 reactivity testing with TCD, acetazolamide testing with TCD, and the breath-holding index (BHI).[16,17] The first 2 modalities require a special gas hookup and an intravenous (IV) medication, respectively. However, the last modality can easily be performed in an outpatient setting provided that the patient is capable of breath holding for 30 seconds. To begin, patients are instructed to hold their breath for 30 seconds and the MFV of the MCA is measured. The MFV is again measured 4 seconds after the breath hold when the patient is allowed to breath. For a breath hold of 30 seconds, the following formula is used to calculate the BHI:

$$BHI = 3.33 \times (MFV_{end} - MFV_{baseline})/MFV_{baseline}$$

Vasomotor reactivity has a variety of applications, including determining the risk for ischemic stroke in individuals with severe asymptomatic carotid artery stenosis or intracranial stenosis, in particular in those with a BHI of less than 0.69.[18] The presence of impaired vasomotor reactivity has also been suggested in individuals following a concussion or those with Alzheimer dementia.[19]

Vasomotor reactivity testing with TCD can also detect paradoxic MFV reduction during increase in CO_2 levels. This intracranial steal phenomenon, termed reversed Robin Hood, can lead to neurologic deterioration and high risk of early stroke recurrence.[20,21]

REAL-TIME PROCEDURAL MONITORING

Neurologic complications of carotid endarterectomy (CEA) and carotid artery stenting (CAS) are commonly related to cerebral hypoperfusion, cerebral hyperperfusion, or most often thrombosis and embolization.[22–26] Real-time detection of such events with TCD monitoring is critical to prevent, diagnose, and reverse procedure-related complications. By monitoring the bilateral MCAs, TCD is the only modality that monitors the intracranial vessels to prevent end-organ damage. Intraoperative TCD allows direct visualization of the patient's intracranial collateral flow, giving patient-specific information to the surgeon performing the CEA. This technique allows surgeons to perform vascular shunting only when necessary, thereby preventing unnecessary complications. By monitoring the amplitude of the diastolic component of the Doppler waveform to ensure that it is approximately half of the peak systolic amplitude, intraoperative TCD also allows anesthesiologists the patient-specific information needed to augment or reduce patients' blood pressure during CEA or CAS to prevent cerebral hypoperfusion and hyperperfusion. The lack of global acceptance of this practice centers on the lack of lucrative reimbursement for this outcome-changing modality (**Figs. 11** and **12**).

OPTIC NERVE SHEATH DIAMETER

Bedside ocular ultrasonography can identify foreign bodies, globe rupture, retinal detachment, and increased intracranial pressure (ICP) as shown by an increased optic nerve sheath diameter.[27] In order to measure optic nerve sheath diameter, a 7.5-MHz to 10-MHz linear array transducer is placed on the patient's closed eye after applying a copious amount of ultrasonography gel. The optic nerve sheath is marked 3 mm behind the posterior aspect of the eye. Two measurements of the transverse diameter of the optic nerve sheath are then obtained at this position. The 2 values are then averaged. If they exceed 5 mm, it is supportive of increased ICP[28] (**Fig. 13**).

In a recent large meta-analysis, Robba and colleagues[29] concluded that optic nerve sheath diameter may be a useful surrogate for increased ICP when standard invasive monitors are not available or indicated. The investigators noted marked heterogeneity in the publications, including variability in the units of ICP measurement and cut points for high ICP.

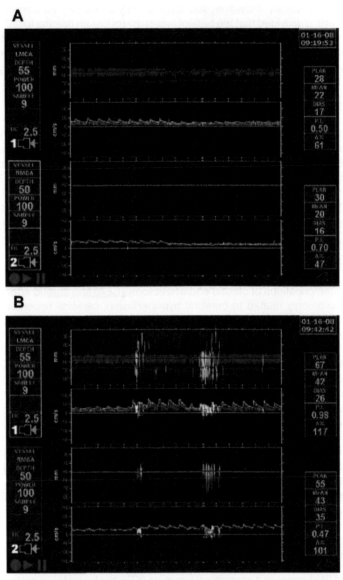

Fig. 11. (A) Bilateral MCA monitoring was performed during left carotid endarterectomy. Clamp placement produced blunted signals in both MCAs. Indirect evidence for bilateral disease clamped carotid feeding the other MCA. (B) Clamp released, producing microembolic signals in both MCAs. Pulsatility restored in the MCA bilaterally. (*From* Garami Z, Alexandrov AV. Neurosonology. Neurol Clin. 2009; 27(1):89-108; with permission.)

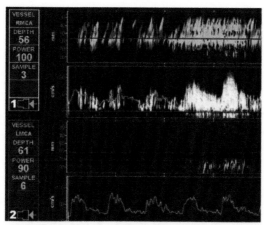

Fig. 12. Bilateral MCA monitoring during right CAS. Stent placement resulted in Micro-embolic signals (MES) only in the ipsilateral MCA. (*From* Garami Z, Alexandrov AV. Neurosonology. Neurol Clin. 2009; 27(1):89-108; with permission.)

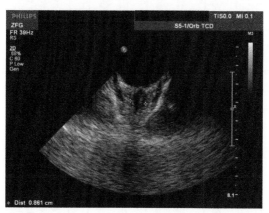

Fig. 13. Two measurements of the transverse diameter of the optic nerve sheath are obtained.

NEUROCRITICAL CARE APPLICATIONS OF BRAIN ULTRASONOGRAPHY

The use of TCD in neurocritical care units continues to grow, and regulatory bodies are beginning to mandate its availability in order for institutions to obtain the highest-level designations, such as level 1 neurointensive care unit (neuro-ICU) and comprehensive stroke center.[30,31] The increasing availability of TCD has led to use outside of standard vasospasm monitoring for aSAH.

Optimization of CBF and oxygen delivery are the goals of neurologic management of patients with traumatic brain injury. Historically, this has been monitored by measuring ICP and monitoring cerebral perfusion pressure (CPP). However, this model is inadequate because some patients have poor neurologic outcomes despite appropriate management of these two parameters. Among noninvasive modalities, TCD is the most accurate tool for measuring brain perfusion at the bedside.[32]

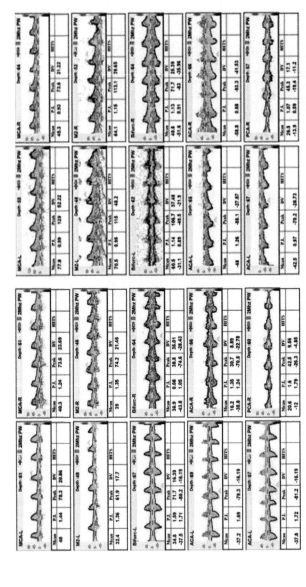

Fig. 14. TCD can non-invasively monitor cerebral perfusion by assessing the diastolic component of the spectral waveform (EDV). Left panel shows high resistance waveforms with EDV less than 50% of the PSV. The patient then had an external ventricular drain placed (right panel) and the pulsatility indices normalized resulting in an increase in the diastolic component of the waveform such that the EDV is greater than 50% of the PSV.

The brain's cerebral perfusion is maintained in both systole and diastole, as shown by the systolic and diastolic component of the TCD waveform. In contrast, the hand is perfused only in systole, as shown by a radial arterial line waveform. This difference is caused by the marked difference in resistance, with the brain being a low-resistance system and the hand being a high-resistance system, as well as the higher energy requirements of the brain compared with the hand. Therefore, the adequacy of CBF can be assessed by evaluating the diastolic component of the TCD waveform and ensuring that its amplitude is approximately half of the peak systolic amplitude. If it is less, the clinician can: a) increase the patient's blood pressure using IV fluids, vasopressors, or by giving a blood transfusion; b) decrease the $Paco_2$ by decreasing the respiratory rate on the ventilator (with intubated patients) or increasing the patient's sedation; c) reducing the patient's ICP by cerebrospinal fluid diversion, increasing sedation, or treating the patient's fever, among other means (**Fig. 14**).

Insonation of the anterior cerebral arteries (ACAs) can be a challenge in neuro-ICU patients because of cerebral edema, recent surgery, or intracranial mass lesions. Frontal bone TCD has previously been described in the pediatric neurology and neuroradiology literature as an alternative window for insonating the ACAs and is a newly described modality for neuro-ICU patients.[33-38]

Hemicraniectomy affords sonographers an excellent window for intracranial imaging. Transporting such patients to the computed tomography (CT) suite poses obvious safety risks to the patients. Serial monitoring of a patient's subdural hematoma and postoperative hygroma can be achieved using a broadband sector array transducer with a 4-MHz to 2-MHz operating frequency range.[39] Bedside ultrasonography also spares the patients radiation exposure and added cost (**Fig. 15**).

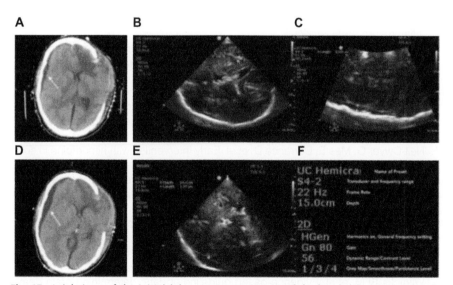

Fig. 15. Axial views of the initial (*A*) noncontrast CT scan of the head; (*B*) ultrasonography (*C*, zoomed to show detail) with follow-up; (*D*) noncontrast CT scan of the head; and (*E*) ultrasonography. The CT scans show the right-sided subdural hygroma (*white arrows*), which corresponds to the near-contemporaneous ultrasonography views of the hygroma (measured by the white plus [+] icons on the ultrasonography images). (*F*) Ultrasonography settings used to obtain images.

DISCLOSURE

Dr R. Hakimi has nothing to disclose. Dr Z. Garami has nothing to disclose. Dr A.V. Alexandrov has received consulting fees from Cerevast Inc and is on the speaker's bureau for Genentech.

REFERENCES

1. Abbott A, et al. Asymptomatic carotid stenosis is associated with circadian and other variability in embolus detection. Front Neurol 2019;10:322. Accessed October 31,2019.
2. Nosal V, et al. Role of TCD emboli-monitoring in evaluation of efficacy of anticoagulant therapy in patients with non-valvular atrial fibrillation. Med Int Rev 2018;28(111).
3. Demchuk AM, Burgin WS, Christou I, et al. Thrombolysis in Brain Ischemia (TIBI) transcranial Doppler flow grades predict clinical severity, early recovery, and mortality in patients treated with tissue plasminogen activator. Stroke 2001;32:89–93.
4. Østergaard L, et al. The role of the microcirculation in delayed cerebral ischemia and chronic degenerative changes after subarachnoid hemorrhage. J Cereb Blood Flow Metab 2013;33:1825–37.
5. Hop JW, et al. Case-fatality rates and functional outcome after subarachnoid hemorrhage: a systematic review. Stroke 1997;28:660–4.
6. Keyrouz SG, et al. Clinical review: prevention and therapy of vasospasm in subarachnoid hemorrhage. Crit Care 2007;11:220.
7. Grosset DG, Straiton J, du Trevou M, et al. Prediction of symptomatic vasospasm after subarachnoid hemorrhage by rapidly increasing transcranial Doppler velocity and cerebral blood flow changes. Stroke 1992;23:674–9.
8. Kassell NF, Haley EC Jr, Apperson-Hansen C, et al. Randomized, double-blind, vehicle-controlled trial of tirilazad mesylate in patients with aneurysmal subarachnoid hemorrhage: a cooperative study in Europe, Australia, and New Zealand. J Neurosurg 1996;84:221–8.
9. Lysakowski C, Walder B, Costanza MC, et al. Transcranial Doppler versus angiography in patients with vasospasm due to a ruptured cerebral aneurysm: a systematic review. Stroke 2001;32:2292–8.
10. Macdonald RL, Kassell NF, Mayer S, et al. Clazosentan to overcome neurological ischemia and infarction occurring after subarachnoid hemorrhage (CONSCIOUS-1): randomized, double-blind, placebo-controlled phase 2 dose-finding trial. Stroke 2008;39:3015–21.
11. Neil-Dwyer G, Mee E, Dorrance D, et al. Early intervention with nimodipine in subarachnoid haemorrhage. Eur Heart J 1987;8(Suppl K):41–7.
12. Kumar G, et al. Vasospasm on transcranial Doppler is predictive of delayed cerebral ischemia in aneurysmal subarachnoid hemorrhage: a systematic review and meta-analysis. J Neurosurg 2016;124(5):1257–64.
13. Osiro S, et al. A review of subclavian steal syndrome with clinical correlation. Med Sci Monit 2012;18(5):RA57–63.
14. Vecera J, Vojtíšek P, Varvarovský I, et al. Non-invasive diagnosis of coronary-subclavian steal: role of the Doppler ultrasound. Eur J Echocardiogr 2010;11(9):E34.
15. Wijdicks EFM, et al. Evidence-based guideline update: determining brain death in adults: report of the Quality Standards Subcommittee of the American Academy of Neurology. Neurology 2010;74:1911–8.
16. Ringelstein EB, Sievers C, Ecker S, et al. Noninvasive assessment of CO_2-induced cerebral vasomotor response in normal individuals and patients with internal carotid artery occlusions. Stroke 1988;19:962–9.

17. Sorteberg W, Lindegaard KF, Rootwelt K, et al. Effect of acetazolamide on cerebral blood flow velocity and regional cerebral blood flow in normal subjects. Acta Neurochir 1989;97:139–45.
18. Kleiser B, Widder B. Course of carotid artery occlusions with impaired cerebrovascular reactivity. Stroke 1992;23:171–4.
19. Gongora-Rivera F, et al. Impaired cerebral vasomotor reactivity in alzheimer's disease. Int J Alzheimers Dis 2018;2018:5 [Article 9328293].
20. Alexandrov AV, Sharma VK, Lao AY, et al. Reversed Robin Hood syndrome in acute ischemic stroke patients. Stroke 2007;38:3045–8.
21. Palazzo P, Balucani C, Barlinn K, et al. Association of reversed Robin Hood syndrome with risk of stroke recurrence. Neurology 2010;75:2003–8.
22. Spencer MP. Transcranial Doppler monitoring and the causes of stroke from carotid endarterectomy. Stroke 1997;28:685–91.
23. Udesh R, et al. Transcranial doppler monitoring in carotid endarterectomy: a systematic review and meta-analysis. J Med Ultrasound 2017;36(3):621–30.
24. Hill MD, et al. Stroke after carotid stenting and endarterectomy in the carotid revascularization endarterectomy versus stenting trial (CREST). Circulation 2012;126(25):3054–61.
25. Garami Z, et al. Simultaneous pre- and post-filter transcranial Doppler monitoring during carotid artery stenting. J Vasc Surg 2009;49(2):340–4.
26. Bismuth J, et al. Transcranial Doppler findings during thoracic endovascular aortic repair. J Vasc Surg 2011;54(2):364–9.
27. Blaivas M. Bedside emergency department ultrasonography in the evaluation of ocular pathology. Acad Emerg Med 2000;7(8):947–50.
28. Available at: https://www.acep.org/sonoguide/smparts_ocular.html#ocularref1. Accessed May 23, 2019.
29. Robba C, et al. Optic nerve sheath diameter measured sonographically as noninvasive estimator of intracranial pressure: a systematic review and meta-analysis. Intensive Care Med 2018;44:1284–94.
30. Moheet A, et al. Standards for Neurologic Critical Care Units: A Statement for Healthcare Professionals from The Neurocritical Care Society. Neurocrit Care 2018. https://doi.org/10.1007/s12028-018-0601-1.
31. The Joint Commission Standards; DSPR 3.4.
32. Bouzat, et al. Ann Intensive Care 2013;3:23.
33. Ben-Ora A, Eddy L, Hatch G, et al. The anterior fontanelle as an acoustic window to the neonatal ventricular system. J Clin Ultrasound 1980;8(1):65–7.
34. Wang HS, Kuo MF. Supraorbital approach of the anterior cerebral artery: a new window for transcranial Doppler sonography. J Ultrasound Med 1995;14(4):259–61.
35. Stolz E, Kaps M, Kern A, et al. Frontal bone windows for transcranial color-coded duplex sonography. Stroke 1999;30(4):814–20.
36. Stolz E, Mendes I, Gerriets T, et al. Assessment of intracranial collateral flow by transcranial color-coded duplex sonography using a temporal and frontal axial insonation plane. J Neuroimaging 2002;12(2):136–43.
37. Yoshimura S, Koga M, Toyoda K, et al. Frontal bone window improves the ability of transcranial color-coded sonography to visualize the anterior cerebral artery of Asian patients with stroke. AJNR Am J Neuroradiol 2009;30(6):1268–9.
38. Sentenac P, et al. The frontal bone window for transcranial doppler ultrasonography in critically-ill patients: validation of a new approach in ICU (manuscript).
39. Srinivasan V, et al. Bedside cranial ultrasonography in patients with hemicraniectomies: a novel window into pathology. Neurocrit Care 2019;31(2):432–3.

Moving?

Make sure your subscription moves with you!

To notify us of your new address, find your **Clinics Account Number** (located on your mailing label above your name), and contact customer service at:

Email: journalscustomerservice-usa@elsevier.com

800-654-2452 (subscribers in the U.S. & Canada)
314-447-8871 (subscribers outside of the U.S. & Canada)

Fax number: 314-447-8029

Elsevier Health Sciences Division
Subscription Customer Service
3251 Riverport Lane
Maryland Heights, MO 63043

*To ensure uninterrupted delivery of your subscription, please notify us at least 4 weeks in advance of move.

Printed and bound by CPI Group (UK) Ltd, Croydon, CR0 4YY

03/10/2024

01040479-0007